DRY BONES BREATHE

"Eric Rofes once again demonstrates that he is one of the rare thoughtful voices commenting on gay life today. His provocative and yet affirming account of gay male culture at the end of the millennium is refreshing after a year of being scolded, chastised, and vilified by other writers. . . . Rather than demonizing aspects of gay culture, he challenges his reader to consider them thoughtfully and to meet today's challenges by building on the legacy of nearly thirty years of the gay movement. Thankfully, Rofes counterweights a discussion that, until now, has seemed decidedly out of balance."

—Bill Mann, author, *The Men From the Boys* and *Wisecracker: The Life and Times of William Haines*

"This book is a must read for every gay man, HIV negative or positive, who is trying to deal with the events of the last two years and the uncertainties that lie ahead . . . Rofes fearlessly strives to define that cultural space between the crisis of AIDS and the present-day thinking that AIDS is over."

—David G. Ostrow, MD, PhD, Professor of Epidemiology, University of Illinois School of Public Health, Chicago, Illinois

"Finally someone has articulated the complex and diverse ways gay men experience the AIDS epidemic . . . Rofes acts as a respectful bridge between groups with vastly different experiences, rather than telling us how we should be feeling and dividing gay men along generational lines . . . In *Dry Bones Breathe,* the goal clearly is not to bicker and moralize, but to help people of all ages and cultures figure out how to create communities for the new millennium."

—Wayne Hoffman, Co-Editor, *Policing Public Sex: Queer Politics and the Future of AIDS Activism*

"Eric Rofes's work will undoubtedly serve as the theoretical underpinning for the inevitable and dramatic struggles we will continue to face in a post-AIDS crisis era. Sure to be met with controversy and surprise, Rofes has fashioned a framework that enables us to breathe new life into the currently stale, barren, and reductive approaches to bettering gay male life. With complexity and passion, *Dry Bones Breathe* carefully maps the terrain of gay male health and identities in a time fraught with political contention and rapid cultural change."

—Michael Scarce, author, *Smearing the Queer: Gay Male Sexual Health and Medical Science*

"*Dry Bones Breathe* is an honest and engaging exposé of gay male life that chronicles the period from the wrenching late 1980s, a time of unrelenting loss of lovers, friends, and political comrades, to the late 1990s' present-day 'Lazarus' experience . . . By exploring the resilient and the ageless desire for a sexual landscape among gay men of diverse generational, geographic, and racial backgrounds, Rofes makes a compelling case for rebuilding a gay male culture replete with sexuality—a case underscored by his powerful personal and political struggles with his own sexual choices."

—Marj Plumb, Director of Public Policy, Gay and Lesbian Medical Association

"This book is important as Rofes raises critical questions about the shifts in people's thinking and responses, from crisis to ongoing epidemic, that need to be articulated in order to create working responses. Expanding on his earlier work, Rofes calls for a long-overdue broadening of the discussion of gay men's health. It is important not only to those in the AIDS service world, but to all who are concerned with the direction and future of the gay community."

—Kevin Cathcart, Executive Director, Lambda Legal Defense and Education Fund

"Drawing on both academic theory and lived experience, *Dry Bones Breathe* pulses with life as it carefully examines post-AIDS living in all its messy and rich variety. Importantly, Rofes refutes the sexual prohibitionists, revisionists, alarmists, and pseudo-scientists with what remains our best tool in gay education and community-building: the truth. A brilliant and provocative book."

—Colin Batrouney, Australian Federation of AIDS Organizations

"Different from the familiar prevention messages and communal battle cries recycled over and over by AIDS service organizations . . . Eric Rofes's groundbreaking new book shows us that today's emerging male subcultures—including the circuit party scene and the revival of sex venues—are life-affirming spaces and rituals."

—Tony Valenzuala, HIV-positive activist, writer, and 1997 Sex Panic Summit convener

"Rofes anticipated the current debate about gay sexual culture when he wrote *Reviving the Tribe*. Now *Dry Bones Breathe* offers more thoughtful, provocative commentary that is bound to be as fiercely debated as his earlier work . . . *Dry Bones Breathe* will fascinate anyone interested in gay community and is required reading for anyone in a position of leadership."

—Mark King, Director of Education, AID Atlanta

Dry Bones Breathe
Gay Men Creating Post-AIDS Identities and Cultures

HAWORTH Gay & Lesbian Studies
John P. De Cecco, PhD
Editor in Chief

New, Recent, and Forthcoming Titles:

Barrack Buddies and Soldier Lovers: Dialogues with Gay Young Men in the U.S. Military by Steven Zeeland

Outing: Shattering the Conspiracy of Silence by Warren Johansson and William A. Percy

The Bisexual Option, Second Edition by Fritz Klein

And the Flag Was Still There: Straight People, Gay People, and Sexuality in the U.S. Military by Lois Shawver

Sailors and Sexual Identity: Crossing the Line Between "Straight" and "Gay" in the U.S. Navy by Steven Zeeland

The Gay Male's Odyssey in the Corporate World: From Disempowerment to Empowerment by Gerald V. Miller

Bisexual Politics: Theories, Queries, and Visions edited by Naomi Tucker

Gay and Gray: The Older Homosexual Man, Second Edition by Raymond M. Berger

Reviving the Tribe: Regenerating Gay Men's Sexuality and Culture in the Ongoing Epidemic by Eric Rofes

Gay and Lesbian Mental Health: A Sourcebook for Practitioners edited by Christopher J. Alexander

Against My Better Judgment: An Intimate Memoir of an Eminent Gay Psychologist by Roger Brown

The Masculine Marine: Homoeroticism in the U.S. Marine Corps by Steven Zeeland

Bisexual Characters in Film: From Anaïs to Zee by Wayne M. Bryant

The Bear Book: Readings in the History and Evolution of a Gay Male Subculture edited by Les Wright

Youths Living with HIV: Self-Evident Truths by G. Cajetan Luna

Growth and Intimacy for Gay Men: A Workbook by Christopher J. Alexander

Our Families, Our Values: Snapshots of Queer Kinship edited by Robert E. Goss and Amy Adams Squire Strongheart

Gay/Lesbian/Bisexual/Transgender Public Policy Issues: A Citizen's and Administrator's Guide to the New Cultural Struggle edited by Wallace Swan

Rough News, Daring Views: 1950s' Pioneer Gay Press Journalism by Jim Kepner

Family Secrets: Gay Sons–A Mother's Story by Jean M. Baker

Twenty Million New Customers: Understanding Gay Men's Consumer Behavior by Steven M. Kates

The Empress Is a Man: Stories from the Life of Jose Sarria by Michael R. Gorman

Acts of Disclosure: The Coming-Out Process of Contemporary Gay Men by Marc E. Vargo

Queer Kids: The Challenges and Promise for Lesbian, Gay, and Bisexual Youth by Robert E. Owens

Dry Bones Breathe: Gay Men Creating Post-AIDS Identities and Cultures by Eric Rofes

Looking Queer: Body Image and Identity in Lesbian, Gay, Bisexual, and Transgender Communities edited by Dawn Atkins

Love and Anger: Essays on AIDS, Activism, and Politics by Peter F. Cohen

Dry Bones Breathe
Gay Men Creating Post-AIDS Identities and Cultures

Eric Rofes

Harrington Park Press
An Imprint of The Haworth Press, Inc.
New York • London

Published by

Harrington Park Press, an imprint of The Haworth Press, Inc., 10 Alice Street, Binghamton, NY
13904-1580

Scripture in Chapter 1 from The Holy Bible, Contemporary English version. Copyright © 1995
by the American Bible Society. Use by permission of the American Bible Society. Text in Chapter
5 has been excerpted from *Writings for a Liberation Psychology* by Ignacio Martin-Baro (edited
by Adrianne Aron and Shawn Corne). Copyright © 1994 by the President and Fellows of Harvard
College. Reprinted by permission of Harvard University Press.

Cover design by Marylouise E. Doyle.

Cover photo by Robert F. Figueroa-Daniel. Used by permission.

The Library of Congress has cataloged the hardcover edition of this book as:

Rofes, Eric E., 1954-
    Dry bones breathe : gay men creating post-AIDS identities and culture / Eric Rofes.
        p.   cm.
    Includes bibliographical references and index.
    ISBN 0-7890-0470-4 (alk. paper).
        1. Gay men—United States—Psychology.   2. Gays—United States—Identity.   3. Gay
men—United States—Attitudes.   4. AIDS (Disease) in mass media.   5. AIDS (Disease) in literature.   6. Proteolytic enzyme inhibitors.   7. Gay communities—United States. I. Title.
HQ76.2.U5R625 1998
305.38'9664—dc21   98-9555
                                                                                                CIP

ISBN 1-56023-934-4 (pbk.)

To William Lopatin Rofes

Also by Eric Rofes

Opposite Sex: Gay Men on Lesbians, Lesbians on Gay Men
(edited with Sara Miles)

*Reviving the Tribe: Regenerating Gay Men's Sexuality and Culture
in the Ongoing Epidemic*

*Gay Life: Leisure, Love, and Living for the Contemporary Gay
Male*

*Socrates, Plato, and Guys Like Me: Confessions of a Gay
Schoolteacher*

*"I Thought People Like That Killed Themselves": Lesbians, Gay
Men, and Suicide*

With students at the Fayerweather Street School

The Kids' Book About Death and Dying: By and For Kids

The Kids' Book About Parents

The Kids' Book of Divorce: By, For, and About Kids

CONTENTS

ABOUT THE AUTHOR

Eric Rofes is the author of the landmark book, *Reviving the Tribe: Regenerating Gay Men's Sexuality and Culture in the Ongoing Epidemic;* is a long-time activist; and is founder of the Boston Lesbian and Gay Political Alliance. He has served as Executive Director of the Los Angeles Gay and Lesbian Community Services Center and San Francisco's Shanti Project, and also served as a board member of the National Gay and Lesbian Task Force and the National Lesbian and Gay Health Association. A former member of the *Gay Community News* collective during the 1970s and early 1980s, Rofes has published nine books, numerous scholarly papers, and journal articles on school reform, race and ethnicity in education, and gay men's culture. He is currently a doctoral student in Social and Cultural Studies at the University of California at Berkeley Graduate School of Education.

Acknowledgments

I am grateful to colleagues who read and commented on all or part of this manuscript and have discussed with me a range of issues important to this book: Michael Scarce, Chris Bartlett, Al Benson, Daniel Geer, Wayne Hoffman, Ross Duffin, Diane Sabin, Margo Okazawa-Rey, Gwyn Kirk, Will Seng, Mark Sponseller, Colin Batrouney, Kevin Cathcart, Terry Miller, and Tony Valenzuela. I value their advice and insight and am grateful for their assistance.

Michael Wright and Deutsche AIDS-Hilfe organized a series of international meetings in Seattle, Vancouver, and Berlin to move forward work on HIV prevention and gay men. I benefited greatly from these discussions, especially from exchanges with Onno de Zwart, Rommel Mendes-Leite, Simon Rosser, David Nimmons, and Wayne Blankenship. The Australian Centre for Lesbian and Gay Research at the University of Sydney invited me to present several papers and I am grateful to Dr. Richard Roberts, Paul Kinder, and Cameron McLean for affording me this opportunity. This book has been greatly influenced by Australian thinking about HIV/AIDS, particularly the work of Gary Dowsett, R.W. Connell, Michael Ross, Daryl O'Donnell, Ross Duffin, Dennis Altman, and Ron Gold.

John Leonard and Steven Plunk of Gay City Health Project in Seattle, and Mark King and David Powers of AID Atlanta kindly organized well-attended town meetings at which I first put forth the analysis recorded in this book and received useful feedback. Reverend Jim Mitulski of MCC/San Francisco and David Lane, PhD, of the Oregon Health Department also organized forums at which I shared my thinking with diverse gay men. Beverly Saunders Biddle and Joyce Hunter of the National Lesbian and Gay Health Association provided important opportunities for me at the National Lesbian and Gay Health Conference in Atlanta in July 1997.

I have benefited from exchanges with Dan Savage, Fran Reich, John Peterson, Marj Plumb, Danny Russo, Beth Kelly, Julie Boler,

David Silvin, Paul Zak, Ron Stall, Tom Moon, Ben Schatz, Mark Behar, Michael Shernoff, Sara Miles, Suzanne Pharr, Allan Bérubé, Richard Burns, Dennis Nix, Janet Ferone, Jonathan Pannor, Jim Rann, Harvey Makadon, Ron Suresha, Tom Hehir, Lawrence Cohen, John Thomas, Bob Crocker, Todd Wohlfarth, Jim Mitulski, Penny Nixon, Gayle Rubin, and Colin Batrouney. Richard Lubrano and the staff of Copymat in my neighborhood have been helpful in countless ways, as has the staff of UC Berkeley's School of Public Health library. I am grateful to Robert Figueroa for providing the photography for the cover. Bill Palmer, Margaret Tatich, Andrew Roy, and the staff of The Haworth Press have again provided invaluable support.

To begin each section of this book, I wanted a pair of quotations—one from disco music of the 1970s and the other from contemporary club music. I needed no help with disco, but much assistance with tunes popular on the circuit. Ray Crossman and Chris Dillehay expeditiously came up with useful lyrics from the Pet Shop Boys, Kama Sutra, D:Ream, Simply Red, Kristine W, New Order, Brian Kennedy, and others. I am responsible for the final selection. Friends who chat with me at the Cove Cafe, Market Street Gym, Pasqua, the Lone Star Saloon, San Francisco Eagle, and Pleasuredome have assisted my work in many ways. The deaths of Frank Kenealy, Dick Nathan, and Greg Bennett occurred while I was preparing this book, and their contributions to my life and understanding of gay politics, sex, and cultures are threaded through its pages.

Thanks to students with whom I work at UC Berkeley who challenge my thinking on many of the issues focused upon in this book. This book is dedicated to my father, who has been an archivist, community organizer, and political worker throughout his life; clearly I follow in his footsteps, even as my work focuses on different issues and communities. Finally, the encouragement and support of Crispin Hollings continues to keep me happy.

SECTION I:
IN THE AFTERMATH OF DECIMATION

Now that our fathers are gone and we've been left to carry on,
What about the age of reason?

—John Farnham, "Age of Reason"

Show no fear . . .
In your hands, the birth of a new day . . .

—Limahl, "The Never Ending Story"

Chapter 1

Now That It's Over

This is a strange and special time for many gay men in America. Rumors and stories about a changing AIDS epidemic swirl around our psyches, leaving us alternately hopeful and disbelieving. Pieces of information drop on us, trapping us in the middle of a jigsaw puzzle of confusion. Whispered conversations among friends and lovers tiptoe up to the question all of us want to ask but none of us feels prepared to address: Is the AIDS epidemic coming to an end?

In 1996, a variety of biomedical developments and cultural shifts came together to create a dramatic change in the communal mindset of gay men throughout the nation. Early reports of the success of protease inhibitors and combination therapies led many to believe that the treatment for which we had yearned for years had arrived. Researchers at the International AIDS Conference in Vancouver hailed the impressive results of early trials. A few dared to use the word "cure," and at least one gay newspaper's front page was emblazoned with the headline, "Activist Says AIDS Is No Longer a Killer."[1] Rumors circulated widely insisting doctors in Amsterdam had published reports on patients who supposedly had HIV fully eradicated from their systems.

During the same time, a variety of subtle, seemingly unrelated changes in urban gay cultural life coalesced to confirm our sense that a transformation was occurring. During our walks through gay neighborhoods and visits to gay venues we saw few young men using canes. When was the last time we saw a man pushing his lover down Castro Street in a wheelchair, once an everyday, poignant reminder of the epidemic? The obituaries that just a few years earlier had filled two or three pages of weekly gay papers had dwindled to half a page; some papers had stopped printing them entirely, eliminating the section, as if declaring it a product of a bygone era. In several cities, AIDS hospices and housing programs began to shut down, close wings, or accept non-AIDS patients, providing many with what seemed like tangible evidence that the epidemic was coming to an end.[2]

Perhaps the most striking sign of a rapidly changing communal landscape—and the one that has triggered a range of powerful and ambivalent feelings—has been the rebirth of sexual cultures in hard-hit cities. The sparse landscape of commercial sex cultures we inhabited in the late 1980s again has bloomed into a diverse garden of sex clubs, bathhouses, and circuit parties, initiating changes unimaginable just a few years ago. A new bathhouse opened in New York, the first since most were ordered closed in 1985. As if deliberately calling attention to the dramatic shift it represents, it was located on a block adjacent to the headquarters of Gay Men's Health Crisis, New York's premiere AIDS organization.[3] A group of gay activists initiated efforts in 1997 to open a bathhouse in San Francisco, the city that closed down such clubs in 1984.[4]

These factors, occurring simultaneously and with greatest impact on urban gay ghettos, have led some to feel AIDS is over. Men infected with HIV who have shown dramatic health improvement and increased energy as a result of combination therapies best exemplify the spirit of hope and optimism. Many are returning to work, resuming careers they had been forced to abandon in a cyclone of infections and exhaustion. Some have declared their AIDS diagnoses relics of the past, and embraced new identities as survivors.[5] Instead of confronting morbidity and mortality, they are being rocked by what the *The New York Times* has called "the jolt of facing a new life."[6] Careers, boyfriends, credit card bills, and plans for old age, the flotsam and jetsam of everyday middle-class life, increasingly seize center stage as the epidemic recedes into the past, fading away like a very bad dream. AIDS seems over, and so we come back to life.

Yet for many people, AIDS is not over. In fact, it's far from over. A discussion of the end of the epidemic strikes these people as bizarre, absurd, and deeply offensive. Those for whom new treatments have not worked, as well as those who do not have the funds, health care resources, inclination, or predictable patterns of living that allow for a strict regimen of pill taking, may react in horror at the suggestion.[7] Will their suffering and human needs be left behind while the culture moves on, writing about AIDS in the past tense? Populations such as African Americans and Latinos, who may be a few years behind epicenter gay communities in the caseload curve, and who currently are experiencing rising numbers of new infections, may be appalled at the suggestion that AIDS is over.[8] Developing nations, now home to the vast numbers of AIDS cases in the world, may be stunned at even the hint that the epidemic is ending.[9] They say, what about *our* people? What about *us?*

HARBINGERS OF A NEW ERA

I first became transfixed by gay men's rapidly shifting conception of the AIDS epidemic during the spring of 1996. I had read bits and pieces about the new treatments but hadn't given them much credence. After a decade of hopeful support for friends on everything from AZT to Compound Q to GP120, I found it difficult to summon up optimism about treatments.

A friend with whom I share tea at one of the ubiquitous queer coffeehouses in the Castro broke through what had become my habitual nonchalance. He had returned from a trip to the East Coast looking robust, energized, and, for the first time in years, happy. Our usual chit-chat of gossip and political griping was replaced by his enthusiastic recounting of what seemed to me to be a remarkable recovery from illnesses that had plagued him for a number of years. He talked about the reappearance of his libido, his return to the gym, and his reentry into local social scenes.

I was struck by the powerful transformation that had occurred in this man in the few months since I'd last seen him. Instead of somberly and with great ambivalence grappling with his approaching death, he was reconceptualizing his life possibilities and reengaging with the world. An escalating tendency toward isolation had been stopped in its tracks and he was now talking with gusto about trips to the Russian River (a Northern California gay resort area), evenings at dance clubs, and visits to the symphony. Like the biblical figure Lazarus, he seemed to have returned from the dead.

I can easily discount evidence of cultural shifts when a solitary informant is the source, so initially I did not take my discussion with this man seriously. I didn't mention his transformation to anyone and, on a deep level of consciousness, I didn't actually believe him. Instead, I viewed him as yet another friend with AIDS on his own path toward making sense and meaning from a senseless and meaningless epidemic. Ever generous of spirit when it costs me nothing, I told myself that, being uninfected myself, it would be wrong to judge him. I remembered the New Age mantra from the days of the early epidemic and repeated it to myself: "Love him, don't judge him. Love him, don't judge him. . . . " Wasn't I a benevolent guy?

Yet within a few weeks, I'd come upon other friends who were telling similar stories. One man whom I thought had died because I hadn't seen him around our usual haunts, surprised me one morning at the gym. Having become accustomed to such weird occurrences over the past dozen years, I wasn't too disturbed to see a ghost. Yet Julio wasn't simply alive, he was his old hunky self—big arms, great legs, solid mass of butt. My first thought was that he'd joined my pal Al and his cronies in their quest to beat wasting syndrome through the use of steroids. But before I knew it, Julio was rattling off lists of drugs of which I'd never heard, singing the praises of his physician, and complaining about having to live by an alarm clock. One ten-minute conversation yanked Julio out of the cemetery of my mind and placed him back in the mad whirl of San Francisco's gym/bar/dance/party/sex culture.

Perhaps the man most responsible for shaking me awake to the changes occurring around me was my friend Tony. Tony was a young man, barely in his thirties, who had been infected with HIV for about ten years. During the first few years, he'd had no illnesses and showed no indication of slowing down his intense social life. On the rare occasion when I'd go to book readings, movie screenings, or fancy restaurants, Tony always seemed to be there, brimming with chatter about the dozens of other engagements he'd had that same week and commenting on this museum opening or that opera. Many people admired his zest for life and his apparently unlimited appetite for upscale dining and high culture.

Many also envied Tony for having an older, uninfected lover of significant wealth and achievement who supported both the socialite and the dilettante in the young man. Hence Tony had the opportunity and means to construct a life that at times seemed to emerge from middle-class fantasies. I'd met the husband only a few times, though they'd been together almost a decade. He was a handsome man in his sixties, enmeshed in a conservative professional career, who clearly adored Tony's zany side and was neither manipulative nor judgmental of the younger man's extravagant, and occasionally quirky, tastes. I felt no sense of exploitation or sugar-daddy power games between them, just enjoyment of each other's company, an identical sense of humor, and a whole lot of love.

When Tony began experiencing AIDS-related illnesses about five years ago, his lover turned into a combination of Florence Nightingale and the Tooth Fairy. He provided constant care and support, while indulging Tony's frequently outlandish requests. One winter when he was struggling with a bout of pneumocystis, Tony sorrowfully whined that he'd never had a fur coat. His lover made sure a full-length ermine coat was under the tree at Christmas.

Imagine my surprise when I ran into a healthy-looking Tony in line at the gay film festival and he told me he'd found a job working in a bookstore and left his lover for a man his own age. It seems Tony was one of the first in the city to be put on combination therapies (perhaps due to his lover's wealth and influence) and his response was rapid and extraordinary. Within six weeks, he'd experienced a full turnaround in his health and his doctor was cautiously using terms like "remission" and calling his condition "manageable." Tony had met Marc, a waiter at one of his favorite restaurants, and quickly reconsidered his current relationship, faced up to its limitations, and decided, in his words, "to go for it." The spurned husband was severely dejected, though not vengeful, and left the door open for Tony's return should life with Marc come to an unhappy ending.

Most of what I recall about seeing Tony at the film festival was that I was outraged at him for leaving his lover. Perhaps because I am the uninfected lover of an infected man, I immediately empathized with Tony's lover and, under the surface, raged at my friend's selfishness and lack of gratitude. The older man took care of his infected lover in sickness while, when health arrived, my friend exited the scene with a handsome younger man. Isn't that what younger men have traditionally done to older men? Will this pattern be replicated by all the Lazaruses of the world, returning from the dead only to get buzz cuts, put on tight jeans and tank tops, and announce to their uninfected partners that, now that they are healthy, it's time to end the relationship?

Yet quite apart from my judgments about Tony's relationships, something was dawning in me, directly below the level of consciousness. I was becoming aware that men who were responding to these new therapies were in for a sea change in their life expectations, relationships, and core identities. This wasn't simply another twist on what had become the roller-coaster ride of having AIDS. No, something new was happening here, something that had the potential to qualitatively change the texture of our collective lives in the epidemic. At that time I was not precisely sure what might happen and I can't pretend I was convinced such changes would be long term or permanent. Yet it was becoming clear to me that the fragile foundation of gay community life amid the epidemic—the assumptions, processes, and understandings we'd collectively come to share—was about to be profoundly shaken.

While friends with AIDS who responded well to combination therapies were the most obvious sign of shifts in the epidemic, more subtle changes in daily life seemed to be harbingers of a new era. Whereas five and ten years earlier, the vast majority of my friends were HIV infected, now the balance had shifted in the other direction. Fewer invitations to memorial services came my way, and fewer phone calls from far-flung friends brought announcements of deaths.

I noticed this shift most dramatically when, over a period of a few weeks, two dear friends who had been long-term AIDS survivors died. I learned of Dick's death in a shocking manner. I'd spoken to him the day I left for a week of travel and set up a lunch date for when I returned. While he'd suffered his first serious HIV-related illnesses over the previous six months, his spirits were good and he'd recently experienced significant improvement in his health. Just a few days later, while thumbing through *The New York Times* over breakfast in Seattle, I came upon his obituary. It felt as if the roof had fallen in.

Frank's death followed, after he'd endured three months of tremendous suffering. Frank had been my closest friend throughout my dozen years' sojourn in California and was the friend with whom I traveled overseas, participated in Gay Games festivities, and rented a house in Provincetown at the end of each summer. Together we shared holidays, went to street fairs, and attended motorcycle runs. He'd had AIDS since 1985 but had bounced back after any number of serious illnesses and was incredibly active and engaged with life.

In the end, cancer got him and got him bad, the same type of cancer that had killed his dad at age thirty-seven. While Frank's friends, family, and caregivers never agreed on the role AIDS played in his final illness and death (we sparred about what should be stated in the obituary), for me his powerful decline over a brief period was marked by most of the maladies and manifestations of AIDS.[10] When he finally allowed himself to die, I felt that familiar awful mixture of gratitude and grief. But I told myself I was doing fine.

A few days after Frank's death, these two losses blindsided me, as if I had been hit by a Mack truck while casually crossing the street. I created mental lists of reasons why these particular deaths might hit me so hard: Frank was my primary link to the disco years, Dick served as a kindly mentor to me for two decades, and both men were among the few surviving gay male pals from my years in Los Angeles.

Yet a few weeks later, something else dawned on me: prior to these losses, I'd gone for a year without a significant death. This had been the longest expanse of time in a dozen years that I'd been free from bedsides and suicides, morbidity and memorials. The deaths of two close friends in a short time, once so commonplace that such occurrences felt normal, now seemed shocking. It was as if the videotape of my life had been rewound and I was jolted back to 1985.

Noting my reaction to these deaths helped me realize changes were occurring. Statistics for cities such as San Francisco and New York clearly indicated that the peak years of deaths for gay men of my generation had been 1989-1995.[11] Somehow I hadn't realized that the contortions in my psyche and the bizarre deformations of daily life could recede. Nothing had prepared me for life after the tidal wave. After spending a dozen years tossed amid rough currents of terror and rage, grief and shock, what happens to the human spirit when it is finally washed back ashore, and rests peaceably in the sunshine?

WHAT IT WAS LIKE AND WHAT IT'S LIKE NOW

I believe many gay men in America today who have survived the first two decades of AIDS share a similar paradoxical situation. We inhabit worlds where suddenly fewer are sick and fewer are dying. The tremendous weight of loss has eased and the terror within has abated. It feels like we are taking our first deep breaths since 1981. It feels like AIDS, as we have known it, is over.

Yet people *are* still dying, not only people from whom middle-class white gay men often separate themselves—Latinos, blacks, drug users, women, poor people—but middle-class white gay men like Dick and Frank.[12] And people *are* still getting infected, including new generations of young gay men. Many infected gay men remain on pins and needles, dreading new health problems, wondering whether their success on protease inhibitors represents the end of the storm or simply the eye of the hurricane. How can some of us have this feeling that AIDS is over when we have the knowledge that it is not? How can two such different understandings of what is happening around us coexist?

My answer here is neither easy nor simple. A stark shift has occurred that has produced conditions out of which these paradoxical feelings emerge. Those who have lived at the center of the cyclone since the early years of the epidemic—gay men in epicenter cities, people involved in AIDS groups, residents of urban gay neighborhoods—are especially likely to harbor these conflicted feelings for one major reason: AIDS, as we have known it, *is* over.

From the outset of the epidemic AIDS emerged as two distinct entities: AIDS the biomedical syndrome and AIDS the event. Some activists fought to prevent this split in the early 1980s, arguing that AIDS was simply a disease, no more, no less. When writers and political leaders would whip the new epidemic into a metaphor or a symbol, we insisted that AIDS was simply a collection of illnesses or a viral-driven sickness, nothing else. It was certainly not the work of a wrathful god. Certainly not a sign of judgment on gay sex. It was just a disease and should not be politicized.[13]

By the late 1980s, however, the swath AIDS cut was so wide and so destructive, it was impossible to stop the media, public health officials, and antigay crusaders from projecting a diverse array of meanings onto the epidemic.[14] Try as we might to prevent AIDS from becoming stigmatized, because of the unexpectedness of its arrival, the fury of its force, and the populations it targeted, we watched helplessly as public health officials and television commentators attached a range of cultural meanings to the epidemic. Once that battle was lost, lesbian and gay communities threw themselves into combat with every powerful sector of the culture—journalists, doctors, politicians, movie stars, religious leaders—over the precise shaping of the event called AIDS.

Before we knew it, AIDS the disease was merely the terrain, the thin layer of topsoil, on which AIDS the sociocultural event was being constructed. AIDS the event overshadowed AIDS the disease, and different communities adapted the event to suit their own needs. Swiftly, AIDS became a magnet for countless anxieties, understandings, and social misgivings. For urban gay men, the event rapidly became marked by three key meanings that emerged from gay ghettos in epicenter cities: (1) AIDS meant a quick and usually ugly death; (2) AIDS meant an end to the sexual revolution and the gay sexual cultures of the 1970s; and (3) AIDS meant most of our friends would be wiped off the face of the earth within a very short time.

All three of these characteristics became the focus of tremendous debate among gay men. Many argued that AIDS was not necessarily fatal, and charismatic leaders of people-with-AIDS groups who had lived for several years with an AIDS diagnosis were pointed out as evidence. Sexual liberationists fought to prevent a medical syndrome from being used to stigmatize sexual practices and moralize against promiscuity. Activists alternately exaggerated and downplayed the estimates of deaths. Despite arguments and the occasional evidence to the contrary, public health leaders and journalists gave powerful symbolic weight to these meanings and drilled them deep into many of our psyches.

I'd argue passionately with friends that AIDS wasn't 100 percent fatal and, the next day, on hearing a friend had been diagnosed, I'd pencil his name onto the death list in my mind. I'd tell myself that I could still be a proud, promiscuous homosexual, but I found fewer places to meet men and fewer men open to casual encounters. After a while I had to admit I could no longer avoid feelings of disgust for my sex life or keep guilt feelings out of my encounters.

For many of us, the event called AIDS and its meanings have become deeply inscribed on our consciousnesses and our bodies and are not easily dislodged. AIDS hit the very foundations of our lives like a tornado, ripping apart assumptions, shredding identities, spinning long-held beliefs about ourselves and our community into the air, like cows and chickens. On a visceral level, we experience AIDS as awful, ugly, powerful, and intransigent. For many gay men throughout America, the acronym "AIDS" resonates powerfully with fatality, sexual repression, and cataclysmic loss.

Yet this no longer is how everyday life in gay communities *feels* to us. Our social practices and daily experiences often have shifted dramatically. We know people with AIDS who have survived fifteen years. We have HIV-positive friends who are healthy, active, and engaged with life. We know Lazaruses who have returned from long periods on the brink of death and now seem filled with energy and activity. On hearing a friend has become infected, we no longer quickly write him off as an inevitable death.

We are no longer in the midst of a time in which vast numbers of our friends are dying. The profound impact we felt in epicenter cities from 1989-1995 has abated. The intensity now is muted, spread out, mitigated. It seems strange to admit, but the experience of losing twenty-five friends, colleagues, and social acquaintances in a single year is qualitatively different from losing them over a ten-year period. Having what felt like an entire generation of gay men die in a single decade is different from having a significant portion of the next generation of gay men die over three decades.

The avalanche of AIDS hit during a cultural moment when gay liberationists, along with other sexual liberationists, had struggled to free ourselves from guilt and repression. We said "Gay is Good" and "Sex is Good," and forced issues of danger, guilt, and religious moralizing to recede into the background. Because of this, many experienced AIDS as an extremely punitive version of a fall from innocence. On a psychic level, the epidemic seemingly confirmed the ugliest predictions of Anita Bryant, Paul Cameron, and Jerry Falwell, antigay crusaders of the 1970s. If AIDS meant an end to the sexual revolution and the gay sexual cultures of the 1970s, its meaning today is extraordinarily different.

During the mid- and late 1980s, in many urban centers, gay male sexual cultures virtually dried up. Some clubs went underground and managed to operate during this dry spell but with significantly fewer participants. There were a few years in San Francisco when it was difficult to find a place to dance on a Friday or Saturday night or anything resembling a legitimate sex club. Fast-forward a decade and San Francisco, Los Angeles, and New York City each offer more than a dozen spaces for men to meet and have sex. The evolution of circuit parties drawing thousands of men to large urban centers over holiday weekends has replaced the disco soirees of the 1970s and early 1980s. Gay ghettos are again active sites for unabashed cruising and sexual pickups.[15]

The surviving men who inhabited sexual spaces in the early 1980s are now in our late thirties, forties, fifties, and older. Our generation does not occupy a dominant position in most contemporary gay male sex venues. Instead our places have been filled by vast numbers of men in their twenties and early thirties. The impact of AIDS on these men's sexualities is extraordinarily different from our own. They came out during the Reagan-Bush-Gingrich years, a time when gay leaders who sought public acceptance through a strategy of conformity to heterosexual norms actively maligned gay liberation's foundational belief that sexual freedom is valuable and life-affirming.[16]

What is more, these young men's entire adult sex lives have been lived under the cloud of the epidemic.[17] From the start, they have had to contend with profound linkages between gay sex and disease. The primary language about sex that has been placed in their mouths and wired into their brains has a vocabulary of "risk," "condoms," and "safer sex." Instead of living through the period of gay liberation and sexual freedom, then having a house fall on them, they've constructed their sexual identities and networks amidst the reality of a rapacious, sexually transmitted virus.

In this book, I argue that although AIDS the biomedical syndrome continues to march forward, the event of AIDS as epicenter gay men came to know it in the 1980s is over. The experience of gay men's everyday lives at the end of the 1990s is qualitatively different than it was as the corpses piled up around us a decade earlier. As one event ends, a new event is emerging that offers distinct experiences and new understandings of the epidemic. Research data drawn from interviews with young gay men have foreshadowed this difference since the early 1990s.[18]

At least three key changes have brought about the changing of the events: (1) AIDS no longer usually means a quick and ugly death; (2) Since 1990, new and highly visible sexual cultures have appeared and taken root in urban centers; and (3) the volume and rate of loss for gay men has declined dramatically. Influencing this powerful yet often unrecognized shift is another matter quite separate from AIDS: the passage of time. A fifteen-year passage of time has been accompanied by a tremendous influx of young gay men into gay circles. The men who comprised the nebulous thing we call "the gay community" in 1980 are no longer numerically and culturally dominant. Not all of us are dead, but many of the survivors have withdrawn due to exhaustion, disaffection, and simple life-cycle shifts. Our lives in middle age may be constructed very differently from our lives in our twenties.

Yet the formal structures of gay community life have not acknowledged this shift. AIDS organizations, gay activists, HIV-prevention campaigns, queer cultural events, and gay men's literature all continue to operate out of assumptions and understandings rooted in the AIDS event of the 1980s. Michael Wright, a social worker and leading prevention theorist, put it this way:

> I still see campaigns for ASOs (AIDS service organizations) which characterize AIDS as an emergency situation. In the beginning AIDS was an emergency, but no emergency lasts seventeen years. Diarrhea continues to be a major cause of death among children in developing countries, as it has been for generations. Why is that not an emergency?
>
> AIDS is, like many other serious diseases and other risk situations, gradually an integrated part of modern life. People

have developed ways of dealing with this reality, some effective, some not so effective. The existence of ASOs cannot be justified by declaring a state of emergency.[19]

This book offers reasons why gay communities must shift their perspectives and fully acknowledge the diverse realities of contemporary gay men's lives. It is critically important that this shift occur soon. Although each new person who becomes infected may experience crisis on a personal level, the collective gay community has left the emergency state. The failure to change with the times and work with gay men in the realities of their present experience of the epidemic is not without cost. Young gay men experience high levels of alienation from formal structures of gay life such as community organizations, political events, cultural rituals, and community-based media. Many feel patronized, lied to, and strangely ignored by gay public officials, organizational leaders, and journalists.[20] This alienation is in large part a response to the tremendous dissonance between their everyday experience of the epidemic and the bizarre ways in which that experience is reflected back to them through lenses as diverse as mainstream movies, HIV-prevention campaigns and mass gay fund-raising events. It leaves young gay men without trust in the leadership and institutions of their communities.

Yet it is not only young gay men who experience this dissonance. Middle-aged and old gay men who have found ways to come to terms with the decimation AIDS has wreaked on their lives find the continuing rhetoric and constructions of AIDS as a crisis to be debilitating and inauthentic. These men are put in a position of either sacrificing their own hard-earned adjustment and acceptance of the epidemic, or exiting community life. Many no longer experience the epidemic as an emergency and are pressured to feel either guilty or wrong for the shift they have made. To remain involved in community life requires them to anesthetize their emotions and deny their perspectives.[21]

The costs of continuing to operate out of a paradigm of AIDS forged in the 1980s go beyond this pervasive alienation from community institutions and leadership. The failure of HIV-prevention efforts to protect large numbers of at-risk gay men from becoming infected is increasingly related to their failure to speak to the realities of gay men's lives.

The campaigns we have crafted in the United States and the paradigms on which we base our work now require reconsideration. There are other ways that our nation could have structured its effort against HIV/AIDS. David Halperin has brilliantly summarized the vast gulf between U.S. and Australian approaches to HIV/AIDS. He shared his lecture notes on this topic with me:

Australia. Since 1984, cooperation with affected communities (gay men; also IV drug users and sex workers); a unified national response (given federal system in which states are responsible for health care delivery). Gay groups had already mobilised to form AIDS Action committees in 1983; by 1985 these became the AIDS Councils, linked by the Australian Federation of AIDS Organisations, funded by Commonwealth (either directly or indirectly). Commonwealth Government responsible for overall policy and funding, nongovernmental organizations for education and prevention in local communities. States help coordinate and distribute federal funds directly to gay community agencies, IV drug user groups, sex worker collectives, etc. Three three-year national strategies, the latest launched in 1996. Nonpartisan issue. Linked to gay law reform: gay sex was still illegal in New South Wales and most states in 1984; now it is legal throughout Australia; Federal sexual privacy law. New South Wales has passed laws criminalising discrimination against lesbians, gay people, transgendered people, and people with AIDS; it has also made antigay hate speech illegal. It has granted greater recognition to homosexual relationships; Federal government treats all unmarried couples alike for the purpose of immigration law (though Howard government has in effect gutted that provision). Needle exchange legal.

United States. No national AIDS strategy. Expenditure of federal government funds on explicit safe sex information is illegal. No national health care/Medicare. Prostitution and needle exchange illegal nearly everywhere (though juries fail to convict violators of needle exchange statutes). Gay sex itself is illegal in about half of the states, but antigay discrimination is legal. In forty-three of the fifty states, it is perfectly legal to sack an employee, or to refuse to sell or lease housing to someone, solely because that person is homosexual. The same-sex partners of U.S. citizens have no right to residency or immigration, and people infected with HIV may not enter the United States, unless granted a waiver.

In Australia, the epidemic has been contained; by the end of March 1997, about 16,400 people had been infected. There have been 7,383 cases of AIDS; 5,325 people have died. Three inner-Sydney health districts together account for about half the national total of AIDS cases. More than 80 percent of HIV infections are in men and are ascribed to transmission through male-to-male sexual contact. In the last two years, new HIV infections have actually been declining in real numbers. According to the 1997 Annual Surveillance Report, produced by Professor John Kaldor of the National Centre in HIV Epidemiology and Clinical Research at the University of New South Wales, the number of diagnosed cases of AIDS per year in Australia peaked at 962 in 1994 and has since declined to 706 in 1996; they are expected to fall steadily to 600 by the year 2000. Currently, about 500 people are infected with HIV each year in Australia.

Compare this to the United States. In the United States, a million people have been infected. More than 500,000 cases of people with AIDS had been officially recorded by 1996, and more than 300,000 people had died (60 times as many deaths from AIDS as in Australia). AIDS has become the leading cause of death in the United States for males aged twenty-five to forty-four years (accounting for 23 percent of deaths in this group) and the third leading cause of death for women in this age group (11 percent of deaths). The number of cases by year has increased tenfold since 1984.[22]

For those who believe the United States' approach to HIV/AIDS is superior to that of the rest of the world, Halperin's stark contrast with Australia's effort may seem startling. While in terms of sheer numbers, the population of the United States dwarfs Australia's, a comparison of statistics on the seroprevalance level of at-risk populations reveals the superior effectiveness of Australia's approach. San Francisco and Sydney both may be identified in the eyes of the world as havens for gay people and share highly visible sex cultures and many sex-oriented commercial spaces, but about 40 percent of the gay men in San Francisco are infected with HIV while only 20 percent of those in Sydney test positive.[23]

AIDS leaders in the United States could learn a great deal from Australians. Instead of considering gay men as empowered agents working diligently to navigate strategically through a hazardous course as do Australians, American prevention leaders condescendingly issue directives, judgments, and manipulative materials.[24] Prevention efforts in the United States largely fail to respect the rights and trust the abilities of many gay men and, instead, treat us like Pavlov's dogs, awaiting the next stimulus.

MASS EXODUS FROM THE STATE OF EMERGENCY

My thinking about the social and cultural context of American gay communities has evolved enormously over the past three years since I wrote *Reviving the Tribe: Regenerating Gay Men's Sexuality and Culture in the Ongoing Epidemic*. Written before the advent of protease inhibitors, the book suggests that surviving gay men who had been out and involved in building community before the avalanche of AIDS have suffered cataclysmic losses. These losses may be counted not only in terms of bodies, but include also icons, identities, social networks, and the spirit of the times. The symbolic losses may be as devastating as the corporeal ones.

I argued that gay men of my generation faced a stark choice in dealing with an epidemic likely to continue throughout our lifetimes. We could continue to be buffeted by intense emotions as the health crisis took an unpredictable course, or we could commit ourselves individually and communally to regenerating community and culture. The final section of the book focuses on a blueprint for community-wide revival amidst a continuing landscape of death and morbidity.

I was heartened when the book received critical acclaim and significant media coverage. Because it was published by a small scholarly press, I thought it likely the book would go unnoticed. Yet my work seemed to speak to some people about issues they'd quietly pondered, yet never discussed. In the space of a year, I traveled to twenty-five cities to engage in discussions about the issues raised in the book. Because I was aware that some of my thinking was controversial and might introduce volatile ideas into the public sphere, my publisher and I chose a touring strategy focused only on queer venues and media. Not only did I do book readings at gay bookstores, but I also gave speeches for both gay and AIDS organizations, facilitated workshops, and participated in small group discussions with gay therapists and educators, focused on the ideas discussed in the book.

One tremendous and unforeseen benefit of this touring was that I came into contact with many, many gay men who were eager to talk about our sexual cultures, experiences in the epidemic, and possibilities for personal and communal regeneration. I was happy to hear men speak about the important issues in their lives and share their understandings of what had happened to us and what might occur in the future. In locations as diverse as Fort Lauderdale, Seattle, Madison, Houston, and rural Oregon, I was privileged to hear the pain and sorrow, as well as the joy, in men's contemporary lives. Even more important, however, was the vast volume of information I received about how men were steering themselves through the confusion and unpredictability of their worlds. During this period of intense exposure to gay men's understandings and analyses of the impact of the epidemic on their lives, my own thinking began to shift in new directions. Five specific groups of gay men were most responsible for informing my thoughts: young gay men; men outside of the large, hard-hit cities; gay men of color; HIV-positive gay men who were "long-term nonprogressors"; and HIV-negative middle-aged men.

To my surprise, large numbers of gay men under the age of twenty-five attended my workshops and readings. What spoke to them in my book seemed to be the book's sense of hope and commitment to recreating dynamic gay communities. As one man in Boston told me, "I came to see you because I wanted to learn more about the 1970s, the last period when anything like a functional gay community existed. I want to learn how you guys did it so I can be part of doing something similar today."

Young gay men were generous in talking with me about their own experiences in the AIDS epidemic. Whether HIV positive or negative, these men's understandings of AIDS were quite different from many men's of my generation. Almost universally, they were critical of current HIV-prevention efforts targeting their age cohort, finding them condescending, manipulative, and, in the view of one man from San Diego, "infantilizing." Most of them felt like nonparticipants in the event of AIDS. Their experiences of the epidemic were neither highly charged nor overarching. AIDS has been a part of their gay worlds since day one, and they insisted that the social and sexual practices they had developed as they came into their gay identities took into account the dangers of AIDS. They felt they neither ignored the reality of HIV in the world nor were held hostage by it.

The second group responsible for changing my thinking were men outside of epicenter cities. I was clear in *Reviving the Tribe* that I was writing about a limited group of surviving gay men who circulated around gay ghettos in New York City, Los Angeles, and San Francisco, and I stated this intent explicitly several times. Yet when I was in small cities and towns in Minnesota, Oregon, and Texas, I met several men who felt that their experiences of loss in the epidemic paralleled those of men in epicenter cities. I received letters from men living in rural Maine and coastal Washington who felt that my twisted narrative of the epidemic matched their own. I no longer so confidently claim that the themes in *Reviving the Tribe* speak only to men inhabiting neighborhoods such as Chelsea in New York or San Francisco's Castro district, although I do feel rural experiences of AIDS *are* different from urban experiences.

Yet many men from midsize and small urban areas shared with me quite different understandings of the epidemic. While over 65 percent of gay men of my generation in San Francisco are HIV positive or dead, this age cohort of men in smaller, nonepicenter cities may be 10 or 20 percent infected or dead.[25] AIDS certainly exists among gay men living in small towns and rural parts of the nation, yet many men from these places articulated an experience of AIDS qualitatively different from my own. One middle-aged man from small-town Indiana had lost no close friends to the epidemic, and he'd been involved in community life since the 1970s.

This man and others spoke movingly of an experience of the epidemic I'd never even imagined. As the tidal wave of AIDS hit epicenter cities in the late 1980s and became highly visible in both the gay and mainstream media, these men initially felt odd, guilty, somehow "less gay." Some talked of facing identity crises around this time. One man told me he'd deliberately moved to the nearest urban area, in part because he felt guilty about not being involved in the AIDS response. By the early 1990s, many of these men talked about coming to terms with the realities of HIV in their areas, but expressed anger that their own experiences were rarely reflected in media discussions of gay men in the epidemic. One group of men from the South argued that safe sex rules disseminated nationally imposed inappropriate restrictions on them that emanated from epicenter cities. They argued that failure to use a condom during anal sex with a stranger in San Francisco (where about 50 percent of the gay men are HIV positive)[26] carried much greater risk than doing likewise in places such as Jackson, Mississippi, or Hot Springs, Arkansas.

Gay men of color constituted the third group powerfully influencing my thinking. While some seemed to embrace *Reviving the Tribe* and saw their own stories in its pages, others insisted the intense state of repeat trauma that I claimed had seized many urban gay men in the late 1980s and early 1990s was "a white thing." These men, primarily African American and Latino, argued that, while their communities were very hard hit by HIV, they saw a resilience among their peers that was not captured in my book. Gay men of color who lived primarily in the mainstream gay community in urban centers seemed to relate more to the repeat trauma state I discussed than those based in communities of color.

Men of color went out of their way to challenge me to open my eyes more broadly to the conditions of their communities. As a white man with limited direct experience with the internal workings of gay communities of color, I was grateful that these men shared with me stories of their lives in the epidemic. At first I only understood more deeply that when AIDS hit certain communities of color, it was striking a population already contending with various crises—racist violence, massive unemployment, political backlashes, entrenched poverty, gang warfare—and AIDS was simply added to the heap. Those who argue that because these communities did not respond to the epidemic as white communities did in the mid- and late 1980s, they did not respond at all, fail to understand the dynamics of communities under siege on several fronts and the extremely limited resources available to gay men of color at that time. They also fail to understand how economic class is deeply implicated in a community's experience of AIDS.

I grew to understand that many of the qualities and resources that communities of color have had to rely on to survive centuries of racism in America have served these communities well during the AIDS epidemic and have provided gay men of color with different experiences and understandings of AIDS than the crisis construct I wrote about. The strength of the black church (despite the institution's continuing antigay practices), Puerto Rican and Chicano families, and Asian immigrant communities have served many men of color as havens of support during a mushrooming AIDS epidemic in their communities. While certainly homophobia had to be contended with in communities-of-origin, to pretend that gay men of color during the 1980s and 1990s did not reap benefits from these foundational institutions is to rewrite many individual gay men's experience of AIDS.

A fourth group of gay men insisted my book was out of date by the time it was published. These were HIV-positive gay men who had been infected for a long time, yet remained healthy and hearty. Many of these men related to the themes in the book because they too had endured years of life in a state of crisis, searching for lesions on a daily basis and mistaking every cold or flu for the first bout of pneumocystis. They knew what it felt like to spend long periods terrorized by a blood-borne virus, and they knew that it was a stretch to think such a state offered any kind of quality of life.

Yet these men, some after a decade of knowing their status and fearing the imminent arrival of illness, had made a conscious decision to move on, to exit the state of emergency. As one man candidly told me:

> I just couldn't live that way any longer. It was too awful and I wasted too much time anticipating my own decline and death. When that didn't happen, I finally had to change my

way of thinking. I couldn't stay trapped in that same state of obsessive fear any longer. Something had to change.[27]

As I traveled around the country I met many men with HIV who had stopped identifying themselves as "people with HIV" and insisted they were not going to allow HIV to claim a central part of their identity and preoccupy the majority of their waking hours. These men affirmed the optimism I expressed in *Reviving the Tribe* that gay men were beginning to regenerate their lives and their cultures and that AIDS no longer held them hostage. Yet these men insisted I underplayed such a revival in my book and that it was far more sweeping than I had indicated. My work on this current book has been triggered largely by the thinking and observations of these men.

The final group who educated me was a group about whom I felt I knew a great deal: uninfected, middle-aged, urban gay men. I count myself a member of this group and have spent the past six years immersing myself in the study of the experiences and social worlds of HIV-negative gay men. Yet some of these men expressed disagreement, even anger, with my representation of them in my writings and speeches. One group of men in my own neighborhood told me they had adopted strategies very early in the AIDS epidemic that allowed them to have the kind of sex they wanted yet minimized their risk for infection. One man told me he'd never stopped having unprotected anal sex, but he'd only get fucked without a condom by a man he knew both intimately and long enough to trust his representation of his serostatus. Another spoke of deliberately shifting from getting fucked to getting fisted as a way to continue anal pleasures but reduce risk.

These men were like me in some important ways. We had all remained sexually active throughout the fifteen years of the epidemic. We lived in a city where a majority of the sexually active gay men were infected, and we'd all reached 1996 and were still HIV negative. We differed in one essential way: whereas I had not emotionally accepted that my strategies for sex were likely to keep me uninfected, these men insisted they felt confident that their choices were unlikely to expose them to HIV. I still cycled through feelings of paranoia and guilt about my sex, while they, in one man's words, were "long over it."

These five groups of men—young gay men, gay men who lived outside epicenter cities, gay men of color, HIV-positive men who had been healthy for a long time, and HIV-negative urban gay men—forced me to begin to reassess my thinking about the evolving social, cultural, and sexual worlds gay communities were creating in the 1990s. But it was not until I was exposed to the thinking of social scientists from halfway around the world that I began to analyze and understand contemporary American gay men from a fresh perspective.

DRY BONES BREATHE

The work of Gary Dowsett, a sociologist at Macquarie University in Australia, blew out of the water my tentative rethinking of these issues. I'd come across Dowsett's early work during my research for *Reviving the Tribe*. He was part of a research team led by R.W. Connell that examined working-class gay men's sexualities and proposed critical alterations in our understandings of prevention issues and the pragmatics of our work with HIV prevention.[28] I had been impressed with the team's sophisticated understandings of the ways in which sexual desires and practices are constituted and the powerful and respectful ways they presented the social and cultural context of working men's lives.

At the International AIDS Conference in Vancouver in July 1996, I was intrigued by a paper Dowsett was scheduled to present, "'Post AIDS': Assessing the Long-Term Social Impact of HIV/ AIDS in Gay Communities."[29] The abstract in the conference book stated, "There is evidence of a 'post-AIDS' culture emerging in Sydney, and the epidemic has still to 'bite' in Adelaide. . . . These findings argue for a re-reading of prevention modes, and throw doubt on the usefulness of a 'national' epidemic in public health planning in Australia. . . . "[30]

I immediately penciled this paper into my already overloaded conference calendar. When I showed up for the presentation, I was not disappointed. Dowsett rapidly summarized the study that he co-authored with David McInnes:

> There is also an emerging phenomenon that we call "post-AIDS." The first glimmer of this appeared among young gay

men in Oxford Street, who had become gay or "come out" after the epidemic had started. In Australia such men are not significantly at higher risk of HIV infection. These young men were mostly experienced in sex and relationships. They had been tested for HIV and were very well-informed about HIV/AIDS. For them, safe sex has always been there; yet almost all had had unprotected anal intercourse in certain sexual contexts. While the epidemic was very present for them, they were not waiting desperately for it to end. They were already "over it." In one sense they were living "post-AIDS."[31]

By this time, the conference hall sat in stunned silence as Dowsett continued presenting their findings:

> The large majority of gay men in Australia are not infected. They know that and have adapted their behaviour for over a decade now to maintain that fact. Even for many gay men in Sydney, HIV/AIDS is no longer a crisis. They daily live with HIV/AIDS in their work, among seropositive friends and lovers, and within a safe sex culture that suffuses community life. These men are already living as they will for the rest of their lives or until the epidemic is over, whichever comes first. Such gay men are already living "post-AIDS." How much longer can we continue to represent the epidemic as crisis, as chaos, as merely an unsafe slip away, in the face of this obviously successful living with HIV/AIDS?[32]

What I liked most about Dowsett and McInnes's paper, and what I found to be in greatest contrast with most U.S. research on gay men's responses to AIDS, was the respect their work held for gay men as active agents attempting to work through the confusion and hazards of our current lives. In arguing for a "different conceptualization" of the current epidemics, the authors insist that practices such as "segregated partner selection," "concordant serostatus relationships," and "debates on unprotected versus unsafe sex" are not "disasters for prevention or safe sex culture." Instead they are "creative 'post-AIDS' responses to current epidemics, and constitute rich resources for new, more sophisticated community work—work no longer mobilising constant fear or a state of siege."[33]

While the media story from the Vancouver conference focused heavily on protease inhibitors and combination therapies, Dowsett and McInnes's work on gay men's post-AIDS cultural responses was, for me, the conference highlight. Immediately my mind began racing through my tentative understandings of what was going on among gay men in the United States. The fact that the Australian paper focused upon young gay men's adaptations to the presence of HIV, the different impact of HIV in smaller cities, and a variety of strategies that were being used by gay men in my own city, immediately provided me with a new framework to begin to consider what was happening around me. At home I'd become used to people reacting in horror upon hearing that an HIV-negative man had chosen to sleep only with other uninfected men, or that an HIV-positive man had placed a personal ad looking to get fucked by other men who had tested positive. Dowsett and McInnes offered a new conceptualization that saw such actions as smart strategies some gay men employ in order to have the kinds of sex they find meaningful and pleasurable while minimizing the risk of transmitting HIV.

There was at least one big difference between such strategies in Sydney and in San Francisco: 20 percent of the gay men having sex in Sydney were infected with HIV in 1995, while in San Francisco about 50 percent of the men were.[34] Hence while "a bit of luck," in Dowsett and McInnes's words, could be part of what keeps Australian men who engage in "some judicious risk-taking" uninfected, a great heap of luck would be necessary in San Francisco. Is post-AIDS living possible in hard-hit American cities?

Not only do I believe post-AIDS living is possible in San Francisco, Los Angeles, New York, and other urban centers, I believe many men have been doing so for quite a few years. Although the contexts of gay male communities in Australia and the United States are quite different, most gay men in the United States, HIV positive and HIV negative, appear to have adapted themselves to the arrival of the epidemic, created strategies to maximize their safety, and have gotten on with their lives. HIV-positive men on combination therapies are among those who remain anxious and may be vulnerable to powerful emotions as they face uncertainty and occasional side effects of the new treatments; ironically, they are the ones viewed by the public as real-life embodiments of the end of AIDS.

This book is titled *Dry Bones Breathe: Gay Men Creating Post-AIDS Identities and Cultures*. I've taken the title from Ezekiel 37 in the Bible, despite my ambivalence about traditional conceptions of god and my rage at the ways the Bible continues to be improperly quoted and used to restrict the rights of women and gay people. The passage captures a spirit of renewal that is sweeping gay male communities:

> Some time later, I felt the Lord's power take control of me, and his Spirit carried me to a valley full of bones. The Lord showed me all around, and everywhere I looked I saw bones that were dried out. He said, "Ezekiel, son of man, can these bones come back to life?"
>
> I replied, "Lord God, only you can answer that."
>
> He then told me to say: Dry bones, listen to what the Lord is saying to you, "I the Lord God, will put breath in you, and once again you will live. I will wrap you with muscles and skin and breathe life into you. Then you will know that I am the Lord."
>
> I did what the Lord said, but before I finished speaking, I heard a rattling noise. The bones were coming together! I saw muscles and skin cover the bones, but they had no life in them.
>
> The Lord said: Ezekiel, now say to the wind, "The Lord God commands you to blow from every direction and to breathe life into these dead bodies, so they can live again."
>
> As soon as I said this, the wind blew among the bodies, and they came back to life! They all stood up, and there were enough to make a large army.
>
> The Lord said, Ezekiel, the people of Israel are like dead bones. They complain that they are dried up and that they have no hope for the future. So tell them, "I, the Lord God, promise to open your graves and set you free. I will bring you back to Israel, and when that happens, you will realize that I am the Lord. My spirit will give you breath, and you will live again. I will bring you home, and you will know that I have kept my promise."[35]

For much of the last two decades, many surviving gay men of all antibody statuses were reduced psychologically, spiritually, and sometimes physically to dry bones, languishing in the hot sun, awaiting destruction or revival. In the aftermath of decimation, we've heard the bones connecting again, and witnessed muscle and skin again covering the skeleton. The dry bones have had life breathed back into them and now stand as giant tribes, eager to move forward, awaiting the new era.

When we look at the emerging cultures that gay men are creating at the end of the 1990s—from rural men's networks to urban circuit parties, black men's discussion groups to conventions of bears, cruisy coffee shops to huge church revivals—we know they rise out of the ruins of a painful past but offer hopeful visions of community beyond crisis. These changes challenge much of the rhetoric produced by AIDS activists and service workers, who argue that gay men must not move forward without keeping AIDS as the sole center of their collective cultures. The everyday lives of gay men throughout the nation demonstrate otherwise, and make clear one thing: AIDS-as-crisis, as defined by epicenter gay men in the 1980s, is over.

Chapter 2

The Protease Moment Takes Hold

After the July 1996 International AIDS Conference in Vancouver, stories about protease inhibitors appeared throughout the media, providing basic information about the new drugs, dancing between countervailing urges of hope and caution, and presenting dramatic stories of lives miraculously snatched from the brink of death. Although these accounts clearly had a huge impact on American conceptions of the path the epidemic was taking, gay men who regularly perused gay publications were exposed to a parallel, equally influential body of texts: multipage glossy advertisements for specific protease inhibitors that appeared in gay magazines and on bus shelters, subway billboards, and street kiosks in gay neighborhoods throughout the nation.

Queer understandings of the appearance and lifespan of people with HIV had been in flux for several years before the dawning of what I term the "Protease Moment," the post-Vancouver period when all social and cultural changes in our experiences of the AIDS epidemic were explained in light of the new therapies, or "the cocktail." The ubiquitous advertisements for Crixivan, Ritonavir, and other new drugs succeeded in consolidating conflicting images into a single, unified representation. People with HIV appeared now as healthy, active people bearing no obvious differences from uninfected people. Assaulted daily with powerful visuals of squeaky-clean, athletic, and hearty people with HIV, is it any wonder gay men throughout America, who at the same time were voraciously consuming journalistic narratives of resurrection, began to declare an end to the epidemic?

Very rapidly, the news out of Vancouver and the images of newly revived people with AIDS were displaced by a third closely related body of discourse. Newspapers and magazines throughout the United States during a four-month period from October 1996 through January 1997 published articles with bold headlines declaring "The End of AIDS." Cover stories in *Newsweek* and *The New York Times Magazine,* urban alternative weekly papers such as *The Village Voice* in New York City and *The Stranger* in Seattle, and gay publications such as *The Advocate* and *Frontiers* barraged Americans with images of a dramatic shift in the course of an epidemic that had held our lives in its tight grip for most of the past dozen years. The headlines seemed to scream at us daily, proclaiming "The Twilight of an Epidemic," "The End of the AIDS Crisis," and "After the 'Cure'."[1]

What were we to make of these pieces: the dawn of a new era or simply another round of media hype intended to salve our flagging spirits and sell tabloids?

Although the authors of these articles were certain to pepper their texts with qualifying statements assuring the reader that the biomedical syndrome of AIDS had not been vanquished, the overall effect of the headlines and the powerful artwork accompanying the pieces outweighed this token gesture. Given the power of the media to shape public understandings in a postmodern age, journalistic declarations of apocalypse now, replete with nods to the long-suffering gay community and descriptions of what I call "protease babies," born-again people with AIDS (PWAs) granted a new lease on life, set into motion powerful shifts in the ways gay men understood the epidemic.

Before this transformation could congeal, an energetic backlash emerged to challenge the media's attempt to declare HIV as chronic and manageable and lower the curtain on the final act of the AIDS drama. Letters to the editor, editorials, and op-ed pieces by gay community leaders appeared in the gay press, determined to put an end to the burgeoning AIDS-is-over rhetoric. AIDS organizations held "Hope or Hype" forums.[2] Attempting to whip the troops back into line and reaffirm the narrow understandings of AIDS embraced by gay men in the 1980s, the voices of the backlash chided the community repeatedly, reminding them "the AIDS crisis is not over," until these words seemed like the mantra of 1997. After all, they insisted, protease inhibitors are unavailable to large numbers of

HIV-positive people, or they don't work for most people with AIDS, or homeless people are too unstable to master the demanding regimens.

Newspapers throughout the nation again became sites of nasty debate over conceptions and representations of the epidemic moment. An inaccurate and dangerous misunderstanding of the changes occurring in gay cultures was foisted upon gay men. As had happened since the earliest days of the epidemic, the success or failure of pharmaceutical drugs became our sole way of explaining the trajectory of the epidemic. We became obsessed with protease inhibitors and used them to explain everything from gay men's unprotected sex to the drop-off in participation at AIDS walks to the near-zero residential vacancy rate in San Francisco. Left unidentified and undiscussed were a range of structural, cultural, and biomedical changes that, independent of the new treatments, had brought tremendous change to the social worlds of urban gay men in the years preceding the Protease Moment.

What makes the situation especially confusing is that both AIDS-the-disease and AIDS-the-event are shifting during the Protease Moment; the two, while not bound firmly together, are closely interrelated. As many begin to experience HIV infection as chronic and manageable, it cannot help but shift how the event of AIDS is understood. Few recognized the changes in everyday social practices for gay male communities in the mid-1990s, before protease inhibitors and combination therapies commanded attention. Only with the arrival of the Protease Moment did the public begin to grapple with powerful material changes in gay communities around the nation. Protease inhibitors have become the convenient explanation for all shifts occurring in this phase of the epidemic. They serve as a powerful magnet, drawing out people's hope, almost encouraging people to spin out fantasy yarns about "cure" and "viral eradication."

People who already had suffered great disappointments by tying their collective hope to a narrative of illness and health produced by Western medical discourse have yet again been set up for dissension, disaffection, and disappointment. The success or failure of the fight against AIDS continues to be evaluated using narrow constructs of "the cure," "the vaccine," and "the end of the epidemic" as the overarching goals. Rather than encouraging gay men to understand changes occurring in our everyday lives in their full complexity, journalists, public health officials, drug company executives, and leaders of AIDS organizations have united to gently coerce the nation's gay male population into misrecognizing what was in front of our faces. Instead of taking advantage of a very real breathing space that is opening up in gay male communities and offering a moment's respite from the constant battles of the past fifteen years, we are being ordered to remain crouched in our bomb shelters, heads tucked between legs, firmly locked in a state of emergency until the *real* cure arrives.

RELIEF, HOPE,
AND PROLIFERATING POSSIBILITIES

Long before scientists and journalists announced changes in the epidemic at the Vancouver conference, the everyday lives of gay men in epicenter cities offered evidence that a profound transformation was occurring in our communal experiences of the AIDS epidemic. Since the early 1990s, many noticed gradual yet meaningful shifts in urban gay spaces, communal sex cultures, and personal and collective social rituals. These changes initially went unacknowledged and unscrutinized by much of the community leadership. As the most intensive period of AIDS death occurred from 1989-1995, there was little room for alternative understandings of the event called AIDS. While the corpses piled up and discussions of a "second wave" of gay male infections became increasingly prevalent, the peprally campaigns launched in the mid-1980s were amplified. We repeatedly reminded one another to "Be Here for the Cure," "Practice Safe Sex Every Time," and "ACT UP, Fight Back, Fight AIDS."[3]

In *Reviving the Tribe* I recount a visit from an East Coast friend in 1993, who, after touring the Castro, helped me see how the neighborhood's depressed spirits had begun to lift. As Tom put it, "It feels like summertime has arrived after a very long and cold winter."[4] This forced me to look afresh at the urban gay ghetto in which I live:

> I gazed down the Castro Street hill toward 18th Street. Tom was right: the neighborhood *had* come alive again. While the

streets never stopped teeming with men, the energy had gone through a series of unsettling shifts. . . . Now it felt upbeat again but not crazed or manic. The district was filled with bookstores, New Age shops, burger joints, and queer clothing markets. Almost a dozen coffee shops had emerged in recent years, replacing bars and discos as the primary site for rendezvous and flirtations. The lesbian owner of a company offering walking tours of gay San Francisco passed by, leading a half dozen tourists wearing pink triangle shirts and carrying disposable cameras.[5]

I argued in *Reviving the Tribe* that these changes occurring in gay men's collective lives were a sign of the resilience of the human spirit. Rather than be defeated by disaster and tragedy, survivors and the communities they constitute commonly revive themselves and experience cultural rebirth and regeneration. If the epidemic continued fiercely throughout our lifetimes, as I suggested was likely, gay men faced a stark choice: to continue to cycle zombie-like through the burnt-out wreckage of our lives or to get off our butts, reclaim our psyches and our sexualities, and reconstruct our identities and communities. I believed gay male culture was reemerging powerfully in the 1990s, as vast numbers of gay men stripped off the sackcloth of the 1980s and reentered the land of the living.

While my understanding of the cultural meanings of the epidemic for gay men has continued to deepen, diversify, and take off in new directions, the changes that have occurred in gay communities since the book was written in 1993 both reinforce and alter my arguments. From the vantage point of 1998, I understand the landscape of those times a bit differently. While the book offers insights into ways the epidemiology of AIDS interacts with the cultural shifts gay men experience, I now believe my analysis of our reemergence from a collective state of trauma fails to capture at least one key concept.

Discussion of "anticipatory grief" has become widespread among mental health practitioners working with gay men who have experienced repeated, catastrophic losses. The term succinctly captures the complex psychosocial process of slowly letting go and entering the grieving process before a loved one actually has died. While I have never heard discussion of "anticipatory joy," I now believe such a process was occurring in the early and mid-1990s, as urban gay men began letting go of the weight of death accompanying our experiences of AIDS in the 1980s and early 1990s. On a mass psychic level, was the regeneration I identified triggered by a bizarre unconscious calculus weighing together infection levels, past deaths, and future losses? Did the charts and graphs that passed in front of our eyes on a weekly basis in the 1980s which showed epicenter AIDS deaths peaking throughout the early 1990s, work their ways into our psyches and set our internal alarm clocks to trigger collective revival in 1995?

Long before protease inhibitors entered public discussion, gay men were forging new understandings of ourselves and creating new cultures in a context of relief, hope, and proliferating possibilities. This was particularly apparent in urban social and sexual spaces, where the generation of gay men who had been involved in community response to the epidemic since its arrival was no longer numerically dominant. Many of the young gay men who came out amid cultural linkages between the erotic and death, gay identity and morbidity, filed into bars, dance parties, and sex clubs and created new rituals and cultural semiotics that, while linked to the epidemic, were increasingly independent of the crisis constructs of the 1980s. Part of the antagonism many gay men of my generation feel toward the muscular circuit party crowd may be triggered by our readings of these semiotics. Shaving chests may be interpreted as deliberate attempts to separate the young from the middle-aged; huge pecs may seem intended to distinguish the healthy from the ill; bodies that appear promiscuously tattooed may seem absurd after our generation fought off proposals to tattoo HIV-infected people just a decade ago.[6]

These young gay men did not experience AIDS as a crisis in their everyday lives. For most, this was not because they were naive, drunk, or in denial, as AIDS prevention workers generally insisted, but because they'd always known AIDS as a part of the terrain of gay male cultural life. Gay men in the 1970s lived through a decade dominated by themes of liberation, joy, and optimism, only to have the avalanche fall on us in the early 1980s. It was this sudden and stark shift in life expectations, and the seemingly powerful confirmation of our worst enemies' declarations that gayness was sick, sinful, and destructive, that made "crisis" an accurate representation of our life experiences.

By 1995, a year before the Protease Moment arrived, queer men ages sixteen to thirty-five were likely to have entered gay communal life with an awareness of the epidemic in the forefront of their psyches. The relationship these men had with the epidemic, one of preexisting hazard rather than shocking and sudden peril, encouraged the creation of an entirely new sector of gay male urban spaces that represented AIDS differently than their surviving counterparts in my generation. To draw on the rhetoric of leather cultures that were experiencing rapid transformation and accompanying conflicts between the "old guard" and the "youthful vision," the daddies and boys of the gay community by the mid-1990s found themselves forging vastly different meanings from the epidemic. A generation gap had emerged, causing twenty-five-year-old queers to acquire an understanding of AIDS radically different from the one held by forty-five-year-old gay men living in the same apartment building.

THE INCREDIBLE SHRINKING OBITUARY PAGES

By 1995, my own experiences of life in the epidemic had changed enormously from just a few years earlier. When *Reviving the Tribe* was published in January 1996, and I toured throughout the country talking about its key themes, I was convinced the analysis set forth in the book was on target. Even before I heard the first informal accounts of men on combination therapies, or read my first articles about protease inhibitors, I noticed significant changes in community life that provided me with a heightened sense of individual and communal regeneration.

Perhaps most notable was the diminution of illness and death around us. At first I told myself I was imagining this shift, that I had simply become so overwhelmed that I withdrew from the world. Yet small pieces of evidence began to accumulate and make me conscious of this shift. Months went by without death in my life. I noticed this because funerals and memorial services had become so damn problematic to me over the course of the epidemic. A friend's funeral would push me into inner conflict: to attend or not to attend? By 1989, I'd found myself cranky and judgmental at people's memorials; it was often a relief for everyone involved if I did not attend as I'd inevitably silently stew over any number of issues. Was the deceased's gay identity prominently and appropriately highlighted? Was the family from Idaho who'd done nothing to care for him given greater status than the lover and caregiving team who wiped the shit off his legs? After a number of months passed when I did not have to wrestle with the decisions and courtesies involved in funeral attendance, I felt great relief.

Early in the epidemic, I'd devised specific rituals to keep me focused and vigilant about AIDS. These activities now began serving as evidence that the epidemic's prominence in my life was changing. I'd been like many urban gay men who, in our twenties or thirties, picked up the understandable but seemingly age-inappropriate habit of obsessively checking the obituary pages of newspapers daily. In fact, because of the geographic shifts in my life and my involvement in several local gay communities (New York, Boston, Los Angeles, and San Francisco), for periods of time I read three daily papers, primarily to scan and tear out appropriate death notices. I developed tremendous skill at rapidly eyeballing the obit pages for evidence of AIDS deaths, necessary sleuthing when newspaper editors unethically collude with families of origin to cover up homosexuality and disguise causes of death.[7] During the early years, I routinely clipped and filed all obituaries that seemed to be AIDS-related. I also read weekly gay papers from over a dozen cities in the nation, in order to note the deaths of cohorts who were queer organizers in far-flung locations.

Maintaining my book of obits was not a meaningless or morbid habit. It was a ritual intended to begin to quantify the losses as I attempted to make sense out of a tragedy. At various stages of the epidemic this ritual served distinct purposes. In the earliest days, it was a way of slicing through denial. With newspaper clippings in hand, it seemed impossible to pretend the deaths were not happening. With an entire file folder brimming with these bits of newspaper, it was impossible to pretend the deaths were not overwhelming my life. What my brain could not immediately accept became real in the recesses of my file cabinet.

Just a few years later, the same ritual became a way to keep track of who had died. A few times a year I would take the clippings from the file folder and paste them into a scrapbook along with programs from memorial services, personal notes I'd received from friends before they died, and snapshots of deceased friends I'd taken during better times. I labeled these scrapbooks my "Good-bye Books," and the simple process of neatly trimming and methodically organizing the clippings, then pasting them into the book, served to remind me who had died and who might still be living.

A recent experience of drawing on my Good-bye Books reinforces their special place in my epidemic narrative. My friend Jane Rosett called from New York because she was assigned to write a story for *POZ* magazine commemorating the June 1, 1987, landmark AIDS demonstration and mass arrest at the White House.[8] This was the first collective national act of AIDS political resistance and united, for one brief moment, the newly established, high-energy New York group called ACT UP and mainstream gay community leadership from groups such as National Gay Rights Advocates, the Human Rights Campaign Fund, Mobilization Against AIDS, and Metropolitan Community Church. It is emblazoned in my mind as a pivotal moment in AIDS activism history. I had participated eagerly in the event and, ever the son of an archivist, had passed a sheet of paper around our jail cells, asking participants to sign it as an artifact of the experience.

In her piece for *POZ*, Jane wanted to list the names of those who had participated in the event who had subsequently died. An AIDS activist and talented photographer experienced at documenting political demonstrations, Jane had wonderful photos of us stopping traffic and sitting down on Pennsylvania Avenue, as well as being carried or led to school buses that had been brought out to carry us to jail. These photos, along with my autographed artifact sheet, reminded us that Leonard Matlovich and Dan Bradley had participated. Prominent gay male leaders who had died of AIDS were fairly easy to recall. But then Jane and I got lost in confusion about not only which people with AIDS had actually been arrested, but who had died and who was still alive. I immediately thought of my Good-

bye Books and gathered them together, reading out of them over the
phone to Jane:

> **Eric:** Was Richard Rector there?
>
> **Jane:** Yes he was. I remember it because he hassled the
> cops. But we're only looking for those activists who have died
> and he hasn't.
>
> **Eric:** I might be wrong, but I think he died a few years ago
> . . . let me check the book and see.
>
> **Jane:** I would have heard if he'd died. I saw him just last
> summer, and he definitely was not dead then. What about Jim
> Ryan? Was he at the demo?
>
> **Eric:** I know that Jim Ryan is dead and I think he was at the
> demonstration but I don't think he got arrested. . . . Oh, here it
> is . . . I found Richard Rector's obituary. He died in October
> 1996 in Denmark. I have a clipping from the *B.A.R.*
>
> **Jane:** I can't believe that I didn't know he died. Maybe I
> did. Maybe I didn't remember.
>
> **Eric:** What about Carlos Moldanado? I found his signature
> on the paper. I didn't remember that he was there. He was
> really sick a few years ago. Do you know if he has died yet? I
> know I don't have anything in the Good-bye Books on him.
>
> **Jane:** I heard that he'd died a few years back. Check the
> "death census" that they passed out at the Quilt in October
> and see if his name is in there . . .

This conversation recounts in authentic (and often bizarre) dialogue the way the volumes of loss experienced in the epidemic
reconfigure thought processes and reveal the limitations of memory
to take in and process morbidity. It also shows how the ritual of
reading, clipping, and filing obituaries, pursued over a fifteen-year
period, itself becomes a social process in which shifts in the epidemic
are inscribed. While in 1990 my files would fill swiftly and every
two or three months I'd be pasting a dozen obituaries into the book,
by 1996, I'd open my files and find only seven or eight obits. Was I
reading fewer newspapers? Had I wearied of the obsessive work of
clipping and filing? Or were fewer friends and colleagues dying?

A related AIDS ritual highlights the diminution of death in my
life. My lover and I preserve Friday evenings as a special time
together. We celebrate the Sabbath by making a special meal, buy-

ing a challah, and lighting the candles in our window. We say blessings over the candles, the challah, and the grape juice (masquerading as wine). Years ago, we began taking time after lighting the candles to name and recall friends, social acquaintances, political colleagues, tricks, and even strangers we'd admired, who had died that week. Most weeks during the early 1990s, we'd find ourselves voicing one or two names, but occasionally the deaths would number up to four or five. We'd rarely linger over this part of the Sabbath; instead we'd take a moment to feel the loss, and then let go of it by turning to the challah, the grape juice, and the comfort of a regular Friday night meal together at home.

Sometime in 1995, we noticed it was becoming difficult to cite a single death after we'd lit the candles. At first I wondered if I had lost touch with reality. People were still dying, I told myself, but maybe I was so fried that I could no longer take it all in. Yet as we found ourselves with no one to memorialize on repeated Friday nights, I began to wrestle with disparate interpretations of the cause of the shift. Was everyone I knew already dead? Had I stopped making friends with gay men, and thus knew fewer people who were dying of AIDS? Was the community so burnt out by the epidemic that we were no longer able to write and submit obituaries of our dead friends to the newspapers?

Gradually it became clear to me that something else was occurring: fewer gay men were dying and, of those dying, fewer still were from my gay generation.[9] I'd long been aware of the graphs that charted the dates of AIDS infections among gay men in San Francisco and, using the "natural history of HIV" studies, predicted the peak years for AIDS deaths would be from 1989 to 1995. Yet nothing prepared me for a shift out of a landscape of voluminous, unceasing death. Nothing prepared us—hard-hit gay male communities throughout the nation—for life beyond disaster, for community beyond suffering.

WHAT WE MEAN WHEN WE SAY "THE AIDS CRISIS IS OVER"

Any discussion of the end of the AIDS crisis is likely to trigger intense response from those involved in AIDS advocacy, prevention, and service delivery. I have found it wise to present my analysis and point-of-view on this topic slowly, with clarity and thoughtfulness. This may prevent some people from becoming belligerent, but it is unlikely to deter many from reacting with confusion, disagreement, and intense feelings. AIDS has accrued powerful meanings for many gay men, some of them symbolic, others quite mundane and visceral, and any attempt to envision a major change in our communal understanding of the epidemic is likely to shake the foundations of our common culture. People, inevitably, will get pissed off.[10]

Discussing the end of the crisis is different from discussing the end of AIDS, yet inevitably the two become closely entwined in many people's minds. Because AIDS-as-crisis has held a monopoly over gay men's public representations of the epidemic, many find it difficult to separate the crisis from the AIDS. This may be particularly true for some HIV-infected gay men who feel the entire discussion of an end to AIDS, or an end to the crisis, is inappropriate and discounts them as active members of the gay community. One man, responding to a presentation I made before a large audience of primarily gay males, criticized my presentation to the host organization:

> I am weary of HIV-negative men heralding the end of [the] AIDS crisis when 25 percent of people with HIV/AIDS do not respond to the drugs. . . . We are being relegated to the status of AIDS war veterans and are somehow looked on (like the veterans of foreign wars) as quaint artifacts. If the "community" Mr. Rofes speaks of is to truly coalesce and survive, the emphasis must be on inclusion, not a class system of HIV+/HIV − which somehow the events and activities [of your group] seems to support. There is more to the health/ well-being of the community than staying HIV negative. And if that is soooooo important, don't you see the message that is giving men who are positive? You failed, you're other, you aren't included in this community of HIV-negative men who are planning the great new communities of the "post-AIDS crisis" future.[11]

It easy for some to hear any discussion of the end of the crisis stage as suggesting the biomedical syndrome of AIDS is over; speakers and writers on this subject must be sensitive to the disparate needs of men of differing serostatuses who make up our audience. Making it clear that the *communal* experience of AIDS-as-crisis has ended, even while individual gay men may find themselves experiencing AIDS or HIV infection as a frightening, terrorizing experience, requires tremendous care.

The tendency to conflate end-of-crisis with end-of-epidemic is not solely due to the linkage of AIDS and crisis in the mind of gay America. Some writers and activists have toyed with this linkage to ignite controversy and draw attention to their work. Writers of articles often acknowledge up front that the epidemic itself is not over, yet their headline writers and editors see great potential sales emerging from playing with this confusion and pasting the title "The End of AIDS" on the piece.

Dan Savage, the quirky, upbeat gay journalist who writes a national sex advice column titled "Savage Love" which appears in alternative weeklies across the nation, published such a cover story in *The Stranger,* a Seattle paper, which was reprinted in *The Village Voice, The Chicago Reader*, and other urban weeklies.[12] The cover of *The Stranger* boldly proclaims "DAN SAVAGE ON THE END OF THE AIDS CRISIS." Savage's piece, however, clearly states:

> AIDS ain't over.
>
> But don't be fooled: Even if AIDS isn't over, the AIDS crisis is.
>
> AIDS and the AIDS Crisis are not the same thing. In America something isn't a "crisis" unless people are dying—and by "people" we Americans typically mean presentable, well-spoken, middle-class Americans, preferably white. AIDS is just a virus that, because of a set of unlucky circumstances, has been allowed to kill hundreds of thousands of unlucky men and women—mostly gay men, heterosexual IV-drug users, and their partners—with little regard for race or class.
>
> But it was the deaths of presentable, middle-class, well-spoken white people that made AIDS a "crisis." And these are the same people who now have access to the new drugs; the same people who—judging from reports in *Newsweek, The New York Times*, and *The Advocate*—don't seem to be dying anymore.[13]

Despite clear presentation and sophisticated analysis of the ways race and class intersect with the crisis construct, those who sent letters to the editor responding to this article expressed alarm that anyone would observe that the crisis had ended. The writers appeared intent on arguing that Savage had declared the epidemic over. The director of Gay City Health Project wrote:

> Dan Savage's article was arrogant, mean-spirited, danger-ous, and wrong. The AIDS crisis is not over. A crisis, accord-ing to *Webster's*, is "the turning point, for better or worse, in an acute disease." The recent advances in AIDS treatment have brought us to that crisis, and there's good cause to believe that we've reached a major turning point for the better. But if we prematurely declare victory, we risk sabotaging all the progress we've made up to this point.[14]

A doctor who directs Seattle's AIDS Control Program also wrote:

> Yes there is some good news, but make no mistake about it: The AIDS crisis is not over. In fact, AIDS is worsening in many groups.[15]

The executive director of the Northwest AIDS Foundation added his voice to the chorus, addressing his comments to the publica-tion's readers:

> The AIDS crisis is not over. There is no cure for AIDS. AIDS can still kill you. Don't allow your frustration with condoms and safe sex messages, coupled with poor advice from others, entice you into making life-threatening choices about unsafe sex . . . [16]

The letters make it clear that leaders within the local AIDS sys-tem, which Savage and others have dubbed "AIDS Inc.," will line up to denounce forcefully anyone arguing that the crisis stage of AIDS among gay men has ended. Another letter writer, incensed that Savage "announced to the world . . . that the AIDS crisis is over," stoops to a new low in his personal attack on Savage:

> What would happen if all the HIV-positive men in Seattle decided to corner Savage in some dark troll bar and gang rape

him on a pinball machine? HIV is quite a selective and picky little virus; all the circumstances would have to be just right for you to get it. But if you did seroconvert, I don't think you'd be singing the praises of your almighty Protease Inhibitors, when you feel like throwing up all the pills you just took at the same time you're experiencing incontinence.[17]

Internal gay community debates over whether we remain in a state of crisis might be expected to get nasty. Urban gay men experienced AIDS as a crisis in the early and middle 1980s, yet we became acutely aware, even frustrated and enraged, that most of our neighbors (including most of the other hard-hit populations) did not share in this understanding. This was not always because other populations were in denial about the epidemic or ignorant of its impact, as gay men commonly insisted in the 1980s. With the exception of hemophiliacs, nongay American populations experienced neither the swift saturation of HIV infection, the volume of loss, nor the public stigma linked to the epidemic that gay men initially suffered.

Because urban gay men emerged as the hardest-hit population early in the 1980s, and because we took on the early tasks of mounting a response to the epidemic, the way our population was coming to understand AIDS slowly influenced the broader mainstream culture. This was expedited by the fact that many of the men who first experienced AIDS-as-crisis were white and middle-class and had the resources and privileges that accompany those statuses. Race and class impacted this population's communal meaning-making in two key ways: (1) white middle-class men authentically experienced AIDS as paramount crisis because our communities-of-origin were shielded from many of the other catastrophic losses common to less privileged populations; (2) these same men had access to sources of power that profoundly shape cultural understandings: journalism, television news production, corporate marketing, and medical care. Our relatives, college roommates, and next-door neighbors could be marshaled occasionally to assist in moving gay men's experiences and understandings of the epidemic into new spheres with great visibility and influence.

AIDS as a disaster demanding a unique response from government, the health care system, and the public-at-large, took hold in the mind of America in the mid- and late 1980s after the death of Rock Hudson. Thousands of people signed up for AIDS walks and celebrities began to wear red ribbons on Oscar night; even homophobic legislators ended up providing significant funding to AIDS services. By allowing white middle-class gay men's experience of AIDS-as-crisis to become culturally dominant, an entire system of housing, social services, prevention programs, and political activism came into being. It is hard to imagine how this could have occurred without the crisis construct.

Much has changed in the dozen years since 1985. As I show in Chapters 3 and 4, most gay men no longer experience AIDS as an authentic emergency, even if we still use crisis rhetoric in our lobbying and street demonstrations. We've integrated the shifting realities of AIDS into our daily lives and accommodated ourselves to their hazards. Gay men do not need to feel bad about this. To expect human beings to remain in an active state of crisis for a period approaching two decades is to introduce an appalling quality of life that might take a powerful and permanent toll on mental health, intellectual development, and the broader psyche.

What do I mean by "crisis"? By arguing that most gay men no longer live their daily lives in a state of emergency, I am not arguing rhetorically. The social practices, subjectivities, and emotional landscapes transversed by most gay men are no longer dominated by elements that constitute a state of crisis. Many of us are not motivated to take extreme measures and make extraordinary sacrifices, as we were in the mid-1980s. We no longer feel intruded upon by an unknown viral agent, moved to disrupt our central pleasures and core meaning-making activities. Feelings of being stalked, pursued, even terrorized by the epidemic are less common. Instead, we have seventeen years of experience with AIDS that allows us to integrate it into our everyday lives, and divest it of much of its intense symbolic power.

The populations who see rising numbers of infections, such as African Americans and Latinos, have been ineffective in attempting to use crisis rhetoric to spark mass mobilization, in large part because their communities already face many other crises. As we approach the third decade of AIDS, it seems impossible to sustain the charade that AIDS is experienced as a communal crisis. Certainly individuals, particularly those recently infected with HIV or currently suffering illness, may experience AIDS as a personal crisis, but this is different from the communal crisis that once dominated gay life.

The experiences of gay men with HIV illustrate the tensions emerging from a continuing state-of-emergency rhetoric. Newly infected men might understandably default to ways of understanding their experience rooted in crisis constructs of the 1980s, especially since few alternatives have been offered. Yet many men who have been infected since the early or mid-1980s readily acknowledge their relationship to their HIV status. What it means to be a person with HIV is markedly different from a decade ago. One urban white gay man told me,

> I can't live on the brink of doom anymore. I can't sustain the crazy state of panic that dominated my life when I first tested positive. At that time, we had little information beyond doom and gloom. Now I have over ten years of living with HIV that have been relatively free from illnesses. That makes it impossible for me to pretend I'm on the eve of destruction. I still get nervous now and then, and I continue to watch my numbers closely. But HIV has been removed from its central position in my life. It's still there, it's just not the engine that's driving everything else.[18]

Men with HIV do not argue that the biomedical syndrome of HIV/AIDS is over; they are living proof that it is still present. They know all too well that HIV courses through their bloodstreams, leaves them vulnerable to a range of illnesses, and may eventually claim their lives. For some men with HIV, it's hard to be a Pollyanna while taking dozens of pills a day that rigidly control their daily eating schedules. Yet many healthy gay men with HIV are aware that they've stepped beyond the crisis stage and moved into new and unexplored territory.[19]

Most urban gay men—infected and uninfected—appear to have made similar moves, and we see the shift reflected in our common

cultures. Flyers posted in my neighborhood announced Christmas
Eve 1996 services at our local Metropolitan Community Church:

> Tonight There Will Be The Celebration of a Miracle
> For the first time in 16 years Christmas Eve in the Castro
> Is About Life, Not Death from AIDS . . .
> Join a community commemorating the birth of Christ
> and acknowledging answered prayers
> in the fight against AIDS and HIV infection.[20]

An advertisement in the local gay paper offers T-shirts stating
"Annoy Them . . . Survive."[21] A flyer available in my doctor's
office advertises a group that few would have taken seriously a
decade ago:

> SURVIVAL
>
> Dealing with the trauma of surviving HIV
> New group forming to help you understand
> what it means to suddenly have
> a potentially normal life expectancy[22]

We read articles about viatical companies suddenly refusing to purchase the life insurance policies of people with HIV/AIDS, and some
of these businesses are going under. Firms that once offered people
with HIV 90 percent of the policy's face value, now offer 50 to 60
percent.[23] A company makes headlines when it agrees to sell life
insurance policies to people infected with HIV.[24] We hear reports in
large cities such as Boston and Los Angeles of AIDS hospices,
created a decade ago primarily through gay men's efforts and
resources, closing their doors. Studies appear showing that the frequency of hospital stays among HIV-infected people has been greatly
reduced. Meanwhile, reports throughout the nation indicate that
long-term housing for people with HIV/AIDS is at a premium.[25]

MARKETING THE PROTEASE MOMENT

Our daily lives in gay communities provide ample evidence that
fewer gay men are sick and fewer gay men are dying than a decade
ago. Yet we find it difficult to take in, digest, and interpret this

evidence because we receive conflicting messages from gay leaders, AIDS advocates, and the mainstream media. Recent reports on the decline in AIDS deaths illustrate the difficulties many experience in interpreting the changing data.

The lead headline in *USA Today* on February 28, 1997 read "AIDS Deaths Drop 13% in First Decline." The first paragraphs of the article read:

> The number of deaths from AIDS in the USA has fallen markedly for the first time in the 16-year epidemic, the government said Thursday. AIDS deaths in the first half of 1996 were down 13% from the first half of 1995, says the Centers for Disease Control and Prevention in Atlanta.
>
> Hard-hit New York recently reported a 30% drop for 1996. Experts credit better drugs to fight the AIDS virus and related infections and cancers. They also cite a slower accumulation of new cases.[26] (Copyright 1997, *USA Today*. Reprinted with permission.)

One gay leader is quoted who adds what was swiftly becoming the requisite cautionary note, urging us not to stroll too far from our bomb shelters:

> "We hope it's a turning point," says Christopher Portelli of the National Lesbian and Gay Health Association, representing 155 AIDS clinics. But he worries that "people are going to read this as some kind of signal that we no longer have an emergency epidemic."[27]

Another doctor offers a view that counters the optimism of the rest of the article:

> "This decline is unfortunately only a lull," Irvin Chen, director of the AIDS Institute at UCLA, told the Associated Press. "Not all patients are responding as effectively as the majority of patients."[28]

What's problematic about both this quotation and the article in itself, as well as most of the front-page stories that appeared in U.S. newspapers following this CDC announcement, is that the decline in AIDS deaths is attributed primarily to the arrival of combination therapies. Nowhere in the piece is the reader informed that this decline in AIDS deaths was predicted in the mid-1980s by epidemiologists and public health planners and is attributable primarily to when people became infected with HIV.

This is particularly true of the large number of AIDS deaths of gay men in epicenter cities. Buried deep in a piece on the CDC announcement that appeared in the *San Francisco Chronicle:*

> The slowdown has long been coming. Last month, health officials in New York City reported a 30% drop in AIDS cases since 1996. In San Francisco, new cases of AIDS as well as deaths from the disease have declined sharply since 1992 . . .
>
> In San Francisco [Dr. Mitch] Katz said, the decline in deaths and new AIDS cases was predicted as far back as 1984, when the number of people newly infected by HIV, the virus that causes AIDS, had dropped from 8,000 to 1,000 in only five years. Since the average lag time between HIV infection and outbreak of AIDS is about 10 years, Katz and his colleagues were able to foresee that new cases would be declining significantly by 1994.[29]

Despite evidence that suggests the epidemic curve is largely responsible for the fall-off in AIDS deaths, the lead paragraph of the *Chronicle*'s story reads:

> For the first time since the AIDS epidemic struck America in 1981, deaths from the disease have begun declining significantly, federal officials reported yesterday. They attributed the favorable trend to more effective drug therapies and improved prevention efforts.[30]

We are witnessing here the machinations of federal officials and the collusion of the press in interpreting the decline of deaths primarily to new drugs rather than the long-predicted scaling of the epidemic hump. Needing to validate requests for funding for new treatments and prevention efforts, and desperate for hard data that could be waved before the eager eyes of policy makers, officials seize on whatever they've got—in this case empirical evidence of a decline in deaths—and simplistically attach to it their latest funding need. This is mirrored in *The Washington Post* story in which Mary Ann Chiasson, a health department physician, argues:

> "Clearly, new treatments have made a big difference," Chiasson said. "But in New York City, clearly new funds are also having a major effect on access to care [for people with AIDS]."[31]

Chiasson is referring to New York's share of funds from the Ryan White CARE Act, which rose from $44 million in 1993 to $100 million in 1994. Despite her claims, included in the same article is evidence that makes it clear the decline in deaths may have little or nothing to do with the new treatments or the new funding. The number of deaths in New York fell from 7,102 in 1994 to 7,046 in 1995, before the advent of protease inhibitors.[32] It fell substantially in 1996, to 4,944, when most people with AIDS in the city were not yet on combination therapies.

The problematic nature of this misuse and manipulation of statistics is evident in an editorial in the March 5, 1997 issue of the *San Francisco Examiner:*

> We hope last week's news of a 12 percent drop in the nationwide number of AIDS fatalities during the first half of 1996 is the first of many confirmations of progress in treating the illness. . . . The shrinking death toll was credited in part to combinations of drug therapies even before the widening use of a promising class of drugs called protease inhibitors. The improvement also may be related to better access to treatment and better financing of care.[33]

Nowhere does the editorial mention that epicenter cities such as San Francisco and New York were seeing declines in death that were long predicted by epidemiologists. An inaccurate impression is given that pharmaceuticals are primarily responsible for the decline in deaths, even when evidence suggests otherwise. This adds to the emerging chorus of voices that obsessively is mistakenly attributing any and all actual changes in the epidemic landscape to the arrival of the miracle treatment, combination therapies. These voices urge us to cling to a narrative wedded to polarized possibilities: crisis or cure. Other possibilities are not even considered.

Would it be possible to believe that protease inhibitors and combination therapies might offer a dramatic improvement in the health and lifespan of people with AIDS, yet fall short of a cure? Perhaps they've only extended PWAs' lives by a year or two and then resistance sets in and health declines suddenly. Could we merely have entered the eye of a hurricane, rather than reached the end of the storm?[34] With the other drugs in the FDA pipeline that we hear whispered about, is it possible we've entered a phase in which HIV infection is becoming chronic and manageable over the long haul? Rather than urging gay men to consider multiple possibilities or enjoy the relief offered by the shifting epidemic moment, we are forced into a corner and given two untenable options: do we continue to occupy a state of emergency or do we declare the battle ended?

MAKING MAGIC OF PHARMACEUTICALS

Articles that sparked debate about "The End of AIDS" appeared over a four-month period from October 1996 through January 1997. Publications ran high-profile pieces with bold headlines and television news shows rushed to replicate the dramatic effects. At the same time, colorful advertisements began appearing in gay newspapers and magazines throughout the nation, urging infected men to sign up for one protease inhibitor or another. An examination of specific texts appearing during this crucial period provides a foundation for understanding rapidly changing conceptions gay men maintained about the epidemic.

On November 10, 1996, readers of *The New York Times* picked up their Sunday magazine to find a stark, eerie cover trumpeting an astonishing message. A bold, white-on-black headline at the bottom of the cover declared, "WHEN AIDS ENDS by Andrew Sullivan." The cover text contains a quotation from Sullivan's essay:

> A difference between the end of AIDS and the end of many other plagues: for the first time in history, a large proportion of the survivors will not simply be those who escaped infection,

or were immune to the virus, but those who contracted the illness, contemplated their own deaths *and still survived.*[35]

Although the cover names the essay "When AIDS Ends," inside the magazine the piece is titled "When Plagues End: Notes on the Twilight of an Epidemic." The table of contents page of the magazine also lists the essay as "When Plagues End."[36] Yet throughout the essay, the shorthand title "After AIDS" appears at the top of every other page. Clearly there were multiple perspectives on the best way to represent the essay in marketing the magazine. Does "After AIDS" provide a more controversial, and more marketable, rhetorical flourish than "When Plagues End"?

Sullivan's piece represents a shift for the writer.[37] His usual analytic tone is softened and interspersed with deep personal meditations on key controversial questions. The essay moves back and forth between summing up the impact of AIDS on the changing position of gay issues in the public sphere and Sullivan's assessment of how successful experiences with combination therapies have altered his life plan and social practices. At once courageous and discreet, intellectually challenging and emotionally powerful, the article may be read from a generational perspective, as the work of an infected man of the under-thirty-five gay cohort. In fact, in this essay, Sullivan struggles to fit his experience with AIDS into the narrative framework crafted by men of my gay generation. How easy it seems for a younger man to mistake his own awful experiences with infection, loss, and grief for our experiences of generational decimation. Sullivan's essay is one of several compelling perspectives on AIDS by gay men under the age of thirty-five that offer insights into the different age-based epidemics experienced by gay men.[38]

Perhaps most interesting about Sullivan's essay is the fact that a cover story titled "When AIDS Ends" is almost entirely written from the perspective that an end will, in fact, arrive and that this salvation will occur through the development of new drugs. While referring to Camus's novel *The Plague*, Sullivan writes,

> The description of how plagues end is particularly masterful. We expect a catharsis, but we find merely a transition; we long for euphoria, but we discover only relief tinged with, in some cases, regret and depression. For some, there is a zeal that

comes with the awareness of unsought liberation, and the need
to turn such arbitrary freedom into meaningful creation. For
many more, there is even—with good reason—a resistance to
the good news itself.[39]

Yet whomever titled the piece "When AIDS Ends" has ensured
that the reader loses any sense of the transition Camus discussed. A
doctor sent a letter to the editor about the piece, emphasizing this
point:

> Drugs do not end epidemics. Plagues abate because of
> changes in human behavior, living conditions, hygiene, resis-
> tance to infection or microbial ecology. In part, this requires
> persistent, global educational efforts in disease prevention.[40]

Thus Sullivan's influential piece steers popular understanding of
changes in the epidemic in an unfortunate direction. Causes for the
changing epidemic beyond the new drugs go unnoticed and un-
analyzed. We are left thinking that the epidemic's end, for this
particular writer and for gay men throughout America, may safely
be attributed to a single factor: the development of new drugs.

With Sullivan's essay fresh on peoples' minds, the December 2
issue of *Newsweek* appeared featuring a four-inch bold headline
asking, while effectively declaring, "The End of AIDS?"[41] Tucked
away on the side, adjacent to the larger headline, is the question's
answer in 3/4-inch print: "Not Yet—But New Drugs Offer Hope."
Below the headlines are graphic designs of AIDS medications 3TC,
Ritonavir and ddI. John Leland's piece inside the magazine appears
not under the headline of "National News" or "Health," but under
"Lifestyle." This may reflect the distinctly human-interest perspective the writer brings to the issue as he focuses on the personal
experiences of infected men and women primarily in their thirties.

In this story, we hear from Jim Howley, a California psychologist
"diagnosed HIV positive in 1983," who had recently completed a
triathlon in Hawaii and appeared centrally in so many pieces on
protease inhibitors that he could be declared the poster child for the
Protease Moment.[42] Numerous photos accompany the piece showing healthy-looking people who, we are informed, also have been
"diagnosed" HIV positive. We're instructed in the real-life chal-

lenges facing people who are responding well to combination therapies, and numerous people returned-from-the-dead are paraded before
our eyes. The text of the article and the cover graphics of the new
drugs support readers' belief that contemporary changes in the epidemic come from a single source: protease inhibitors. Any larger
sense of how the epidemic was changing before the development of
the new treatments and how it continues to change independent of
them is omitted.

As might be expected, energetic responses to this "End of
AIDS" discourse appeared in the gay press. John D'Emilio, director of the National Gay and Lesbian Task Force's Policy Institute,
wrote a response titled "The End of AIDS? Not Exactly," which
appeared in dozens of queer publications throughout the nation.
D'Emilio argued, "The pious intoning of phrases like 'the end of
AIDS' won't get us there. Political mobilization and moral courage
will."[43] Author and activist Urvashi Vaid published a piece in *The
Advocate* astutely titled "Hope versus Hype," insisting that "media-
constructed hype and our own earnest hopes led us to conclusions
that neither the facts nor the tea leaves bear out," and tossing off a
list of current statistics on AIDS infections to prove the epidemic
still raging.[44] Bruce Mirken, a San Francisco-based writer, in a piece
titled "Hope, Hype and Survival," offered a particularly insightful
look at both the protease inhibitors and the media representations of
combination therapies.[45]

Such pieces by queer social critics go a long way toward separat-
ing rhetoric from reality and provide a more nuanced understanding
of media representations of medical matters. Yet none of the authors
steps outside the narrative of cure/crisis that has dominated gay
understandings of AIDS. Vaid comes closest when she discusses the
impact of the Clinton administration's policies on health care, welfare, and insurance, as well as homophobia and AIDSphobia, on the
trajectory of the epidemic. And none of the pieces offers a critical
look at how AIDS was and is changing, distinct from the Protease
Moment. Clearly the authors had other purposes in writing these
essays, yet thoughtful rebuttals to media representations of the epidemic that do not challenge the terms of the debate set by mainstream writers appear to be as far as the gay press will go. Independent analyses and alternative interpretations of our communities

and the changing circumstances in which we experience HIV seem beyond their purview. The ability to distinguish the event of AIDS from the biomedical syndrome appears absent in much of the gay press coverage of these debates.

A separate body of discourse targeting gay men appeared during this same time and further reinforced the impression that the epidemic was ending. Ambitious marketing campaigns advertising individual protease inhibitors appeared everywhere one looked during the fall and winter of 1996 and 1997, barraging readers of gay publications and habitués of gay neighborhoods with visual images of people with HIV who were hearty, robust, and engaged with life. The drug company Merck even took out ads for Crixivan in mainstream publications such as *Men's Health, Vibe, Spin,* and *Details.*[46]

The advertisement for Invirase (saquinavir mesylate) from Roche Laboratories runs five pages in one issue of *The Advocate* and, on its first page, shows a handsome, beaming white man in denim shirt and shorts, sitting on a rocky beach staring directly at the reader.[47] "When Considering an HIV Protease Inhibitor . . . " reads copy that continues on the next page with "Consider a Protease Inhibitor You Can Live With." Additional messages are pitched to the viewer: "Because treatment is a long-term commitment," "Because AIDS-free survival *can* be improved," and "Because effective therapy should also be practical for everyday living." In an attempt to strengthen the credibility of the ads, the reader is told, "All individuals depicted are HIV positive," and is shown snapshots of HIV-positive people with trim bodies, smiling faces, and outfits from L.L. Bean or J. Press, doing sit-ups, sitting on swings, or shaving in the bathroom mirror. The advertisement aims to exhibit normal people doing normal things in its efforts to normalize HIV seropositivity. A mixed-gender couple is shown cuddling one another on a beach. The lone male couple is pictured more discreetly, arms around one another's shoulders. These "saquinavir babies" of many races and ethnicities do the work they were hired to do: they illustrate clearly that AIDS-free survival can be a happy time.

A campaign conducted by the National Minority AIDS Council and the National Lesbian and Gay Health Association, and funded by Glaxo Wellcome, makers of AZT, makes use of different images to provide a similar message.[48] This campaign's theme is "Be

Smart About HIV," and insists "New Research Suggests that Reducing the Amount of Virus May Help You Live Longer." It's intended to motivate people with HIV to consult their health care providers about the new treatments. The glossy images again show multiracial groups of people smiling, having fun, and being productive participants in the world. A central image here is of a young male couple hugging, one man grinning through his goatee as he rests against the chest of his clean-shaven, blond boyfriend. A black woman and child, presumably mother and son, are also hugging. Three men of different races appear on a volleyball court, while another group dressed neatly in business attire appears to be scrutinizing architectural plans.

Other advertisements for the new treatments use similar images. Bristol-Myers Squibb's campaign for Zerit (stavudine) stresses the convenience of their product, one capsule taken twice a day with or without food, and is headlined "Put Some Freedom into Your HIV-Medication Schedule." The image utilized is a handsome African-American man wearing a bright yellow and blue cycling shirt and smiling as he rests on his bicycle.[49] Merck promotes Crixivan (indinavir sulfate) with images of a young man rock climbing and finally standing atop a precipice, gazing out over the valley.[50] An advertisement for Norvir (ritonavir) features a white man in shorts and T-shirt, playing with his Irish setter in a park, with his mountain bike resting nearby. This advertisement tells us about the person featured: "Chris Crays is a person living with AIDS who is using NORVIR."[51]

There's a lot I like about these advertisements: the upbeat message intended to support infected people in managing their health status; the multiracial, gay-positive groupings; the sense that people with HIV engage in the same daily activities (reading, shaving, doing sit-ups) as other middle-class people. While some have expressed concern about the linkage of gay and AIDS community-based groups with drug companies, and others have critiqued the campaigns as part of a drive to get all people with HIV onto one protease inhibitor or another, my concerns here are different. When I first saw these advertisements, I thought, "Who are these people?" Unable to come up with much of an answer to that question, I examined the advertisements more closely.

I began to wonder how repeated bursts of these images exploding onto the pages of queer publications interact with the journalistic discourse about the end of AIDS. Do the powerful visual images of people with HIV, active and engaged with life, encourage people to believe that AIDS is over and drug companies deserve credit for its demise? I would like to see similar images of people with HIV who are not on combination therapies, and yet are active, healthy people. Where's the snapshot of my lover, infected for almost a decade, with no serious ailments, and no Western medicines? Let's have photos of him in his yoga class, or riding his bicycle up Mt. Tamalpais. Or simply hugging and kissing me.

THE MIXED-STATUS COUPLE
FACES THE PROTEASE MOMENT

As an HIV-negative gay man, I expected to be the last person significantly affected by the Protease Moment. Yet my life shifted dramatically during this time as a direct result of the cultural changes occurring in urban gay communities in response to the publicity surrounding early successes of combination therapies and the changing epidemic moment. Because my lover is HIV positive, I observed firsthand that every HIV-infected person may be affected by the new treatments, even those who are not taking them.

My lover treats his HIV through an overall program of health maintenance focused on diet, yoga, rest, and happiness. Because Crispin works at the airport with a team of other engineers and mechanics who ensure the reliability of airplane engines, he has a fair amount of excitement in his work life. He tries to keep the rest of his life free of conflict, crisis, and drama. He's better at doing this than I ever imagined. My own life, while calmer than when I worked within gay and AIDS community organizations, retains more than a modicum of pressure. I use a variety of tools—psychotherapy, twelve-step groups, the Stairmaster, dancing on Sunday nights at Pleasuredome—to release the steam as it builds in the pressure-cooker of my psyche. Generally, most of my days are peaceful.

When the news out of Vancouver hit the general population, my lover and I noticed subtle but important changes in communication from those who know his HIV status. His mother clipped articles about the new treatments, enclosing a brief note of optimism along with the clipping. My mother's weekly inquiry continued ("How is Crispin's health?"), but was accompanied on two occasions by questions about whether he was on the new drugs. One day, in yoga class, my lover flirted with an attractive man and the two began to share stories about yoga and their statuses as HIV-positive men. The man talked about how well he was doing on his protease inhibitor, then turned and asked, "Which one are you on?" My lover told his yoga pal that he does not treat his HIV infection with Western medicines. He was left with the impression, now commonly felt by people with HIV who are not on combination therapies, that there is a growing assumption that people with HIV will be on these treatments. If you're not on them these days, people expect an explanation.

Two major issues arose in our relationship that I did not at first understand to be related to the Protease Moment. We had long held different views of where we wanted to live. For years, I had wanted to return to the Northeast to be closer to old friends and enjoy the four seasons in Massachusetts, the area I'd long considered my home. When I applied to graduate programs and gained entrance to both Berkeley and Harvard, we faced this conflict head-on. My lover offered a deal: if I stayed in San Francisco, commuted across the Bay, and received my PhD from Berkeley, he agreed to move wherever I found a teaching job once I completed the program.

This seemed like a good deal to me for several reasons. First, I knew the academic job market was tight and realized I could easily end up joining the faculty of a university far from either San Francisco or Boston. Having my lover agree early on to join me anywhere, especially if a job offer came from such places as New Mexico, South Dakota, or Alabama, struck me as fortunate and a way to avoid a future conflict. This was also a good deal because Berkeley is a public institution and the costs are minimal compared to attending Harvard. I could go through four or five years of a doctoral program at Berkeley without going into significant debt; my calculations led me to believe that spending a similar period of time at Harvard might leave me $50,000 in the hole. These reasons, along with the quality of the program I'd been accepted into at Berkeley, made turning down an East Coast move fairly easy.

Three years later, after I'd finished coursework at Berkeley, begun preparations for my oral examinations, and initiated early inquiries about potential jobs in New England, my lover confessed he'd had a change of heart. He could no longer imagine uprooting himself from San Francisco. He liked his life here too much: his new pack of friends, the airport job, involvement in his church. While he acknowledged the agreement we'd struck several years earlier, he was ready to renege on his offer of that time.

I was furious. A range of emotions overwhelmed me and left me confused. The relationship was loving, fun, and rooted in honest communication. After six years, I continued to enjoy my lover's company, be grateful for his willingness to put up with my occasionally impassioned ways, and treasure the daily routines of life together. Yet I felt duped into making a deal which, after living three additional years in California, was now being declared invalid. What bothered me most was I felt Crispin was unwilling to step outside the traditional male role and give up the assumption that his career was more important than my own. I understood that the kind of work he does is not easily found in most parts of the country and that his job fulfilled his childhood dreams. But two-career couples struggle with these questions all the time. I'm embarrassed to admit it, but I felt like the wife being told I have to live where my husband's job is located and sacrifice my career for the marriage.

When similar conflicts had arisen in the past, I gave in all too easily. Sometimes I've understood this as codependence, encouraged, as many of my generation have been, to pathologize generosity of spirit as a disease and attend twelve-step meetings to tone down the intensity of my self-sacrificing; at other times, I've viewed giving in to my lover as reasonable and appropriate. After all, he's got the long-term stable job that pays good benefits and will reward him in retirement. Why risk it to join me at a job in Idaho, when it's likely I'd have second thoughts immediately after the moving vans departed?

This time I was not willing to accept Crispin's change of heart. I was empathetic and understanding, but a deal was a deal. I was unwilling to stay in San Francisco and he was unwilling to leave. Yet neither wanted to break up the relationship. We needed help. So we turned to a therapist who'd helped us through a difficult period early in the relationship when we were negotiating outside sex arrangements, and began counseling focused on work, geography, and the power dynamics within our relationship.

Within the first few sessions, it became apparent I was asserting my desires and needs in a new way. While many of my friends see me as bossy, in my primary relationships I've often struggled to maintain a sense of myself as an autonomous person and place my needs on parity with my lovers'. In my current relationship this tendency was intensified by the antibody status difference between us. Because Crispin is HIV positive and I am not, I often found myself deferring to him on a range of issues that had little direct connection to HIV. When I had to make the decision about where to go to graduate school, I told myself I didn't want to force my lover to go through the lengthy and burdensome process of finding new health providers. He was already happy with his chiropractor, acupuncturist, herbalist, physician, and HIV-positive support group. How could I rip him out of his network of care and support in San Francisco and demand he find new providers in Boston? If he believed his T-cell level was kept strong by his regular bicycle rides over the Golden Gate Bridge to Mt. Tamalpais in Marin, how could I force him to live in a climate where cycling was impossible for a major portion of the year?

These thoughts were playing out in my mind because I maintained a common underlying assumption about people infected with HIV. When we met in 1990, he told me he was HIV positive from the get-go. Calculating the years from infection to death, I told myself I'd be lucky to enjoy five years with this man. Since my other relationships had lasted the same length of time, it felt like a good deal to me. When I was considering doctoral programs, I recall hoping Crispin would live long enough to see me graduate. In all kinds of subtle ways, my understandings of the meaning of HIV determined many of the decisions I reached about our life together.

The Protease Moment changed everything between us. After living with him for six years and watching his T-cells remain in the 1,000 range, I began to realize I was not going to be a widow anytime soon. When viral load testing became popular and his test came back marked "undetectable," the antibody status difference between us began to have much less weight. Suddenly, on a subconscious level, I was no longer constantly preparing for his decline and death. I had to face the possibility that he'd be walking this earth as long as I and that we might have the chance to become two old guys together.

This made me happy, but also shifted the foundational assumptions I brought to our negotiations as a couple. I no longer had to cede my right to assert the desire to move to New England. Suddenly, it felt like we stood together on an even playing field, HIV-negative and HIV-positive men together. I insisted that we engage in a reevaluation of our long-term plans as a couple and the processes with which we negotiated our differences.

The second major issue triggered by the Protease Moment involved sex. Like many male couples, we had reached an agreement early on that we would enjoy sexual encounters with men outside our relationship. While my lover preferred casual dalliances and was adept at meeting similarly minded men at the gym, in yoga class, on a computer bulletin board, and at sex clubs, my own style tended toward the development of long-term, ongoing, fuckbuddy relationships. We both enjoyed fairly vigorous sex lives and could usually manage to share stories without inciting possessiveness or jealousy.

Our problem was that we had different levels of interest in sex together. I had long ago made it clear that keeping sex alive in our relationship was important to me. While I knew many couples, male, female, and mixed gender, for whom sex receded into the background after the first year or two together, it felt vital to me to continue to engage in erotic activity with my lover. The situation was complicated by Crispin's waning sexual interest in me, caused in part by his erotic attraction to activities over which a shadow of transgression loomed. Sex with one's lover was difficult to construe as outlaw sex.

When we first met, the sexual charge between us was intense and our encounters were passionate and satisfying. We shared an interest in role-playing aspects of the leather scene, and delved into new and kinky areas. Yet as we moved toward a committed relationship, it became more difficult to keep things hot for both of us. Making the leap from being one another's "honey" or "sweet baboo" to fantasy scenes of police brutality or forced captivity became impossible. As the kinks straightened out, we settled into a comfortable, loving sex life without the intense energy that crackled between us when we'd first met. He would occasionally still force my arms over my head in simulated bondage, or talk a bit dirty as I approached orgasm, but our sex had calmed down significantly from the first rushes of passion.

I understood the sexual differences between us in various ways. Sometimes I thought this was a matter of cultural difference: his Catholic versus my Jewish upbringing left him with obsessions with jerking off and other "bad-boy" behavior and me with hang-ups about anal sex. I occasionally thought my fascination with bondage and S/M and my limited sex drive left us incompatible sexually. Sometimes I thought we were two tops in search of a bottom. At other times, I believed the difference in antibody status made our sex extremely problematic. He was determined not to infect me, so he put some firm boundaries on our activities together. I was obsessed with AIDS for long periods of time and, even during safe-sex activities with Crispin, could not keep it out of my head.

It didn't help that my lover's handsome face and tight body made me feel his appeal was frequently greater than mine in the sexual marketplace. I've considered him a classically attractive gay man and seen myself as a narrower "type," eminently marketable in the leather scene or the bear bars, but not always able to cross over into mainstream gay sex cultures. This was exacerbated by the age difference between us: he is in his mid-thirties and I am in my early forties. When he began joining me three mornings a week as my workout partner, I watched his formerly lithe body become buff overnight. When a local producer invited him to star in a porn video, I had many mixed feelings: protection, envy, anger, pride, excitement.

I enjoy having a lover who strikes many gay men as attractive. Long ago I became accustomed to seeing men aggressively cruise him on the street, come on to him in front of me, and slip their phone numbers into his pocket. The way we've constructed our life together permits such activities. We do not pretend there aren't risks involved and on a regular basis we work hard to negotiate boundaries and process feelings that our lives in gay sex cultures kick up.

My concern about my lover's limited sexual interest in me, the tensions that emerged from our different "looks," and the challenges of establishing boundaries in an open relationship, came to a head during Gay Pride Week in 1997. A number of nagging issues—it had been months since my lover initiated sex with me, his smooching a guy on the street for longer than I liked, and a flirtation with a man that he started during our visit to the Pride March—caused me to boil over. When he began making out on the dance floor at Pleasuredome with a man from our gym, I hit the ceiling.

This precipitated the first energetic fight we'd had in almost five years. I felt angry, hurt, and abandoned. He felt misunderstood and unfairly judged. I demanded that something had to change or I couldn't envision continuing with such tensions. He argued that I was overreacting and going to extremes that were not warranted. We spent a few uncomfortable days together, trying to understand what was happening between us and how this tempest had arisen so quickly.

I came to understand that a variety of factors had triggered my reaction: some difficulty making the transition to middle-aged gay identity, long-standing insecurities about my attractiveness, my fear of losing the affection and desire of my lover, and a sense of the growing gap in sex appeal between us in the marketplace of the Castro. Perhaps most important, however, was my dramatically altered sense of my lover as an HIV-positive person in a rapidly changing epidemic environment.

Before the Protease Moment, I viewed my lover's outside sex with some generosity. In the back of my mind, I'd tell myself it was nice he could have such a good time, since bad times were likely to be right around the corner. I felt supportive of his efforts to stay sexual and healthy in a world where many thought HIV-positive gay men should become eunuchs or limit their sex to other pariahs. I also felt secure in the relationship, in part because I'd married him during a time when the messages we received about HIV/AIDS led us to believe it unlikely he would lead a long life. I imagined that his gratitude for my willingness to be with him despite his HIV status would keep him forever bound to the relationship.

The cultural shifts occurring during this moment of optimism called my assumptions into question. It was one thing to be in relationship with this sexy guy when I didn't expect it to last more than a few years; it was quite another thing to imagine dealing with his popular appeal for a decade or two. Rather than see his outside sexual activities as a triumph for the rights of people with HIV to be sexual beings, I began to view his dalliances with disgust and consider them trashy, careless, and insulting to my status as his lover. I also began to feel insecure in the relationship. Would I suffer being thrown over by an HIV-positive lover who has decided, now that he's going to live, that he wants a younger, sexier boyfriend?

The Protease Moment forced us to look at our relationship in new ways because the underlying assumptions I'd brought to the partnership—that we'd have just a few years together, my lover's health would decline precipitously, and I'd have to be prepared to be his caregiver—had been abandoned. This did not mean my earlier fears would never be realized. Instead, our relationship was like a blackboard that had been wiped clean, and we were ready to chalk up new visions for the future.

Whether tackling matters such as our location, work, sex together, sex apart, and long-term commitment to one another, the changes in what it means for him to be HIV positive and me to be HIV negative had radically altered the dynamics between us. We knew there were no easy answers to pressing concerns about where we'd be living and whether we could keep sex alive between us. We hoped, as the fallout from the Protease Moment settled, things would become clearer for both of us.

PUTTING ALL OUR EGGS
IN THE PROTEASE BASKET

The gay AIDS epidemic that preceded the Protease Moment is rapidly being written into history as a static and unitary fifteen-year block of time suffused with illness, death, and the heroic response of the community. Limited, unidimensional narratives are recycled and served up as our central understanding of what's happened. Discrete and distinct stages of community response, diverse gay AIDS epidemics affecting different subcultures and locations, and competing social and cultural forces interacting with shifting empirical data all simplistically are reduced to a singular gay male experience of AIDS.

Gay men's experiences of AIDS have been complex and variegated. The epidemic facing gay men in Omaha has long been quite different from that confronted by gay men in San Francisco. Our collective faith that drugs ("the cure") would lead to the termination of the horror show was quite different in 1985 than it was in 1994, after the International AIDS Conference in Berlin trounced our AZT-induced fantasies that "the cure" had arrived. As the popularized narratives appear in the history books, the rich sociocultural context of the times is simplified and we focus only on the stories of heroic individuals. We see the trees rather than the forest, and make of the recent past whatever suits our current purposes.

The failure to bring together epidemiology, sociology, community psychology, anthropology, and social theory and create a textured understanding of the changes occurring for gay men in the late 1990s is evident in the essays and articles that raise questions about the end of the AIDS crisis. Most of the articles of this period focus narrowly on gay men who are finding renewed energy and improved health status thanks to combination therapies. This individualized approach is compelling to many and creates intensely dramatic stories of life after death that appeal to a Judeo-Christian worldview deeply interwoven into the collective consciousness of American culture. We hear about men regaining weight, returning to jobs, beginning to envision a future. It all sounds great, but it turns the focus away from changes in gay communities that occurred separate from protease inhibitors.

It is dangerous to consider protease inhibitors as the sole cause of growing gay awareness of a changing epidemic, yet we are asked repeatedly to put all our fragile eggs into the protease basket. We've done this before and our communal psyche has paid a heavy price. If protease inhibitors don't work for many people, or fail to be effective after a year or two, or end up doing more harm than good, the roller coaster we've been riding for fifteen years is likely to snap and whip us all into another sudden and sharp decline. The impact would likely be devastating.

Yet there are at least two other reasons why the current obsession with protease inhibitors and the accompanying determination to see all gay-related phenomena through the lenses of the cocktail are problematic. First, discussion of protease inhibitors consistently affirms traditional understandings of the epidemic that see HIV as the sole cause of AIDS, insist that infection inevitably leads to illness and death, and ignore the realities of many people who have been HIV positive for a long time and have remained healthy and active. By 1997, many of us knew people who'd been infected for well over a decade and had experienced no significant illnesses. The obsession with protease inhibitors fails to explain—or even consider—the experiences of large numbers of people exposed to HIV through unprotected anal or vaginal sex or through needle-stick injuries who do not become HIV infected. It also has opened a moment when AIDS dissidents, those who do not believe HIV causes the syndrome known popularly as AIDS, are prominently calling into question foundational assumptions about gay men's health, risk factors, and treatment.[52] While we have significantly more data in 1997 than we had in 1985 indicating that infection with HIV does not lead inevitably to death, discussions of protease inhibitors are being used to buttress hegemonic understandings of the epidemic that were introduced in 1985.[53]

Second, we do people with HIV a disservice when we insist that the epidemic will remain static until the miracle of medical research serves up a cure. Discussions of protease inhibitors almost always include a token caveat that they are "not the cure," but the surrounding rhetoric and the first-person stories and photographs that accompany most of the journalistic accounts and media advertising represent the situation otherwise. Protease inhibitors might not be the cure, but they sure sound like one in the words of Andrew Sullivan. HIV-infected subjects certainly have the right to draw whatever meaning they choose from the new drug therapies. Yet by offering gay men only two possibilities, a continuing crisis of illness and death or a vaccine and a cure, we force them into an untenable and unrealistic position. Why aren't we aiming to support a narrative that focuses on the diminution of AIDS' impact in our individual and collective lives, a respite from the AIDS-as-crisis story, rather than clinging obsessively to a less realistic goal of total elimination?

My argument is not that combination therapies should have no impact on gay men's collective understanding of the epidemic. Instead, I am suggesting that other changes—structural, cultural, and biomedical—have occurred independent of protease inhibitors. Although neglected in most analyses of this epidemic moment, these changes are actually central to the shifts in our everyday experience of AIDS. The structural changes include the presence of a population of long-term nonprogressors, the declining number of AIDS deaths, and the influx into gay community spaces of large numbers of young men with vastly different understandings of the epidemic. The cultural shifts include the post-1990 revival of sexual cultures in urban centers, the decentering of AIDS in gay community rituals and institutions, and the increasing presence of gay male couples raising children. The biomedical include the development of several new treatments and their effectiveness at countering opportunistic infection and wasting syndrome.

Yet thoughtful, experienced gay leaders are considering supporting major policy changes based on the supposed effectiveness of the new treatments, even before long-term empirical data is available. Jeff Levi, in an essay titled "Rethinking HIV Counseling and Testing," has argued "we are sitting on top of a public health failure," and "policies about testing and treatment should shift due to the promising new treatments."[54] Levi is among the voices calling for a thorough reconsideration of ways to draw at-risk populations into the AIDS testing and treatment system. Some gay men are using the Protease Moment to argue for mandatory testing, contact tracing, partner notification, and centralized reporting of HIV-positive people, ironically at the same time a conservative Republican in Congress has put forward a bill that would codify such practices.[55] Attorney Catherine Hanssens of Lambda Legal Defense has offered compelling arguments that counter the assumption contained in these proposals that discrimination against people with HIV is no longer a pressing problem. She suggests legal protections for people with HIV might be eroded due to the amelioration of people's symptoms and the potential loss of disability status.[56]

The appearance of the new drugs has served to make visible, accentuate, and extend changes already underway in gay men's experience of the epidemic. By crediting changes as diverse as the decline in AIDS deaths, the lengthening life spans of people with HIV, and the revival of hope among gay men solely to the new drug combinations, we invest them with unreasonable power and make magic out of pharmaceuticals. By reacting too swiftly to this epidemic moment, and making major, irreversible policy shifts while flush with hope over the new drugs, we risk creating an AIDS system that might prove more punitive than helpful. Rather than respond narrowly to the Protease Moment or remain rigidly locked in the past, it may be worthwhile to engage in a thorough evaluation of how the epidemic has changed—medically, socially, culturally, and politically—and how our care systems might best respond to all of the changes.

BETWEEN AIDS-AS-CRISIS AND AIDS-AS-OVER

The AIDS crisis is not over! The AIDS crisis is not over! People are dying! People are dying! The AIDS crisis is not over! The AIDS crisis is not over!"

—Activist chant, 1997

ACT UP and other activist groups shouted these words in the late 1980s, and surviving activists continue to shout them a decade later. The concept of AIDS as a crisis was born very early in the epidemic as a lethal, sexually transmitted disease suddenly appeared among homosexual men. As much of the world twiddled their thumbs, attentive writers, health care providers, activists, and people with HIV sounded the alarm, as if to say, "This is not business as usual. This is not small and unimportant. This is not without ramifications for the entire world. Wake up! Pull the alarm! Do something before it's too late!"

The American Heritage Dictionary of the English Language (Third Edition) offers several definitions for crisis: "a crucial or decisive point or situation; a turning point," "an emotionally stressful event or a traumatic change in a person's life," "a point in a story or drama when a conflict reaches its highest tension and must be resolved." It is "a problem coming to a head," "a critical juncture," "things rapidly coming to a desperate pass." Perhaps most appropriate to gay men's experience in the 1980s is crisis as "an unstable condition, as in political, social, or economic affairs, involving an impending abrupt or decisive change."[57]

From the beginning, AIDS-as-crisis was more than rhetoric or a clever strategic move. Gay men during the 1980s experienced the epidemic as triggering abrupt and decisive changes. In epicenter cities and in the sexually active networks of smaller urban centers, a large portion of gay men started to suffer quick and ugly deaths. The burgeoning sex cultures that gay men created in the 1970s and early 1980s were truncated, snuffed out, or forced underground. The everyday assumptions and rituals that made life meaningful were cast aside suddenly, supplanted by new understandings and social processes. Sexual liaisons became places of terror rather than sites of comfort and pleasure. We referred to AIDS as the "health crisis" and gave organizations names such as "Gay Men's Health Crisis," because, to many who had their eyes open and their heads pulled out of the sand, it was a crisis.

By the early 1990s, signs began appearing that indicated that AIDS as a crisis was beginning to wane as an authentic representation of our communal experience of the epidemic. Large AIDS organizations purchased buildings, sometimes spending several million dollars to secure a "permanent home." The sexual cultures of cities such as New York, San Francisco, and Los Angeles began to come alive again as new dance clubs and sex spaces began to fill to capacity. The red ribbon, once a daring sign of support for besieged communities, became kitsch, an Oscar-night emblem for the hip, the socially aware, the chic.[58]

Yet AIDS activists continued to repeat the same chants and attempted to replenish their ranks by hammering home the state-of-emergency construct. AIDS service groups, among the primary beneficiaries of panic and guilt-induced financial giving based on the crisis construct, continued to find new ways to repackage the epidemic-as-emergency and keep the dollars and volunteers flowing.[59] Anyone who questioned the reigning crisis mentality was shunned as a heretic. "The AIDS crisis is not over!" they were told.

Thus we find ourselves approaching the third decade of AIDS with the primary voices speaking for AIDS activists and service groups continuing to frame the epidemic as it was first framed almost two decades ago. If the Left can be considered tired, chanting the same stale chants at demonstrations that were chanted fifty years ago, AIDS activism isn't far behind!

When I interviewed gay men of various ages, races, and geographic locations about the epidemic while preparing this book, I asked whether AIDS was a crisis.[60] Most commonly, men initially would answer affirmatively, yet soon begin to backpedal and qualify their earlier statements. One man told me:

> Of course it's a crisis—it's an awful thing that continues to happen to people like us. . . . I can still get myself into a frame of mind that captures that feeling of crisis: we have to do something! But the reality is, these days, the epidemic doesn't feel much like a crisis, even if I want it to. It feels like it's been with us a long time and is probably going to continue to be with us for a long time. To me it seems to be just the way things are . . . [61]

After several subjects answered my question about crisis in this way, I came to interpret this backpedaling as men engaging in thinking-in-process while they verbally responded to the question. When first asked if they believe AIDS is a crisis, the men responded "Certainly!" as they had lived through a dozen years of this construct being voiced prominently by community leadership and the media. Yet as their thoughts continued to evolve, they realized their lives provided little evidence of the current experience of AIDS as a "traumatic change" or "a problem coming to a head." As one man said, "If you are asking me if fighting AIDS is important, I'd say yes. But if you are asking if I'm freaked about AIDS or if it occupies a large place in my life, I'd be lying if I didn't say no."[62]

One survey of 1,459 gay men conducted in October 1997 found that one-third of the subjects no longer experience AIDS as a crisis.[63] This may be in line with my own findings because survey methods register primarily the initial reaction of the subject to the question, not the mulled-over, well-considered response that was the stage of the interview process in which my subjects began equivocating.

I believe most gay men, HIV positive, HIV negative, and HIV indeterminate, do not experience AIDS as a crisis on a daily basis. A twenty-five-year-old uninfected gay man told me, "AIDS is always what I've known about being gay and having gay sex. AIDS was there when I started having sex with guys and it's still there. I've never known a world without AIDS, so it is hard for me to get agitated and all riled up about the epidemic."[64] An HIV-positive man said, "I've got better things to do than to sit around and wait

for AIDS to get me. I've got my friends, my job, my dogs. I don't
have time to be in crisis mode. It's as simple as that."[65]

A fifty-four-year-old gay man living in Los Angeles told me:

> I just can't pretend anymore that AIDS is the focus of my
> life and that fighting the epidemic is my top priority. Sure, I
> continue to do volunteer work and attend fund-raisers. But
> I've gotten on with my life and have other things to do. AIDS
> took away my lover, my friends, and about a decade of my
> own life and I'm not letting it take away anything else![66]

Many AIDS activists and service providers fear, as the public
normalizes or accepts AIDS and moves beyond crisis, financial and
volunteer support for people with HIV will rapidly diminish. Will
hundreds of thousands still attend AIDS walks if we reframe the
epidemic? Who will care for the sick and indigent people with
AIDS if we don't present the epidemic to the public as a crisis?
Why would the government continue to fund the Ryan White
CARE Act if AIDS becomes simply a normal, undistinguished part
of the landscape?

A crisis paradigm is designed in a tidy way: crisis occurs and
crisis ends. There is little room for other scenarios that reflect the
complex genesis of the crisis or options for resolving it short of total
elimination or termination. I believe that continuing to present
AIDS-as-crisis after more than fifteen years of AIDS organizing is
the single most formidable barrier we have to effectively combating
AIDS and caring for sick people. This is not simply a rhetorical
issue: it is a matter of ethics and effectiveness. By continuing to
willfully misrepresent the epidemic in this way, the communal
psyche is held hostage by a siege mentality that perpetuates many
unfortunate aspects of the epidemic.

I wonder what happens to gay men who buy into the rhetoric and
lock themselves up in the state of emergency for fifteen years. By
stretching a crisis into two decades, well-intentioned activists might
contribute to the current deluge of media reports that suggest that
AIDS is over. The masses may now be simply taking their cues
from years of repeated representation of the epidemic as crisis. We
insisted AIDS could soon be over. We demanded a cure. We did
everything possible to encourage people to fit AIDS into a war

paradigm, and share in a determination to win victory before the boys are sent home.

By not providing more options to the public, have we, in fact, brought the "End of AIDS" construct on ourselves? Once people no longer could sustain the experience of a crisis, did they have no other choice but to fold up their tents and go home? Are there ways of understanding and representing the epidemic among gay men that move beyond the siege mentality? Is it possible to step outside the crisis—or beyond the crisis—and still have viable organizations that are adequately funded and receive strong support from volunteers?

I believe there are no more important questions for those concerned about AIDS to be asking these days. The epidemic has lasted much longer than we anticipated and the pull toward declaring it over poses tremendous risk to communities—including gay men of color, white gay men, and young gay men of all colors—who continue to sustain significant levels of HIV infection. Now might be precisely the time to reconceptualize the epidemic and carve out a new way to represent it in the queer public sphere. If new treatments prove half as successful as the media has proclaimed them to be, we have entered a new era. If they fail two years down the line, we will have shared in a communal moment of hope and possibility and move to a new epidemic moment. Someplace between AIDS-as-crisis and AIDS-as-over lies a useful understanding of the way the epidemic currently manifests in our lives, and a pathway to follow in charting new directions.

OUR FIRST DEEP BREATH IN TWENTY YEARS

There are many ways gay men can mark this shift. It might be useful to take advantage of the bit of breathing time that current shifts in the epidemic afford us. For many gay men, this might seem like the first moment we've had in over seventeen years to take a step back and calmly reassess our lives and the social worlds we inhabit, activities difficult to initiate during a state of siege. This could be a time to reflect on our involvement in the fight against AIDS, feel good about how we've directed our energies, and forgive ourselves for our failings and mistakes. Likewise, this could be a valuable time to appreciate the work of others, pardon their errors or limited involvement, and let go of the weight of angst we've borne during the epidemic. We could use this as an opportunity to recommit ourselves to AIDS work or shift our priorities in some way. We could use this as a time to show gratitude to the veteran workers in AIDS groups.

Organizations that have been heavily enmeshed in epidemic culture might initiate rituals, recounting their collective experience of the epidemic, assessing the organization's achievements and limitations, and charting continued or new directions for the future.[67] Entire local gay communities might undergo a similar process of honest, ritualized self-assessment, as we leave one stage of the epidemic and enter a new one.

There is another way to mark this shift that, however controversial, merits examination. It may be time for gay men to abandon the acronym "AIDS" altogether. On one hand, the acronym stands for "Acquired Immune Deficiency Syndrome," words that continue to capture the central medical experience of the malady and do not impose permanence or lethality on the infected subject. Yet for many of us, these four simple capital letters are permanently stained with the blood of our lovers and comrades in gay liberation. The meanings of the 1980s—quick death, sexual repression and shame, cataclysmic loss—will cling to the term forever. Efforts to recreate and revive community may be assisted by letting go of this term, eradicating it from our daily lives, and using the phrase "HIV disease" or creating a new acronym, one that is invested with the meanings of the new millennium.

This suggestion may sound to many people like an extreme measure that is neither necessary nor useful. Instead they might argue the meaning of "AIDS" will shift on its own in time, following the changes in medical research and disease progression. While I agree that language is neither static nor invulnerable to advances in science, I believe the abandonment of this acronym might serve to accelerate gay men's awareness of life beyond crisis and improve the health and well-being of men previously categorized as "people with AIDS." As men construct new identities for themselves in a post-AIDS period, finding new language that captures our experience will be a critically important activity.

Chapter 3

Creating Post-AIDS Lives

When leaders of gay and AIDS organizations appeal to gay men for participation or financial support, they often ground their appeal in an AIDS-as-crisis understanding of the epidemic. Whether marketing an AIDS fund-raising walkathon, beseeching people to attend a political demonstration concerning new treatments, or encouraging continuing vigilance around safer sex practices, both the rhetoric of the appeal and its underlying assumptions continue to recycle notions of AIDS as out of control, crashing like a sudden avalanche on the gay village.

In the late 1990s, such approaches do not seem to be working. There is considerable talk that AIDS fund-raising is in a precipitous decline.[1] Many argue that we're long past the heyday of AIDS activism.[2] Some AIDS prevention workers privately acknowledge that although they've succeeded in reducing the frequency of unprotected anal sex, they've been unable to keep a large segment of their local gay male population from occasionally engaging in the practice.

Yet few leaders have taken a step back from their work and considered how the messages and methods they employ with gay men may be partially responsible for the drop-off in gay men's engagement with efforts against AIDS. Instead, most working within the AIDS system dig in their heels and redouble their efforts, raise their voices louder and redesign the AIDS-as-crisis construct in an attempt to inject it into the late 1990s consciousness of gay men. Advertisements in the gay press reflect gay and AIDS organizations' sincere attempts to maintain community involvement in the effort against AIDS by employing the crisis construct and reminding gay men that the epidemic has not ended.

One advertisement for the 1997 AIDS Walk in San Francisco exhorted readers to "Join with 25,000 Bay Area walkers who know the AIDS crisis is not over!"[3] A similar advertisement in the *San Francisco Chronicle* boldly stated, "When AIDS has stopped, so can we."[4] During the final weeks before the event, a sticker saying "Keep Walking . . . We're Not There Yet," was placed on the ubiquitous AIDS Walk posters throughout the Bay Area.[5] The campaign succeeded in raising more money during the 1997 walk than in any previous year.[6]

Other nonprofit groups have created similar campaigns reminding gay communities that the epidemic has not ended. The ARIS Project in Santa Clara County (California), took out full-page advertisements displaying a condom along with the headline, "Hang in there. AIDS isn't over yet."[7] One of the Names Project's advertisements insisted "The Great American Sewing Bee Continues," while another, under stark white-on-black letters reading "How To Tell If You're Immune To AIDS," included the following text:

> You may be over it. But it's not over. People are still dying. Still contracting the virus. They need you. We need you. The AIDS Memorial Quilt.[8]

San Francisco's Shanti Project launched an advertising campaign in newspapers and subway stations featuring photographs of people with AIDS under the headline, "We *still* need your help, because they *still* have AIDS." The text designed to recruit donors and volunteers states:

> Promising new treatments are helping some people to live longer, healthier lives. But for others, these drugs are ineffective—or too expensive. And for everyone living with HIV/AIDS, the need for support services remains urgent.[9]

At least one bathhouse has joined the rush to ensure gay men understand that the epidemic isn't over. An advertisement for the Watergarden, a "gay and bisexual men's club and baths" in San Jose features a tattooed, pierced, and goateed stud smiling at the viewer along with the clever text, "The Fat Lady Hasn't Sung Yet . . . Play Safe."[10]

These campaigns reflect advertisers' realization that the changing epidemic moment has to be taken into account if marketing efforts are going to remain meaningful and effective. Although this is a step in the right direction, few organizations and businesses have closely analyzed some gay men's changing involvement in AIDS work. They grasp aimlessly to find explanations for many gay men's lack of interest in the work of AIDS organizations, alternately arguing the gay population is "burnt out" on AIDS, new drugs have made men feel the epidemic is over, young gay men inherently believe they are invulnerable to lethal disease, or all gay men are in deep denial.

This chapter and the following chapter offer alternative ways to understand the shifting involvement of gay men in AIDS work. First, I argue that most men who currently are out and involved in gay community life do not personally understand or emotionally experience AIDS as a simple, discrete crisis, except in the narrowest intellectual sense. Instead, many have accepted the reality of the epidemic in their lives and gotten on with the business of living. Their everyday social practices are generating identities and cultures that could be categorized as post-AIDS. Other men may experience AIDS as one crisis among several facing their community and have difficulty unravelling AIDS from other scourges or seeing it as special. These gay men are helping redefine our communal understanding of AIDS and taking us into a post-AIDS era where AIDS is not seen as the central, overarching trauma visited on gay communities.

When I say "post-AIDS," I draw on Gary Dowsett's work indicating that the event of AIDS generated by urban gay communities in the 1980s is no longer dominant in men's social worlds. This admittedly controversial term claims that the communal experience of AIDS-as-crisis has ended, but does not imply that the epidemic of AIDS is over. As Gary Dowsett has stated about post-AIDS life among uninfected gay men in Australia:

> Post-AIDS is with us now, as uninfected men live with HIV/AIDS over its increasingly prolonged time line. How can we continue to pretend a crisis here? How can we continue to create crisis as the basis for prevention education? Sustaining safe sex strategies often rely on keeping the crisis alive. I

believe we can no longer do that for men who have lived so long and so successfully without HIV in the midst of HIV.[11]

Second, I argue that a dissonance has emerged between the leadership of gay and AIDS organizations and broad populations of gay men throughout the United States, arising from the continuing use of the AIDS-as-crisis construct with people for whom such a representation does not ring true. Community leadership frequently has resisted any attempt to allow the AIDS event of the 1980s to metamorphose into an AIDS event of the 1990s that might resonate as authentic to contemporary gay men. Diminished participation by gay men might be interpreted in several ways: as a sign of (a) resistance to continuing efforts to lock us in a permanent state of emergency; (b) deeper, more complex concerns about "health" and "community" held by gay men than are often acknowledged; (c) a serious misreading of the priorities of gay communities that is fully out of touch with life as gay men live it in the final years of the twentieth century.

These two chapters are intended to encourage all gay men to think deeply about the position HIV currently holds in our lives and the lives of men with whom we share community, and to reconsider strategies utilized in our work on the epidemic. Rather than throw in the towel and claim it's "natural" for gay men to lose interest in AIDS and move on to other endeavors, I believe reenergizing gay male communities in efforts against HIV is possible, but only if our organizations forsake top-down, we-know-what's-best-for-you dictates. Instead, now is the time for organizations to engage in a protracted period of inquiry into the social worlds of gay men, and see our emerging cultures for what they often are: healthy, adaptive, and sometimes highly imaginative responses to the way AIDS manifests itself in our lives at this particular epidemic moment.

DEATH, DEPARTURE, AND DIVERSIFICATION CREATE NEW EPIDEMIC EVENTS

Men who identify as gay and inhabit gay neighborhoods, bars, political organizations, and cultural venues no longer experience the communities they inhabit as existing in a state of crisis. These men might consider AIDS a critically important issue and some might be infected with HIV, yet the worlds they inhabit in the late 1990s are no longer either terrorized by the epidemic or ignorant of its hazards. AIDS has become a significant part of gay men's collective understanding of the world but may not be central to our identities or prominent in our everyday experiences of gay male cultures. Through a complex and protracted cultural process, various realities of AIDS have been integrated into our consciousness, inscribed onto our bodies, and we've moved forward.

Many gay men worked tirelessly in the 1980s and 1990s to create lives beyond crisis and construct communities beyond suffering. They've done so, not because they are uncaring or seek to avoid the epidemic—many of these men are HIV positive—but because they are aware that people defined by terror and loss cannot build viable forms of community over the long haul. Their collective ability to reinvent communities and reconfigure identities is impressive because the leadership of various gay communities—the voices that speak through the gay media, AIDS organizations, and gay activist groups—rarely encouraged or supported such shifts. Interviews with gay men living in various parts of the country highlight the profound ways gay men have shifted their relationship with the epidemic.

Five groups of men seem especially important to examine in considering post-AIDS gay male identities:

1. Gay men who have remained uninfected with HIV throughout the entire course of the epidemic
2. Gay men of color
3. Young gay men for whom AIDS has always been a part of the cultural landscape
4. Gay men living in small cities, towns, and rural areas
5. Gay men with HIV, including long-term nonprogressors, men having successful experiences on combination therapies, and men who are not finding the new treatments helpful

In this chapter and the next, I am not suggesting that *all* rural gay men share a singular experience or that *all* long-term HIV survivors claim common understandings of the epidemic. This would be inaccurate and is not a part of this book's premise. Neither am I saying all young gay men are white or all gay men of color are situated in urban areas. I understand that various identities may intersect and interact. By making use of these categories, I aim to show how some gay male subcultures are thriving outside the crisis construct and others are coping with multiple challenges that make it difficult for AIDS to appear as the single, dominating crisis in the life of a community. My primary aim is to illustrate how communities of men are taking an active role in reshaping and reconfiguring their identities and everyday practices in order to step beyond the crazed mindset and manic routines of epidemic culture.

Some of the men I interviewed have made these changes consciously and deliberately, but most have not. More often, leaving behind a crisis psyche has seemed simply to happen to men over a lengthy time period. For others at this point in the epidemic, daily life may move in and out of crisis stages. Few seem able to sustain life in a bomb shelter for long periods of time. While this might have been the reigning model of life at ground zero for gay men during the first dozen years of the epidemic, these days it appears much less common.

Many of the men with whom I spoke questioned whether the narrative of AIDS created in movies such as *Philadelphia, Longtime Companion,* and *And the Band Played On* was ever the way most gay men lived their lives, even in the 1980s. They felt the media have become adept at taking localized, dramatic situations affecting a narrow population and making them appear universal. During the early years of the epidemic, this functioned to popularize one particular way of experiencing AIDS, while simultaneously silencing other experiences. As one man from a small, Midwestern city put it:

I've always been grateful for the intense response to AIDS that came out of big cities like New York, because that kind of activism has ultimately helped all of us who have HIV, even in backwaters like my town. At the same time, I've always felt disturbed that other responses to the epidemic by less visible gay communities, have gone unacknowledged. Our struggle here has been as much about coming out of the closet as homosexuals as it has been about dealing with sick people. I've seen many more gay men who have been beaten up for being queer than gay men who have developed AIDS. So while groups like ACT-UP have been important to me from a distance, the lives of New York ACT-UP leaders are really different from the lives of men who live here. Why aren't our experiences seen as just as valuable as theirs?[12]

I believe the epidemic moment of the mid-1980s understandably defined AIDS as disaster and triggered gay men to mount a crisis-based response in the areas of prevention, service delivery, and activism. While not every gay man's experience in 1985, this crisis construct was not a marginal viewpoint. Most of the men who were out of the closet and involved in building gay community—whether in San Francisco or San Antonio, West Hollywood or West Hartford—shared in the shock, terror, grief, and panic of those early days. While acknowledging that differences of location, generation, race, and class produced different shapings of that epidemic moment, commonalities did emerge. This occurred precisely because different kinds of losses, some of the most salient forms of AIDS loss, struck all of us.

We didn't all lose our entire network of gay male friends, but we all felt the spirit of optimism of the 1970s yanked out from under us. We didn't all bury lovers and best friends, but we all lost icons who united us across boundaries of geography and ethnicity, such as Sylvester, John Preston, and Al Parker. We didn't all find out we were infected in 1985, but we all felt the fears of wondering, as HIV testing became widely available, whether we already had been infected with the as-yet-unidentified virus. These symbolic losses and intangible experiences encircled a major portion of the gay-identified men of the 1980s and early 1990s and bound us tightly into a state of crisis. Whether in the gay ghetto or in small-town America, most of us had a core part of our identities stamped once again with the brand of sickness, contagion, and pathology.

My own experience in epicenter cities is revealing of this particular epidemic moment. In 1985, I moved to California and became executive director of the Los Angeles Gay and Lesbian Community Services Center, the largest gay nonprofit in the nation. Working with an impressive staff and board of directors, we responded to the arrival of the epidemic as did many similar groups of lesbians, gay men, and bisexuals throughout the nation: we organized our activities based on our collective experience of emergency, crisis, a war besieging our people. In the wake of Rock Hudson's death that year, most of us rapidly worked through stages of denial, shock, and fear, and were ready for action and outrage.

What did this look like? We crafted prevention programs such as Stop AIDS/Los Angeles aiming to keep men safe from "the AIDS virus" until a cure could be developed. We took leadership against the LaRouche Initiative, which aimed to quarantine people with AIDS. We opened the largest HIV test site in the nation because we felt that the volatile politics surrounding AIDS meant it was critically important for our community to handle this sensitive process (and the confidential information that came out of it) our own way. Our work responded to crisis because crises—mounting death tolls, quarantine, and the scapegoating of people with HIV—were in our faces daily.

The AIDS-related ties that bind us together in the late 1990s are quite different and more fragile, because the contexts are so different. The rank and file of contemporary community life is composed primarily of men who do not share in an understanding that AIDS is shocking, terrifying, and cataclysmic. How has this come to be? What happened to the rank and file of the mid-1980s who forged the crisis construct? How did their experience become marginalized?

Three key factors are responsible for marginalizing these men's experience of AIDS in today's worlds: death, diversification of community membership, and the departure of many of these 1980s men from the spaces in which gay men continue to forge collective meanings. When I look at photos from my years at the Los Angeles Center—I departed ten years ago—I'm overwhelmed with the realization that death has claimed almost two-thirds of my male board members and staff management team.[13] The experiences of men who lived through the arrival of AIDS have become marginal in large part because, in one brief decade, an enormous portion of these men died.

Many of the surviving members of this lost generation departed from active involvement in the community during the late 1980s and early 1990s. Some were epidemic casualties of a sort different from corpses: men burnt out from the scorching intensity of the epidemic or toxic interpersonal politics common to queer organizations. Others left without being destroyed or discouraged: they'd simply achieved what they'd hoped to accomplish through their years of involvement and gone on to other activities that provided new meaning to their lives. I know a few men who found lovers and moved to the suburbs and now socialize primarily with other suburban folks, straight and gay. As some men aged, they found some gay male subcultures hostile to middle-aged men, and headed toward other spaces—some specifically involving gay men and some not—that offered sustenance. One man who'd been heavily involved in AIDS services and gay politics now avoids the community altogether and spends his time at car shows and bridge tournaments. Another left the AIDS scene after intense participation for a decade and spends his time in a gay chorus and a gay bowling league. I know several who withdrew to isolated rural areas. This exodus of survivors from epicenter cities has yet to be adequately documented and quantified.

This "emigration" of gay men from pre-AIDS gay cultures to places entirely out of the queer public sphere has been more than balanced numerically with an influx. Diversification of gay communities is the primary reason the crisis construct of the 1980s has moved into a less central position in the life of our communities. There's been an enormous influx into gay communities since 1985, as the public's understanding of issues of sexual identity and representation of our lives has become somewhat kinder. Coming out in 1998 may still require a certain amount of courage, but it's a qualitatively different kind of courage than that reflected in the comings-out of the 1970s and early 1980s. The men who have come into community life since 1985 are diverse and have a broad range of understandings of the epidemic. As the rank and file became filled by young gay men who never knew worlds without AIDS, rural and suburban men whose experience of the epidemic was not the same as that of men in urban centers, and newly-out men who'd spent their twenties and thirties in the closet (and sometimes in heterosexual marriages), new meanings evolved and took hold.

Where are the protease babies in all of this, those men who have been taking combination therapies for a brief period of time? Aren't they regaining health and energy, going back to work and returning to the gym? Don't they exemplify post-AIDS lives better than any other group?

My initial research into the experience of men on protease inhibitors leads me to classify most of them as creating post-AIDS identities, but not in an easy and simple way. While men on protease inhibitors may be the most visible sign of dry bones breathing again, their psychological states may be quite precarious. Many no longer believe they will die of AIDS in the next few years, although most are uncertain *what* to believe. Initial reports are indicating that, quite separate from the relative success or failure of the new treatments, people taking them seem to be walking on eggshells. Powerful shifts in life expectancies and the uncertain nature of the future make it difficult for these people to let down their guard and relax their vigilance. Despite the challenges they face, even these gay men break the mold of the crisis construct of the 1980s because they no longer expect a quick or certain death, and their engagement in life and the social and sexual worlds of gay men often has returned.

I believe creating lives beyond crisis is the way to create sustainable forms of community. As I talked with men throughout the nation in preparing this book, I heard a great desire for revitalized gay communities. The voices and lives of the men in this chapter are intended to serve as starting points from which we might consider new ways of situating ourselves in relation to the epidemic.

The three groups discussed in this chapter do not currently respond to AIDS in the way the broader gay community did in the mid-1980s. Yet none of these groups is ignoring AIDS or pretending the epidemic does not continue to take its toll. Their work at this point in time is focused on inventing post-AIDS identities and forging cultures under rapidly evolving epidemic conditions.

LONG-TERM UNINFECTED GAY MEN: LOST GENERATION OR POST-AIDS PIONEERS?

Men involved in gay social and sexual worlds since the 1970s who remain uninfected with HIV are an understudied population. Researchers may be interested in learning how their sexual practices kept them from becoming infected or what kinds of genes they carry that may have kept HIV from taking hold in their systems, but rarely have researchers investigated the social, cultural, and psychological experiences of uninfected men during the epidemic.

Over the past three years, articles, research papers, and books have started to appear that begin to address a range of issues facing this population. Will Johnston's *HIV-Negative: How the Uninfected Are Affected by AIDS* and Walt Odets' *In the Shadow of the Epidemic: Being HIV-Negative in the Age of AIDS* are landmark works probing issues such as survivor guilt, repeat trauma, sexual safety, and relationships between HIV-negative and HIV-positive men.[14] While these books were both well-received and reviewed, they do not appear to have initiated long-term qualitative studies aimed at understanding the continuing challenges faced by HIV-negative gay men as they attempt to make meaning of the epidemic. *A Crisis of Meaning: How Gay Men Are Making Sense of AIDS,* an excellent book by Steven Schwartzberg, is focused specifically on the meaning-making practices of HIV-positive gay men.[15] We need similar research on uninfected men.

Men who have inhabited gay communities since the 1970s, yet remain uninfected, often maintain bizarre dual identities as both witnesses to and survivors of the epidemic. In *Reviving the Tribe,* I insisted that many of these men had experienced cataclysmic losses yet were expected to be doing fine in the eyes of the world. A huge backlog of unaddressed grief, terror, and rage forced many of these men to walk zombielike through their everyday routines. Michael Wright has written about this condition as the "AIDS survivor syndrome."[16] Unless a concerted effort were made to support these survivors in reengaging with life, I argued, many could be written off as simply another sort of casualty of the AIDS epidemic.

Over the past few years, hundreds of peer support and therapy groups for HIV-negative gay men have been formed that have assisted men as they return to the land of the living. These groups exist not only in San Francisco, New York and Boston, but in Tulsa, Tucson, and Toledo.[17] There are now groups for HIV-negative men of color, uninfected men under the age of twenty-five, and uninfected men over forty. The shift in both consciousness concerning the issues faced by this population and resources devoted to their support has spurred a powerful revival of activity among these men, particularly among midlife HIV-negative gay men. Although some uninfected men remain tightly constrained by survivor guilt or repeat trauma and others have withdrawn from gay community, many others are again emerging as active participants in community life.

For the most part, these uninfected men are *not* creating isolated, separatist cultures. The primary struggle many of them face is not focused on antibody status. Rather, these men are doing the work of creating spaces within gay communities that are welcoming to middle-aged gay men. Many of them spent the greater part of their twenties and thirties responding to the overwhelming demands of the epidemic, only to find themselves in their forties and fifties situated in communities where not only has the number of their generational peers been significantly reduced, but the ageism common to many American cultures devalues their bodies and their lives. Many uninfected midlife men of all races and classes have approached post-AIDS life with a firm determination to create social spaces in which they can survive as whole human beings.

This was reflected recently at the National Forum On and For HIV-Negative Gay Men, held in Atlanta in July 1997, preceding the National Lesbian and Gay Health Conference. Over 200 people gathered to discuss a range of mental health issues facing HIV-negative gay men and meet in small group sessions to probe men's experiences in the current epidemic moment. In his introductory remarks, Andy Humm, an organizer of the institute, identified himself as a "forty-three-year-old member of a lost generation," and provocatively asked participants to struggle with the question, "Can we now consider less than a full-time obsession with HIV?"[18] Alex Carballo-Dieguez from the HIV Center for Clinical and Behavioral Studies in New York presented the results of a survey showing a sharp increase in the number of organizations providing services focused on HIV-negative gay men since 1994, including outreach, peer counseling, individual counseling, and group psychotherapy.[19]

Many of the speeches came from midlife HIV-negative gay men who were wrestling with issues of community building, sexuality, and masculinity. A rough cut of a video was screened that depicted HIV-negative gay men of various races and ethnicities struggling to make sense of their shifting identities. The image of the AIDS Quilt was used repeatedly during the video, effectively framing HIV-negative gay men's experiences as those of traumatic loss and over-whelming grief.

During a break in the forum, I sat with a small group of HIV-negative gay men and reflected on the speeches and video. One man was angered by the tone reflected throughout the program:

> The conversation reflects a very narrow view of what it means to be HIV negative. I went through that state of trauma they're talking about, but it lasted about a year or a year and a half. These days, being HIV negative doesn't often feel over-whelming or traumatic. I resent my experience being framed by the Quilt. Where is the joy? Where is the humor? Where is the fun in our lives? We've been to hell and back, let's talk about what we've learned and how we are moving forward.[20]

This man exemplifies a spirit increasingly common among HIV-negative gay men. Many of us enter a phase of overwhelming loss and frozen feelings, but do not remain there a long time. We work through the pain, guilt, grief, and shock and return to a functional level of participation in the world. While some might remain locked in the "AIDS survivor syndrome" for long periods of time, this is no longer how many HIV-negative men understand our lives. We hunger to see reflected back to us our authentic struggles to create new, meaningful identities and cultures as the epidemic moment shifts, and as we become entrenched in the issues of midlife.

GAY MEN OF COLOR:
BUILDING COMMUNITY AMID MULTIPLE THREATS

People of color were among the earliest and loudest critics of the representation of AIDS-as-crisis put forth by primarily white AIDS and gay organizations. While sharing in the commitment to fight AIDS, many gay men of color—particularly African-American gay men—argued that the crisis construct as scripted by white AIDS organizations did not ring true in their communities of origin. Not only were their communities under-resourced from the start of the epidemic, but for communities of color to acquire funding for men who have sex with men they frequently had to squeeze into white gay male conceptions of the epidemic, public health, community education, and sexual identity.

Concerns voiced by gay men of color were frequently ignored or marginalized. Many white gay men, unable to understand how powerfully the crisis construct was linked to the cultural worlds of white, middle-class gay men, shrugged off the articulate challenges of gay men of color. We often mistook sincere critiques by men of color of our representations of the epidemic for internal community race wars. The understanding of AIDS produced in the mid-1980s by the gay (white) community was a culture-bound understanding, representative of one privileged sector of the larger gay male population. Tony Valenzuela, a Chicano gay man from San Diego, explained it this way:

> As a person of color who has always integrated race into my work, I have found it difficult to consider one issue a crisis over another. Chicanos on the border will always see the abuse of immigrants as a crisis and other problems such as the end of affirmative action, Proposition 187, racism in our everyday lives, financial struggle as personal assaults, to a greater or lesser degree, with AIDS as another major category. I think gay Chicanos . . . we all walk around with *all* these issues under our skin simultaneously, with different ones surfacing at different times.[21]

John Peterson, PhD, spoke about the complex ways the crisis constructs intersect with African-American gay men and men who have sex with men and argues that age plays a distinct role in men of color's relationship to the crisis construct:

> Do African-American gay men experience AIDS as a crisis? It depends on the location and the cohort. Among the men who are in our generation [currently in their forties] and who were hit by the epidemic, crisis—yes. The only crisis? No. The most important crisis? Depends. The most important crisis to men who have sex with men? Possibly. The most important crisis to the African-American community, probably not. I think for the African-American men who have sex with men population in leading epicenters, it is a crisis for the men in the

older cohorts. For the younger men, it's similar to that of the younger men in the mainstream community.

A grandmother said to me once, after I talked about the reticence of the African-American community to respond to the AIDS epidemic . . . she said AIDS would just have to wait in line. She meant there are competing other crises in the African-American community that will have to be dealt with before we can divert our attention to HIV.[22]

Gay men of color understood something in the mid-1980s that took many gay white men an additional decade to learn: work in the epidemic must be deeply and authentically rooted in the cultures of the communities we intend to reach. By insisting, for instance, that the lives of many black gay men of poor and working class origins were embedded in cultures that were already contending with a number of crises (e.g., poverty, racism, violence, drug abuse), they argued that the appearance of AIDS did not suddenly propel their communities into a state of emergency. Likewise, Latino AIDS activists argued that issues of immigration status and poverty made it difficult for many Latino gay men to see a sexually transmitted disease, even a potentially lethal one, as the initiation of a crisis state. Their communities were already suffering under the strain of crisis.

Gay men of color have suffered a large volume of loss due to AIDS. AIDS has brought about the early deaths of many gay men of color and robbed nascent communities of many of their most experienced leaders. In fact, the black gay community nationwide has suffered cataclysmic losses, with much of its visible leadership—including leaders in black gay political, cultural, and social circles as well as black gay men who were leaders in mainstream gay efforts—dying of AIDS-related causes by 1995. Despite this decimation, gay men of color frequently found themselves caught between AIDS groups dominated by white gay men who discounted the importance of race and ethnicity-based cultures in their prevention work, and AIDS groups situated in ostensibly heterosexual communities of color that discounted the importance of sexuality-based cultures in education work.

Yet during the years of the AIDS epidemic, queer communities of color have become home to tremendous institution building and rich cultural production. While this work clearly began during the first decade of the epidemic, these efforts continue to bear fruit in the late 1990s. Today, most urban centers have thriving queer communities of color, often with their own venues, organizations, publications, and rituals.[23]

Gay men of color have been living what could be understood as post-AIDS lives for quite some time. The event of AIDS constructed primarily by white gay men in the mid-1980s never rang true for gay men of color rooted in their communities of origin. They offer a powerful example of how it is possible to marshal forces to fight the epidemic, care for the sick, and launch effective prevention campaigns, without seeing AIDS as the only crisis on the agenda or viewing AIDS as independent from a variety of other important health concerns.

YOUNG GAY MEN: CONSTRUCTING IDENTITIES BEYOND CRISIS

In 1985, when those of us concerned with developing HIV-prevention programs for gay male youth met to exchange ideas, strategies, and funding contacts, our discussions targeted gay men under the age of twenty-three. The category "young gay men" that we developed included very diverse populations: homeless, runaway, and "throwaway" youth from twelve to nineteen years old who found themselves on the streets of large cities; "in-school" youth attending high schools in urban, suburban, and rural areas; street hustlers, escorts, and other sex workers; urban school dropouts who, while of diverse races and ethnicities, usually came from working class and poor families and were struggling to find jobs in a declining economy. Recognizing that these youth had a different relationship to the epidemic than adult gay men, we designed HIV prevention programs that acknowledged their "unique needs."

Fast-forward over a dozen years to 1998. This same population with "unique needs" now ranges in age up to thirty-five years old. The groups that, in 1985, we insisted had very different prevention needs than their cohorts just a few years older are now a dominant population in gay male cultures. In urban centers, the thirty-five-and-under crowd fill dance clubs and sex clubs and gyms and coffeehouses. Yet prevention efforts with these men mistakenly assume, because they've now grown up and become the same age gay men of my generation were when the epidemic hit, their relationship to the epidemic is the same as ours of a dozen years ago. Prevention groups, with rare exception, attempt to foist crisis-focused campaigns onto these men who have never experienced AIDS as the crisis it was for my gay generation.

In 1985, we were unaware precisely why this population had unique prevention needs. Some of us assumed it was because they were young and imagined themselves impervious to illness and death. We wove together a romanticized narrative of young gay men who found it difficult to practice safer sex because life at seventeen meant being carefree, invulnerable, having one's entire life stretched out in front of one. Weren't we untroubled and filled with youthful exuberance at seventeen? Our understanding of why the programs we created for these men were different from our programs for older men was rooted in our social constructions of "youth" as a category and our limited experience of current youth cultures. As this population aged its way to twenty-three, then twenty-seven, then thirty, we simply removed them from the list of men needing unique prevention programs, merged them into the "adult gay men" category, and refocused those programs on the young queer men now occupying the under-twenty-three age slots.

I believe there are at least five generational cohort groups of gay men who have radically different experiences and understandings of AIDS and subsequently require very different approaches in prevention work:

1. Young gay men born after 1977 who are coming out amid the Protease Moment, when understandings of AIDS are undergoing rapid transformation.
2. Gay men born between 1965 and 1977 who entered gay worlds in the mid- to late 1980s and have never known gay communities without the firmly fixed imprint of AIDS.
3. "Cusp" men, born between 1960 and 1965 who were coming out into gay cultures as the epidemic was coming out in the early 1980s and occupy the cusp between pre-AIDS and post-AIDS coming-out experiences.

4. Surviving members of what I have come to consider a "lost generation": gay men born from 1938 to 1960 who were out and involved in community before AIDS and are still walking this earth.

5. Gay men born prior to 1938 who were approaching midlife as AIDS dawned, and experienced their own losses—both symbolic and material—during the tidal wave of the epidemic.

My purpose here is to argue that a population we once readily acknowledged had a very different understanding of the epidemic than older cohorts, gay men born between 1965 and 1977, are now considered no different from the older cohorts and are simply blended in with that group in our prevention efforts.

Just as gay men from small cities, towns, and rural areas have their own stories of life in an epidemic quite different from those of epicenter gay men, so too do these young gay men, now age twenty-three to thirty-five. Theirs is a powerful and complex story that includes the entangling of gay identity with HIV, the constituting, manipulation, and policing of bodies and desires through safer-sex discourse, and the creation of a new legacy of guilt due to "knowing better" yet becoming another gay generation of infection and morbidity. What's rarely been explored about the identity of this cohort is their relationship to the crisis construct of epidemic life that emerged from my gay generation.

Interviews with men under thirty-five highlight some very sharp distinctions between this cohort and older men. As I talked with men throughout the nation, I found their relationships to the epidemic could be categorized in one of three ways: (1) men who joined AIDS efforts and took up an AIDS-crisis rhetoric but wondered why so few of the other men of their generation responded likewise; (2) men who seemed deeply alienated from AIDS work, and often the formal structures of gay community life, and felt those involved in AIDS efforts were, in one man's words, "screwed-up drama queens who need to get a life"; (3) men who contributed to AIDS efforts from a distance and were grateful such services existed but did not feel highly charged about the epidemic or connected to the AIDS system.

Few of the men with whom I spoke—both HIV positive and negative—experienced the epidemic as a crisis, and most had quite a bit to say about men who did. One twenty-eight-year-old white gay man from Chicago said,

> AIDS may be a crisis in a certain sense, but it is not one in my life or the life of my friends. I understand why we need to explain it as an emergency, in order to get funding and stuff like that. But no one I know buys into the intensity and drama that the AIDS groups want us to feel. It just doesn't seem real to us. I mean, I live in Chicago, I know people my age who have died from AIDS, but I've spent my entire homosexual life coming to terms with the virus and, if I haven't gotten infected yet, I don't think I ever will. Knock on wood.[24]

A twenty-six-year-old Latino gay man who is HIV positive saw things a bit differently.

> Before I got infected, I knew a lot about AIDS. I even had worked on a few HIV-prevention teams. But I guess I didn't take it seriously and kept doing things I shouldn't do and then I ended up testing positive at age twenty-four. When that happened, at first I felt nothing. It seemed like no big deal. Then I moved into a period of panic. I tell you, it felt like a crisis then. It sure did. I came out of that phase about a year ago, and I must admit that most days having HIV doesn't seem like all that big a deal. I don't know if it's because of the new drugs, or because I know guys who have been infected for ten years and are still doing fine, but it's unusual for me to get into a state of agitation about having HIV. Most of the time it is not a big deal.[25]

A twenty-four-year-old white man from Massachusetts was highly judgmental of the gay community's focus on AIDS:

> I don't like people telling me what to do or how to feel and I think that every time I pick up a gay paper or go to some kind of event, I get the very strong impression that this thing called "the gay community" wants me to think that AIDS is the

worst thing that has ever happened on earth. It just doesn't
register with me. AIDS is out there, so you try to be safe. But
you don't let it rule your life and you don't stop having sex
with guys. It just feels like a lot of guilting. That's it, the crisis
stuff seems like just another tactic to get guys to keep their
pants on. I don't want anything to do with it.[26]

My interviews with a twenty-nine-year-old gay man living in
rural east Texas place in high relief the various ways some gay men
of his generation experience the epidemic. Mason is a white gay
man working at a local AIDS organization and attending college.
He was raised in a very small town with no supermarket and a
population of less than 2,000. He came out to his family when he
was sixteen years old, and spent the remainder of his high school
years in conflict with his minister father over his sexuality. This
motivated Mason to get out of the family home and join the Army
when he was nineteen, and he spent most of his five years stationed
in Colorado.

When Mason attempts to fit his life and his understanding of
AIDS into the representations of the epidemic he sees in movies
such as *Longtime Companion* or *Philadelphia*, he notices a key
difference between his life and those of urban, coastal gay men of a
different generation:

> I don't think that I have seen the volume of loss that a lot of
> other gay men have seen personally. I know some of my older
> friends who are not HIV positive talk about seeing ten or
> twelve of their friends die. In my case, I've only had one
> person in my age group, a peer, who had HIV. And he killed
> himself . . . so I know no one who's personally died of AIDS
> that's in my age group in my area.[27]

When Mason looks at his peer group of friends of his generation,
he realizes they are experiencing AIDS in ways that are significantly different from older gay men in epicenter cities:

> I probably have eight gay friends that are really close to me,
> and I don't see us being in that state of loss that's captured at
> the end of *Longtime Companion*. At the end of that movie,

when everyone comes back, I just don't see that happening for my friends or my generation.[28]

When asked directly, "Do you experience the AIDS epidemic as a crisis?" Mason responds:

> From a personal level, no. From where I work, yes. But then, a lot of our clients are not necessarily gay men, so I look at it as a crisis, but not necessarily just for the gay community. . . . At some point, I do feel that I'm not having the same experience as some of the other people. Because, obviously, AIDS is a very big issue, especially in big cities, but since I don't live there and since I am younger, my life is not identified with all that loss and death.[29]

Mason's sense of his generation as different from older gay men was shared by most of the men in their mid- to late twenties and early thirties whom I interviewed. They do not feel that the cultures they are creating are destructive or in denial about AIDS, and they are angry that they are expected to make the epidemic an overarching concern. Wayne Hoffman, a twenty-six-year-old gay journalist in New York City, has captured this spirit in an essay titled "Skipping the Life Fantastic: Coming of Age in the Sexual Devolution":

> A new backroom in 1996 cannot truly imitate a backroom from 1976; it is not possible today for most men to view public sex (or any sex, for that matter) except through the viral veil of safety and risk. The public sex venues opening anew are not simply a nostalgic retreat to pre-AIDS times. They are operating in a new milieu—in an epidemic.
>
> The distinction is particularly salient for us younger men, who *cannot* retreat to the backrooms of 1976—because we were in grade school, or even diapers, at the time. For us the new sex venues represent the dawning of a new sexual culture we have never experienced on such a wide scale. Today's public sexual renewal does not represent a step backward in gay men's sexual development—either *to* the days of liberation or *from* the horrors of the epidemic—but rather a step ahead in time toward a new kind of sexual and political expression.

For young men in particular, who have never known a time when our sexuality has not been intertwined with fatalism, mortality, doom, and danger, creating new public spheres where the fantastic can flourish allows the possibility for fantasy to enter into our sexuality on a broad scale. Young men can find the space to start imagining what a new queer sexuality might look like without opportunistic infections, without anti-sex censorship, without legal and societal restrictions, without anti-gay violence.[30]

Perhaps more than anything else, it is this spirit of possibility and reinvention that drives community-building efforts among contemporary young gay men. Finding themselves in an evolving relationship to the epidemic distinct from the relationship thrust among older gay men, they struggle to do justice to their own experiences and create a meaningful sense of community.

Chapter 4

Vacating the Bomb Shelters

In the United States, we have rarely given more than lip-service acknowledgment to different manifestations of AIDS in distinct geographic areas. We readily identify the different populations that constitute "people with AIDS/HIV" in San Francisco and Newark, New Jersey, but we rarely discuss how gay men's experiences of the epidemic are different in these two cities. At national AIDS conferences, one hears speakers insist that AIDS work in such places as Omaha or Galveston is ten years behind big city organizing, suggesting there is a single epidemic trajectory and that small cities are simply less far along this trajectory than larger urban centers. We might debate patterns of equitable distribution of federal AIDS dollars among rural, small town, suburban, urban, and epicenter areas, but most of us have little understanding of the ways AIDS is manifested in these distinct environments and the different resources appropriate to each site. Rarely have we affirmed that the precise trajectory and meanings of AIDS are context-dependent and that comparing AIDS in New York City and AIDS in Wyoming is comparing apples and oranges.[1]

Ignoring geographic differences over the past fifteen years has been key to the development of a belief that there is a singular gay experience of the epidemic in the United States. Many believe gay men's experience of AIDS in Milwaukee or Wichita or Tucson is identical to gay men's experience of AIDS in Los Angeles, New York, or San Francisco, albeit a bit muted, toned-down, or somewhat less intense. We've created an understanding of "gay AIDS" that universalizes the epicenter experience of the 1980s and projects its narratives onto gay men everywhere.[2] Many believe that the communal experience of emergency that overcame men in the Castro or Greenwich Village in 1984 also overcame gay men in Missoula or Bangor or El Paso.

From the onset of the epidemic, gay men in small cities, towns, and rural areas, while often sharing many of the symbolic losses epicenter gay men felt, experienced the epidemic in their own ways. While specific urban communities may have lost hundreds of gay men to AIDS between 1981 and 1987, the losses in smaller cities, towns, and rural communities were much fewer and often more obscured. The variance in the volume and visibility of death, while important to an understanding of nonurban gay men's AIDS experiences, played out differently in each of the thousands of rural and small town gay communities dotting the nation.

RURAL GAY MEN: FORGING CONNECTIONS WITHIN LOCAL EPIDEMIC CONTEXTS

Rural areas, small towns, and small cities in the early 1980s were not always void of openly gay men or organized gay communities, as some appear to believe. Certain vacation spots popular among gay men, such as Provincetown, Key West, Saugatuck (Michigan), Laguna Beach, and Northern California's Russian River area, had prominent communities of gay men and lesbians. College towns, such as Madison, Wisconsin; Columbus, Ohio; Athens, Georgia; Austin, Texas; Bloomington, Indiana; Amherst, Massachusetts; and Ames, Iowa, maintained informal social networks of gay men as well as formal gay organizations. Communities of gay men had taken root in places as diverse as Aroostock County, Maine, and Wolf Creek, Oregon.

Few urban gay men have heard stories about gay communities' experience of AIDS outside of big-city America. From the urban centers hardest hit by the epidemic, we gaze out over the rest of the nation, oblivious to the distinct challenges our counterparts, the small-town boys, have faced. When asked for unique aspects of the epidemic facing rural gay men, we might be cognizant of the "returning-home" factor, gay men who developed AIDS in New York City or San Francisco but went home to rural New Hampshire or Idaho when they became sick, but have little additional knowledge. One friend, when asked about his thoughts on rural gay men's experience of

AIDS, told me that he assumed few of the AIDS cases in such areas were gay men.

The lack of knowledge of rural AIDS has been accompanied by many problems for rural gay men throughout the nation. As the organizers of an institute on rural men who have sex with men noted, "There are still many places in rural America where there are no gay/lesbian/bisexual HIV/AIDS services available. Nothing. And any help from an experienced worker can be enough to get a program started."[3] This problem is exacerbated by many people's ignorance of the rural poor and the mistaken belief that gay men living outside metropolitan areas are primarily middle-class urban refugees.

Some men outside large cities with whom I spoke insisted the majority of gay men outside the hardest-hit cities *never* experienced AIDS-as-crisis in the way urban men did. Sure they saw the movies, read the newsletters, wore the red ribbons, but their experience of AIDS at that time was symbolic and at a distance, rather than visceral and directly engaged. Living in a city where 10 percent of the gay men became infected with HIV during the 1980s is qualitatively different than living in cities where 50 percent or more of the gay men tested positive. This is not to say that Tulsa's gay community, for example, hasn't experienced AIDS as significant and powerful. Yet that city's experience of AIDS could be expected to produce significantly different meanings and collective understandings of the epidemic than West Hollywood's. Not only has the event of AIDS in the 1980s been different in these cities, but the identities and social position of gay men, before, during, and after the arrival of AIDS, have also been quite different.

In my interviews with gay men from five different states (California, Massachusetts, Oregon, Texas, and Wisconsin) who live apart from urban centers, I grew to understand how conflating gay men's geographically disparate experiences of the epidemic does a disservice to rural gay men. Perhaps most important, it demeans the authentic experiences of gay men in smaller cities, towns, and rural areas, and suggests that their losses and their responses, when distinct from the urban narratives of cataclysmic grief or mass heroism, are somehow less important.

It also presents nonepicenter gay men with unfortunate organizing challenges. At national AIDS conferences, they attend workshops on fund-raising, or organizing support groups, or wooing volunteers, presented by the major epicenter organizations. They ricochet between envy at what's possible in the big cities and rage at the assumption that those possibilities in any way apply to their own area. Gay Men's Health Crisis might think of themselves as "First in the Fight Against AIDS," the problematic slogan they unabashedly tack onto their public relations materials, yet in *whose* fight against AIDS are they first and what do they truly have to offer organizing efforts in Fargo, Little Rock, or Bakersfield?

Gay men in rural areas sometimes attempt to emulate big-city AIDS organizing, with disastrous and disheartening results. As one gay man from a small town in the Midwest said:

> Our county AIDS task force put on an AIDS walk for a fund-raiser and we had five people show up. We spent a lot of money on advertising and newspapers and on radio and TV spots and everything. Five people showed up for this walk and they were all related to either the AIDS task force or the county AIDS department.[4]

Another man from rural California discussed a similar experience in his community:

> We've worked hard to put together a major fund-raiser, like a variety show type of thing. We held it in a 308-seat community theater. Forty-three thousand people live in our county over I don't know how many square miles. We had about 250 people show up for the fund-raiser. We can't even fill a 300-seat theater![5]

Nonurban gay men note another problem that arises from denying the different geographic-based gay AIDS epidemics: prevention paradigms and campaigns are frequently transferred with minor alterations from epicenter cities to smaller cities with little serious attempt to understand the context-bound epicenter assumptions. In a city such as San Francisco, we've learned that what works for white gay men in the Castro might not work for Asian immigrant gay men in Chinatown, or white gay men in the working class neighborhoods of the city. This hasn't stopped big-city prevention leaders from disseminating their models (as well as their buttons, T-shirts, posters, and television spots) throughout the nation, in a social marketing form of neocolonialism. As one man from a small town in Texas told me:

> It just doesn't work in my area to pretend that many gay men will buy into the terror of infection that dominates many urban gay men's thinking about sex. There's just not that much HIV out here. If I have sex behind the barn in a town sixty miles outside Laredo—if I get fucked by a guy without using a condom—you'd have a hard time convincing me that the risk is anywhere near as significant as it is if the same act occurred at a bathhouse in San Francisco. It's not that we don't know HIV can be transmitted through unprotected fucking, we simply have a location-based sense of risk and sometimes you just want to do it without a condom so badly that you go ahead and you don't worry so much.[6]

Nonurban gay men's awareness of geographical implications of unprotected sex practices is sometimes so detailed and so deeply considered, one wonders whether awareness of location doesn't reflect a resourceful and creative strategy for safer sex. A man in Northern California said:

> The town I live in is five hours from San Francisco and four hours from Portland, Oregon. But we're also on a major artery. I-5 is a major highway going right through our county. Whereas if you're living off in Modoc County, or a county that does not have a major artery running through it, that makes all the difference in terms of risk. In Siskiyou County, for example, you've got all this traffic that's coming through going north and south, and people stopping off in truck stops and rest areas where the locals go for contact.
> Someone in an isolated county that doesn't have a major artery running through it, they're not gonna have the same access to sex, nor the same risk for HIV when they do find public sex. You're less likely to come across someone who is HIV positive. I mean it's like placing bets. It's like gambling, you know. You play the odds. I'd say in San Francisco the

odds are a lot less in my favor of *not* becoming infected if I
choose *not* to practice safe sex than in Modoc County.[7]

A man from rural Wisconsin had a similar observation:

> If you're talking about a town like Stone Creek, that is in the
> region I live in, it's not located on the interstate corridor. So
> you're talking about a lot of gay men who are having sex in
> public sex environments and I don't think they usually are
> using safer sex guidelines, because they just don't see the
> crisis there. . . . Some men are living pre-AIDS, as if the
> epidemic hasn't ever happened, and some are living post-
> AIDS, as if they've learned after fucking around without con-
> doms for fifteen years that it's unlikely they'll now get
> infected. It really makes a difference where you are located.[8]

If community identity and meanings are forged in epicenter cities
around powerful threats such as AIDS, in smaller cities and towns,
issues of homophobia and violence often loom much larger than
HIV in gay men's everyday lives. As one Texan put it, "In the
county where I live, you don't even mention homosexuals. The
word is taboo, literally." Perhaps one reason many gay men outside
big cities claim never to have experienced AIDS as a crisis is that,
unlike men living in urban gay ghettos, homophobia and violence
are by far the greatest risk facing these men. It is easy for men who
live in large, coastal cities to think the gays in the military debates
or Ellen DeGeneres's coming out of the closet translate into greater
acceptance for queers everywhere. Yet organizers from nonurban,
noncoastal places for years have insisted that social viewpoint shifts
do not necessarily quickly transfer to the hinterlands.

The most exciting queer organizing in the 1990s may not be
going on in Chicago, San Francisco, or Washington, DC, but in
Idaho, where activists successfully defeated an antigay ballot initiative, or Utah, where queer youth organized to keep gay-straight
alliances active in the public schools, or Wisconsin, where gay
youth Jamie Nabozny won a one million dollar settlement from the
school that allowed him to be victimized throughout his high school
experience.[9] Gay men from such areas are not paranoid when they

discuss real incidents of homophobia and violence in their areas. One man from a small town in Oregon said:

> I have peers in my community who would not be caught dead at this [statewide gay] conference. Because if somebody saw them, their whole lives would be changed. They would no longer be able to associate with people in their community. They would be ostracized. I know one guy who's a really, really nice guy, and he'd been with his lover for several years before the lover died of AIDS. He would not be caught dead here because he works as a contractor and if somebody found out about him and brought it back to the community half—no, I think he said 90 percent—of his business would be gone. That's his livelihood and so he's not about to come and jeopardize that.[10]

A man from eastern Oregon talked about how Ballot Measure 9— the antigay statewide initiative in 1993—affected their local AIDS organization:

> We actually have a support group in our county for people with HIV, but we have never been very public about it till two years ago. Our board of directors decided to make a change. We've had an office for years but did not have a sign out on the street. When the ballot measures came about we did not want to have people who needed to come to us for services feeling like they might be harassed or their cars vandalized in some way, whether they were gay or not. We decided to make a change about two years ago, long after the ballot measures stopped.[11]

Another man from Oregon discussed how antigay violence over-rides AIDS as a threat in his town:

> I think the major issue in my county is safety issues, about how to self-identify as gay and not get your ass kicked. At this point, I think AIDS is really far down the list, if it comes up at all. We're just not at the point where it's safe enough to even identify as gay. You have to cover your ass. You can't take the risk.[12]

This sentiment also was raised by a man from southeastern California:

> In our county our main problem is basically rednecks. We don't have the AIDS problem. We have two people within our county that I know of who have AIDS, and they moved back here from San Diego or L.A. If there was a real epidemic among gay men here—if all of a sudden everyone started to get infected and the whole thing blew open—it would be far easier to do AIDS work like they do it in the city. Here we've gotta deal with the rednecks coming after us.[13]

Members of the rural caucus at a national prevention summit for gay men argued that many urban gay activists and AIDS organizers patronize rural men by applying urban standards of "outness" to rural areas and judging rural men as unnecessarily closeted:

> In rural areas and small towns and cities, the dynamics between the closet, out gays, and the larger society can be very complex and certainly shouldn't be inadvertently trivialized with knee-jerk political correctness about being out of the closet. Prevention programs in these areas must take into account the survival needs (not the same as internalized homophobia) of the people to be reached, and respect the fact that rampaging homophobia may very well be an external reality to be understood and faced, not just an internal psychological state.[14]

A number of factors suggest that these areas may not accurately be thought of as five or ten years behind epicenter cities in their gay AIDS epidemics; something qualitatively different is occurring. While some nonurban areas have similarities to large cities—one HIV-positive man from Provincetown, Massachusetts, made a compelling argument that his tiny town (and popular gay resort) is an epicenter of the epidemic—these tend to be small cities and towns that develop tolerant cultures, often due to the presence of gay tourism or a liberal university culture. One man from Montana explained it this way:

> I've lived in two rural communities that were like night and day. In Montana, I was in the closet. I had come from Missoula

where I was just coming out and enjoying all the privileges and acknowledgment of being a gay man and feeling good about it to a community. Because of economic necessity, I moved to a small town and had to go back in the closet. I couldn't discuss my homosexuality and I had to deal with it in the confines of this very small, provincial town. I'm not going to sit here and say that it was hell, because obviously I stayed for three years and I must have enjoyed some other aspects. After about three years, I knew it was time for a change.[15]

A range of structural and cultural factors make gay men's experience of AIDS in nonurban, noncoastal areas different from that experienced in epicenter "AIDS communities." One of the structural factors involves the small queer population and the lack of publicly identified queer spaces. This creates an extraordinary sense of isolation for some men. As one HIV-positive man from rural Oregon said:

In our area, it's not like you can reach out like you can in San Francisco where there's so many resources and the numbers are really intense. To keep a support group going here is so hard. I really feel the sense of isolation in trying to get together with other gay men. The people I know in my county who're HIV positive are straight people. There's not a sense of support like you have in a city.[16]

This isolation is often accompanied by a lack of resources that urban gay men take for granted. A man from a small city in Wisconsin said:

Our AIDS organization's been around for eight years and it's only been in the past two years that a doctor came to us and said he wanted to treat AIDS patients. We have five counties in our region and there are a number of people with AIDS whose family doctors have been willing to take care of them, but never a doctor who said up front, "Send me AIDS patients." Two years ago, a doctor moved from Milwaukee and called our agency and said, "Please send me your patients. I have always had a certain number of patients in my practice with AIDS and I don't want to stop that." Previous to this, the doctor that cared for the most people in our area was the oncology specialist and it just kind of fell in his lap.[17]

Some of the AIDS cases in rural areas involve gay men who had moved to urban centers, become infected or ill, and moved home to their families-of-origin. These men often have a very different relationship to their gay identities and community than small-town or rural men. One man from southeast Washington said:

> We have a big "coming-home syndrome" in my area. Lots of guys, especially in the 1980s, were coming home to the country to die. Sometimes these guys try to hook up with the local community, organize it in some ways, but because it's different here and they don't understand the differences, it really hasn't worked. Basically, we don't have much of a sense of "gay community" in my area.[18]

While AIDS organizations in nonurban areas often serve as a magnet for local queers, the experience of being HIV positive and gay often carries its own sense of isolation with it. Urban gay men can sometimes find advertisements for support groups for "black gay men who have recently tested HIV positive." The situation outside big cities is usually quite different. A man in rural Texas said:

> I believe there are certain issues that cross in rural areas, but I've found it hard to connect with other people with AIDS in my county because of the difference. If there's only four of you who are HIV positive and you all get together and have a support group, it might not work. It didn't work for me. We had two people in the group who are still using [drugs]—a man and a woman—I'm sorry but I simply could not relate. Trying to find other HIV-positive gay men in my area has been the challenge.[19]

Inevitably during interviews with nonurban gay men about the epidemic, views about popular media depictions of AIDS would surface. Men raised a number of issues about such books and movies. A man from Oregon said:

> Looking at movies like *It's My Party*, I relate more from the life that I lived when I lived in Boston, as a positive man for the few years I was there. What I experience being positive and

being open about it in my area, is different. Sure there've been a few people who have wanted to treat me as their missionary project, but on the whole I get more of a sense of awe and honor and people want to come up and gush about how grateful they are that I have given them this information. . . . As far as people condescending and wanting to take care of me like Little Orphan Annie, I haven't experienced too much of that here.[20]

A man living in the Sierras in eastern California had a similar viewpoint:

> I look at those movies like *Philadelphia* and I say, "Oh, that's nice, but it really doesn't pertain to what's happening here." First of all, you'll be lucky to find any company that'd be willing to support you if you are HIV positive. If most of them find out about it you are out the door. You're history. They're not going to deal with you working there and having HIV and they are not going to deal with the fact that their insurance is going to go up astronomically. It's different here, period, across the board.[21]

Ultimately, gay men's experiences of the epidemic are different outside big cities because gay identity and community are quite different from those reflected in the mainstream gay press. Comparing a publication such as *RFD,* a national journal for rural gay men, with *OUT* magazine highlights some of these differences—different gay masculinities, relationships to the commodification of gay identities and urban commercial spaces, and experiences of the natural environment. What it means to be a gay man in Minneapolis may be quite different in Mankato, Minnesota, or Rice Lake, Wisconsin. Nonurban men consistently discuss dominant subpopulations of gay men who are less prominent in white, middle-class urban centers: heterosexually married gay men who have sex with men and male monogamous couples. Gay-identified men who are open about being sexually active outside primary relationships are less visible than in cities. The distinct ways men construct their relational and sexual identities has resulted in greatly different epidemics, as one man from Texas indicated:

When the first wave hit here, it hit a few gay men. In that sense, it did devastate the "gay community," because it took two gay men out of the community . . . I'm using the term "community" loosely here. Here it's a study in dichotomy. It devastated one segment, but it didn't have any effect on the vast, vast, very large segment of gay men who are closeted, who are living with their married spouses but just kind of trick on the side. Because the prevalence rates in rural areas are nowhere near as high as urban areas, by the law of statistics these men who have sex maybe once every six months aren't necessarily getting hit by this. Now, in the second wave, there are a lot of gay men finding out they are HIV positive because they're just starting to get tested, and it's affecting these other segments of the population.[22]

These factors—isolation, limited HIV infection rates, hate violence, scarce AIDS resources, the closet—seemed to cause most men whom I interviewed from small cities, towns, and rural areas to maintain understandings and interpretations of the AIDS epidemic different from those of urban men. While not always unified in their viewpoints, a large majority agreed that they did not experience it as a crisis. One man from an isolated part of Massachusetts said:

It could only be considered a crisis here because we don't know what it's all about yet. It's still a mystery. It's something they're dealing with, not us.[23]

When asked if gay men in his county experience AIDS as a crisis, one rural Wisconsin man active in AIDS work said:

Not in our county, no. They know people, friends, who have died over a period of time, but they don't think of AIDS as a crisis in the community. When I ask them to come to an AIDS vigil or help with a potluck, for this they might come. Overall, though, I don't get a lot of support from gay men when it comes to AIDS, because they don't believe that it is really an issue in our county.[24]

Another man from a coastal community in Oregon said:

> I think the experience I've had in my town is that the issue of AIDS is something for people from the city—like Portland—to come here to get away from. Some of them move here as a way to recover from the crisis. I have two friends who lived in Portland and then Miami and San Francisco in the seventies. They've experienced death on an astronomical level. Three hundred of their closest friends have died from AIDS. So they come to the country to escape and there's a lot of people moving in so they don't have to deal with AIDS issues.[25]

One gay man from rural Texas clearly understood that AIDS was situated in his life in quite a different position than it was for urban men:

> I'm from west Texas. Lived there most of my life. I did get out and see the world in the military, but I'm only twenty-six years old and haven't been to Dallas, let alone New York City. AIDS here is not something that every gay man is living with every day. As a gay man in west Texas, I don't deal with it. I'm not HIV positive. I don't know too many people who are. I know there are several people in the county that have it, but I don't have the statistics and I don't have to deal with it much.[26]

This is how life in the epidemic is for countless men throughout the nation who must be considered part of the gay community. Whether living on dairy farms or working in sawmills, fishing off the coast of Alaska or working as migrant farm workers in California's Central Valley, gay men's experiences of AIDS in the 1990s are rooted more in their local context than in the intangible losses of the 1980s. While prevention leaders might want to infuse a spirit of crisis in men to create a demand for increased attention to rural AIDS prevention and care services, it seems unlikely that large numbers of men from these areas will be inspired to step into the crisis mode. It's not that they refuse to face the realities of the epidemic; rather, they have confronted the realities of AIDS in their local contexts, integrated those realities into their lives, and created post-AIDS identities and social and sexual practices.

There is evidence that organizing among rural gay and bisexual men is flourishing as the post-AIDS era dawns.[27] Rural men have organized social networks in southern Illinois and Indiana, east Texas, and throughout the state of Oregon. In Northern California, the Billy Club, a network of primarily rural gay men stretching from the Oregon border to San Francisco, meets regularly for monthly potluck meals, weekend gatherings, and "heart circles" that one journalist described this way:

> The Billys, sitting in a circle, are encouraged to feel safe and let whatever they need to say come from their heart and not from their intellectual side. The person speaking traditionally holds some kind of talisman (which can be any object, sometimes silly). And when a person is speaking, it's understood they have the floor; the rest listen without interrupting.[28]

Since 1995, the group has grown significantly and successfully struggled to remain true to its original mission of providing a sense of community to rural men. Between 80 and 200 men attend the five annual rural gatherings that the group organizes; weekends include workshops on massage, intimacy among men, art therapy, and "being a warrior without having to be patriarchal."[29] A recent issue of *The Billy Times* discussed the July Fourth weekend gathering, requested submissions for the upcoming *Billy Journal,* and offered a report from the "Task Force on Community and Structure."[30] In the course of a year, thousands of men from throughout Northern California attend one of the Billy events and forge community with other rural gay men.

HIV-POSITIVE GAY MEN:
POSTCRISIS, AWAITING CRISIS, AND IN CRISIS

Articles in gay newspapers and discussions among gay men sometimes discuss shifts caused by combination therapies as a "new birth" for gay communities and, at other times, declare them largely overrated.[31] While usually careful to express caution and to qualify hopeful statements with clauses like "for as long as it lasts," or "if these treatments are able to keep people healthy for a long period of time," in some sectors, community discussion appears eager to declare the epidemic over and bring the troops home. Alternately, letters to the editor, editorials, and feature stories appear that, while cautious not to squelch all hope, insist these treatments should not be mistaken for the cure. Combination therapies and protease inhibitors have profoundly shaken the precarious foundation of community life and tossed many things up in the air. At this point in time many of us bounce back and fall between optimism, pessimism, and boredom with the whole thing. Omitted from the entire discussion are ways in which ongoing advances against opportunistic infections and wasting syndrome are also affecting people with HIV in diverse ways.

For at least a decade, few have wanted to face the way that AIDS has fragmented and caused divisions among gay men. We hear grumbling about splits between HIV-positive and HIV-negative men, but many have embraced a romanticized version of disaster response that insists lesbians, gay men, and bisexuals have "pulled together" to face the challenge of AIDS and, through years of caregiving and funerals, finally forged authentic community for ourselves. This same narrative insists pre-AIDS divisions between lesbians and gay men have been healed, and fears of fragmentation discussed early in the epidemic were simply the paranoid cries of Chicken Littles anticipating the worst.

When divisiveness within gay communities is referenced, most people immediately think of divisions based on antibody status, assuming that the epidemic has funneled gay men into two separate social worlds, one for the infected and the other for the uninfected. I recently observed a meeting convened at a local gay church intended to uncover issues needing to be resolved between HIV-positive and HIV-negative gay men. Almost thirty gay men gathered in a small room and shared perspectives on life in the epidemic. Even among these men who participated in the same church, significant issues and experiences caused divisions. Anger flared from one uninfected man who had long felt positive men stereotyped and held unfair assumptions about uninfected gay men. Some positive men shared their continuing experiences of being rejected in the dating arena by uninfected men unwilling to partner with HIV-positive men. While many men shared a long-term confrontation with issues of loss, grief, and

death, living with HIV in one's bloodstream produced an experience quite different from that of uninfected men.

I came away from the evening with a few surprising realizations.
While many of the men in the room were in their late thirties,
forties, and fifties, a few of the men in their twenties and early
thirties articulated a profoundly different experience of the epidemic than one might assume could be held by a gay man in San
Francisco's Castro district. One man talked of knowing no one who
has died from AIDS and having only one friend who was HIV
positive. A young man who had recently moved to the area from the
rural Midwest shared his own curiosity about the epidemic, as well
as his feelings of embarrassment at his limited experiences, though
he's been an openly gay man involved in community for more than
a decade. Generational differences loomed as one of the major
divisions within this gay community.

Long-term unaddressed conflicts within gay men's communities
may be seriously exacerbated by post-AIDS discussions, just as new
splits may be emerging. Nowhere is this more apparent than in the
fragmentation occurring among HIV-positive gay men. Ironically,
many see HIV-positive people as the embodiment of the end of
AIDS, rescued from death by the new treatments. Yet people with
HIV may be the primary gay male population still inhabiting a space
of crisis. Some live precariously day-to-day, praying that successful
experiences on the new treatments continue. Others find the treatments fail them, or produce significant side effects that reduce quality of life. All men who are "doing well" on protease inhibitors are
not "doing well" at the same level and in the same ways.

Changes occurring during the Protease Moment have presented
new challenges to many people with HIV and introduced other
divisions that are not easily healed.[32] These rifts include:

Divisions based on the efficacy of new treatments. Combination
therapies and protease inhibitors do not work effectively for all people
with HIV. Some gay men on protease inhibitors are unable to tolerate
them or do not show improved health.[33] This has created tension among
people with HIV: those for whom combination therapies do not work
may feel as if the parade is passing them by. One gay man told me that
his mother, on hearing he could not tolerate any of the protease

inhibitors, chided, "That's just great! All my friends think the epidemic's ending, and once again you've gotta find a way to be different!"

Divisions based on financial resources. While many people with HIV are able to cover the costs of treatments through medical insurance, drug assistance programs, public benefits programs, or out-of-pocket expenditures, many poor and working-class gay men living in areas that do not offer adequate financial assistance are not able to afford combination therapies. A long-unacknowledged split among gay men based on economic class has deepened at a critically important moment. The anger some poor men with HIV feel about this disparity becomes exacerbated by cultural messages insisting, "AIDS is over for all but you tragic poor people."

Divisions based on ability to comply with treatments. Current protocols for the new treatments frequently involve taking large numbers of pills at precise times during the day. While this might change as new drugs emerge from the research pipeline, failure to comply with the current recommended schedule and dosage can have detrimental effects on one's health and on future possibilities for treatment. The complicated regimens of pill-taking assume people live stable lives that help them remember which pills to take at which times. Men of all classes, including middle-class men considered "stable," have found themselves unable to remember to take their medications or comply with certain requirements accompanying the treatments. One man in this situation told me, "These treatments are simply creating a new way to divide people with HIV into 'good people with HIV' and 'bad people with HIV.' I'm one of the baddies because I screwed up my regimen and killed my chances for participating in what many people are seeing as the cure."

Divisions based on willingness to take these treatments. Many believe combination therapies are so successful that all people with HIV are eagerly trying to get these medications. Yet some infected people are not scrambling to take protease inhibitors or combination therapies. Many of these people do not support Western medical treatments and are skeptical of the long-term impact of such medications on their health. When AZT was invested with the community's greatest hopes a few years ago, many people refused to jump on the bandwagon and had their views confirmed just a few years later. One friend who is HIV positive yet has high T-cells and no detectable viral load is asked at least weekly whether he is on protease inhibitors. He has occasionally been told he is "foolish" or "crazy" for rejecting the miracle treatments.

Perhaps no group of homosexual men in America is as deeply conflicted about creating post-AIDS identities and cultures as HIV-positive men who are responding positively to protease inhibitors. A cursory read through the pages of popular magazines leaves the impression that life for gay men on protease inhibitors is a series of celebrations and parties. In reality, these men often face an enormous psychological challenge that has been simplistically reduced in many media accounts.

On one level, men on combination therapies often *are* doing fine. If they have been fortunate enough to experience a diminution of viral load, increased T-cells, and revitalized energy, most men superficially appear hopeful and eager to reengage with life. Because the pool of people in this category tends to be those who have not been heavily treated with other medications and who are able to comply with drug regimens, it should surprise no one that many of them are beginning to regain gusto for living.[34] Many of the gay men who are responding well to the new treatments fit the profile depicted in much of the media coverage: they are leaving public assistance, returning to work, and rethinking life goals and career options.

Dig a bit deeper, however, and it is easy to discover a more complex side of these protease babies. Many of the gay men who experience revitalized health also confront serious, sometimes acute, depression. At first, this sounds ridiculous: men snatched from the jaws of death should be exhilarated at their newfound vitality and lengthened life expectancy. Yet protease inhibitors have shaken these men's worldviews profoundly. After spending years adjusting to being HIV positive and struggling to create meaning from that experience, all of a sudden they are presented with a radically different task. Some had found themselves proceeding through Elizabeth Kübler-Ross's stages of coming to terms with dying, only to be rescued at the last minute and yanked out of the entire process.

I spoke with one man who expressed this dilemma in an articulate and moving manner. Joe is forty-four years old, a former civil service office worker, and had been HIV positive for almost a dozen years. He has responded rapidly and powerfully to combination therapies and first experienced his improved health as exhilarating and liberating. "Then I found myself isolating, turning inward, avoiding social situations," he told me. "It was a month before I realized I was exhibiting all the signs of depression—I'd stop eating for days, slept a lot, and found myself moping around the apartment. Finally, my doctor suggested I go and get some counseling."

It was through counseling that Joe came to terms with the depression he was facing:

> At first I felt embarrassed, even in front of the shrink! Here I was, one of the lucky ones who has survived the past decade, at the dawn of an era of optimism. Yet I was feeling bummed out instead of joyous. By talking to my therapist, I realized a lot was going on for me. I was having a lot of difficulty shifting the horizon of my expectations. While I was experiencing improved health, I was fighting it at the same time. I realized I was having a tough time trusting that these changes could last a while. In a way, I kept waiting for the other shoe to drop, I expected the AIDS symptoms to return. It was hard to trust that the protease's effects could last for a while. In a way, I was asking myself to get on that highway of hope I'd been on before and I was afraid to do it . . . afraid I'd make a fool of myself by believing it could ever be over.[35]

Depression is not the only challenge facing these men. Many wrestle with boredom. When they were ill, their lives narrowed greatly and they had fewer friends, social contacts, and activities. Their daily routines had been scaled back to simple activities like errands or picking up the mail. All of a sudden, with energy levels booming, many face a new set of problems. One man told me that boredom is the largest challenge he now faces. "Before combination therapies, I was lucky to do two or three things in a single day," he recalled. "Now I do two or three things after breakfast and have nothing to do for the rest of the day except watch game shows on television. I'm just scared to create a new life for myself—scared that I'll create a new life only to have it snatched out of my hands before I can enjoy it."

Considering returning to work is a powerful dilemma for many men.[36] Before protease inhibitors, they often discussed former jobs longingly; now a range of very real concerns about work confronts them: Will the energy last long enough to get through a work day? Is the former job the best way to expend my energies? Will I be able to maintain my benefits if I return to work? What happens if I take the risk to return, become ill again, and find myself without the benefits I enjoy now?

It surprised me to talk with men responding well to protease inhibitors who seethe with anger. Ricardo, a thirty-eight-year-old artist, told me, "I'm mad at a system that let so many of my friends die while the solution was right under their noses," he said. "And I find myself mad at hope, for tempting me again to imagine a life and a future that, I know, could be snatched away from me again at any time. I know I'm supposed to be grateful at these medical miracles—and I am—but I'm also furious at how this epidemic was allowed to happen."

A range of other issues are emerging as HIV-positive men respond to the new therapies:

Credit card nightmares. Many men ran up huge credit card bills when they thought they wouldn't live long enough to worry about paying them off. Other debt also may have accumulated as immediate gratification or pressing medical needs took precedent over prudent fiscal planning. The revived health associated with combination therapies forces some people with HIV to come eye-to-eye with their spending patterns. One man with HIV I interviewed used five credit cards to their limits and now realizes, if he returns to work, his efforts will largely go into paying off debt.

Confronting the reality of a relationship. Some HIV-positive men remained in less-than-satisfying relationships while they dealt with critical health problems against a backdrop of a short life expectancy. For some male couples, the restored health associated with protease inhibitors is a time of great joy as couples are able to engage in long-range planning for the first time. Some infected men, however, on experiencing renewed health, make the decision to leave their lovers and seek more satisfying relationships. As one man told me, "I feel a bit like a heel leaving him because, had I gotten sick and unable to care for myself, he would have taken great care of me. But now I am not going to die anytime soon and I no longer need a caregiver. What I want is romance and sex and he really doesn't offer me either."

Substance use relapse. Many gay male alcoholics and addicts experience their sobriety as fragile, something that might be easily upset or undermined by changes in the circumstances of their lives. Recent shifts in the epidemic's trajectory may have contributed to some men's resumption of substance abuse. Infected men who are responding well to the new treatments, those who are not responding well, and uninfected men who are entrenched in gay cultures may all find themselves at risk for relapse. Several gay-focused alcoholism and drug abuse treatment programs throughout the nation noted an upswing in demands for services during 1996, perhaps reflecting the ways powerful cultural shifts affect men's ability to stay clean and sober.[37]

Changing relationships with HIV-negative men. As combination therapies change what it means to be HIV-positive, the status of HIV-negative men shifts as well, sometimes in unpredictable and surprising ways. One positive man told me, "I feel like uninfected men treat me as less of a pariah now. All of a sudden the gap between us isn't as large as it used to be. I guess dating a positive man doesn't have to mean you're signing up for inevitable loss anymore." An HIV-negative gay man who is in a long-term relationship with an HIV-positive man saw things a bit differently. "I feel much more comfortable asserting my own needs," he told me. "Before I felt my lover should have his way when we got into disputes about important items. It was like, so he wants to live in the suburbs, I can do that for a few years. He'll be dead soon anyway, then I can do what I want.

Now that he's so much better healthwise and that his prognosis is so good, I feel quite comfortable asserting my own needs."

Reentering the sexual marketplace. Many infected men who'd gotten sick or lost energy withdrew from the bars, dance clubs, and sexualized sites of gay community life. As one forty-two-year-old told me, "I had neither the energy nor the looks that I once had and going cruising just became incredibly painful to me. I had to make a change." Yet this same man has regained his health, gained weight, and lost the pale demeanor that had come over him a few years earlier. He's returned to swimming and aerobic classes, and has begun to frequent gay bars again. He faces a range of unexpected issues: "First of all, I'm no longer in my early thirties. Now I'm middle aged; that is itself an incredible challenge. Also I find that I've lost that protective defensive covering I'd built up over the years that allowed me to survive in this kind of scene without getting my feelings hurt. Now I find, when guys treat me badly or simply reject me, that my feelings get hurt easily. I'm more vulnerable to the games and the attitude that many gay men give off."

The challenges facing HIV-positive men who are on the new treatments are major factors contributing to many men's continuing personal experience of HIV disease as a precarious, frightening condition. This leaves HIV-positive gay men as a population with many different contemporary experiences and understandings of AIDS. Some infected men, particularly those who have been infected for a long time and have developed no illnesses and maintain high T-cell counts and low viral loads, may have shifted into post-AIDS living. This experience might be shared by many who are having successful experiences on the new treatments and exhibiting no side effects. Other infected men may be in a state of crisis-anticipation, walking on eggshells because of side effects caused by the new drugs, declining health, or the anxiety that accompanies uncertainty. And many infected men may remain solidly locked in crisis, as they find themselves failing at treatments yet again, only this time they are failing what many understand as the "miracle cure."

Five years ago, the experience of people with HIV was understood to fall within a narrow range of possibilities. While some became sick quicker than others, many people believed it likely that HIV-infected people would succumb to AIDS. This encouraged a spiritual unity among people with HIV that allowed differences to be overlooked and divisions to go unaddressed. AIDS organizations often benefited greatly from this enforced unity.

The Protease Moment has changed all of this. If all gay men with HIV continued to experience AIDS as a personal crisis, it would be difficult for uninfected men's post-AIDS understandings to dominate community discourse. Because HIV-positive men are having disparate experiences—some remaining in crisis, others on the brink of crisis, many moving beyond crisis—it will be increasingly difficult to rein in forces driving the communal mindset of gay communities in a post-AIDS direction.

SCRUTINIZING SPACE ALIENS

Hence many gay men inhabiting gay communities throughout the nation no longer experience AIDS as a crisis except in the narrowest sense, as a political call-to-arms in order to garner energy and resources for continuing efforts against the epidemic. We increasingly inhabit post-AIDS social and cultural worlds and psychologically and emotionally adjust to lives that include AIDS as a continuing material reality. We are vacating the bomb shelters some of us have crouched in for fifteen years. While some AIDS workers interpret this shift as a problem and offer numerous pathologizing explanations, an alternative possibility exists that problematizes the mind-set of AIDS leadership rather than the rank and file gay male population.

Throughout the epidemic, gay men have been told our reactions to the rapidly changing realities in our individual lives and collective cultures are misguided, inappropriate, or examples of "false consciousness." We were told condoms were fun, when most gay men experienced them otherwise. We were told we were responding beautifully to the challenges of the epidemic, when we knew we were tearing at each other's throats. We were told being uninfected meant we were doing just fine—and we even repeated this over and over to each other—when we could barely keep our guts from spilling out as we read the obituary pages.

Where were we getting these messages that made us discount or question our authentic experiences of our bodies, subjectivities, and social practices? The leadership of AIDS and gay organizations, as well as countless gay male doctors, psychologists, counselors, authors, editors, journalists, activists, and prevention workers, have functioned as a collective community-based brain trust. This brain trust generated understandings of "the gay experience of AIDS" that have been reproduced at political demonstrations, in gay newspapers, and through the formal organizational life of our communities. This brain trust has *not* functioned as a conspiracy, nefariously manipulating gay men and profiting from their suffering. Indeed the brain trusts and our communities coconstitute themselves in a dialectical cultural process. They are we; we are they. This wasn't about who was doing what to whom. It was about what we were all doing together.

Alienation has emerged in the form of an ever-increasing gap between that brain trust and the rank and file of gay male communities throughout the nation. A disagreement over how the epidemic "should" be experienced, conceptualized, and represented has flared that, in the late 1990s, may be responsible for widespread disenchantment gay men feel toward the leadership of the community. Driven by highly politicized funding processes, and often addicted to the drama and terror of the event of AIDS as conceived in the 1980s, the leadership of some AIDS and gay organizations seems unable to seriously consider creating cultures and putting forward understandings of AIDS that let go of the crisis construct.

Gay men now live on two different planets. One is occupied by those who continue to experience AIDS as an ongoing emergency demanding continuing hypervigilance. Occupants of this planet are primarily those people with HIV who are experiencing powerful fears and anxieties about their health. They are joined by many staff members and volunteers of AIDS organizations. The other planet is populated by gay men who have integrated AIDS into their everyday lives and gotten on with the business of living. While there is significant traffic between these two worlds and some men migrate from one planet to the other and set down roots, current community debates appearing in the gay press clearly assign raconteurs to one of these two planets.

We gaze at each other across the distance as if we are scrutinizing space aliens. Citizens of Planet Crisis look at men who have stopped volunteering in AIDS groups or started to attend sex clubs or get fucked without condoms as insane maniacs out of touch with reality. They explain the paltry turnout at political demonstrations as a product of "AIDS burnout" and the drop off in participation at AIDS walks as caused by men's denial-based belief that the epidemic is over. Citizens of Planet Post-AIDS hear leaders demanding that sex clubs and bathhouses be regulated or closed as deranged, moralistic crusaders, filled with self-loathing. They scoff at writers proposing monogamy as a central tenet of gay male community life, trashing them as deeply disconnected from contemporary gay men, and consider institutionalized AIDS organizations to be self-perpetuating death cults populated by burnt-out automatons.

Welcome to the interplanetary wars of the 1990s! Gay men creating post-AIDS identities and cultures may experience intense judgments from community leaders and institutions because our perspectives have diverged greatly. The massive attack on AIDS organizations launched by some activists, journalists, and people with AIDS who depict the groups as bloated bureaucracies useful to no one may be attributed partly to this disaffection. The sniping at symbols of AIDS vigilance created by the community in the 1980s such as the AIDS Quilt or red ribbons is another manifestation of the dissidence. Perhaps most troublesome is the widespread alienation from gay male spaces, cultures, and communities cited repeatedly by gay men in their teens and twenties.

However unpleasant and disruptive the trashing, sniping, and alienation might be, they indicate that the rank and file of gay male communities is largely unwilling to remain locked in a state of emergency as we approach the third decade of AIDS. The resistance to leadership suggests a growing maturation in our communities and a burgeoning movement of gay men intent on reclaiming and redirecting the brain trusts toward a wider, more diverse agenda that considers AIDS one among several important concerns facing gay men as a class. Post-AIDS movements are demanding an expanded understanding of gay men's health incorporating not only a wider spectrum of threats faced by gay men (other sexually transmitted diseases, addictions, violence, and mental health issues) but also attention and resources directed toward our social, cultural, and spiritual lives as we rebuild existing communities and invent new ones.

Why is it important to note that significant portions of contemporary gay men do not experience AIDS as a terrible crisis befalling their communities? At least three key reasons make it important to achieve this recognition at a community level: (1) Most of our efforts to encourage gay men to contribute time and money to AIDS groups are presented utilizing the crisis construct; diminished success in these areas may, in part, be attributed to a mismatch between audience and message; (2) Our work with gay men's sexual practices and cultures usually assumes a foundational belief that we remain locked in a state of emergency; we might improve our effectiveness in this work if we meet men where they actually are, rather than where some want them to be; (3) Gay men's authentic understandings of AIDS in the late 1990s are being ignored and largely unaddressed by our community organizations; because most organizations have not shifted with the times, they are unable to meet the current needs of gay men of all antibody statuses.

My efforts to demonstrate that large portions of gay communities have abandoned the bomb shelter and stepped onto terra firma are aimed at transforming the foundation from which we consider gay men in relationship to HIV/AIDS. By realizing most gay men are no longer overwhelmed, terrorized, stunned, or terribly disheartened by AIDS, our work with gay men on a broad range of meaningful issues may be greatly enhanced. This can be done in ways that strengthen efforts to support people with HIV, and make prevention work more effective with gay men.

SECTION II:
SEX AFTER CRISIS

Though we never thought that we could lose, there's no regret.
If I had to do the same again, I would . . .

—Abba, "Fernando"

Have you noticed that people are still having sex?
All the denouncement has absolutely no effect.

—La Tour, "People Are Still Having Sex"

Chapter 5

Don't Fuck with Gay Culture

This is a test. It is only a test. Which statement was made in 1978 by Anita Bryant, and which was made by Larry Kramer in an essay published in 1997?[1]

- "It is an indisputable fact that the homosexual lifestyle is incapable of reproduction and doomed to certain extinction. In a real sense, it is not a lifestyle but a 'death-style'."

- "We've all been partners in our destruction. AIDS has killed us, and while we certainly did not invite it in, we certainly did invite it in. We still invite it in. . . . We have been the cause of our own victimization."

One of these statements appeared in Dr. Timothy LaHaye's *The Unhappy Gays* in 1978, and one appeared in Michelangelo Signorile's 1997 book, *Life Outside*:[2]

- "It is impossible for a straight person to imagine the preoccupation with sex that obsesses many young homosexuals. In fact, they are regularly disinterested in gainful employment— their interest is sex, not work."

- "It is my hope . . . that many gay men within the culture of narcissism and hedonism that envelops much of the gay world will follow in the footsteps of a great many others, gay men who have discovered a more rewarding, fuller, and richer life, outside."

Which statement was made by Anita Bryant and which is part of a collective manifesto signed by 125 therapists, substance abuse counselors, and HIV prevention leaders—primarily lesbians and gay men—in San Francisco in 1997?[3]

- "The homosexual is promiscuous and his attachments fleeting. He is always cruising, looking for fresh young partners. . . . Youth and good looks are the *sine qua non* of the homosexual . . ."

- "Gay male culture appears to place value on youth and physical perfection above most other aspects of a man's personal characteristics. . . . Gay culture is also marked by a reverence for youth."

Which of these quotations were written by antigay crusaders in the 1970s and which were written by gay male writers during the late 1990s?

- "Nature always extracts a price for sexual promiscuity."[4]

- "Serious consequences to health, resulting from a promiscuous homosexual lifestyle, bear testimony to the inviolability of biological laws."[5]

- "We have made sex the cornerstone of gay liberation and gay culture, and it has killed us."[6]

- "As one indulges in homosexuality, God warns, he receives in his own person the due penalty of his error. The Bible teaches that there is physical as well as psychological deterioration in the man or woman who violates the sexual boundaries God has set up. Homosexuality will destroy the whole person."[7]

- "There is an overriding, mostly white, youth-focused, and often drug-fueled social and sexual gay male scene that is highly commercialized and demands conformity to a very specific body ideal."[8]

- "The quest for the 'fountain of youth' is all but universal . . . but with the homosexual, youth is an obsession. Their entire life style is based on physical attraction."[9]

- "Gay liberation has unleashed what seems to be an endless epidemic that swallows up its own . . ."[10]

- "Under the banner of democratic freedoms, they push against the boundaries of biological reality itself."[11]

- "Ultimately to understand sexual ecology is to understand that the gay sexual revolution of the seventies was profoundly anti-ecological."[12]

The answers to this test are in the notes at the end of this book. The answers to the problems emerging from a dynamic in which statements made by contemporary gay writers sound increasingly like the statements of antigay crusaders are the focus of this chapter.

SPRINGTIME IN SAN FRANCISCO

The month of May 1997 brought spring to San Francisco, balmy evenings that send people in my neighborhood out to Castro Street at 10 p.m. looking for ice cream or onto their front porches, looking for company. Ten months after the Protease Moment dawned, shook our lives, and made us realize our communal worlds were changing, we survived a different kind of onslaught. Thanks to Ellen DeGeneres staring us down with that "Yep, I'm gay" grin from the cover of *Time,* we endured an intense period of public obsession with homosexuality. Allen Ginsberg may have died, gay men might continue to become infected with HIV, state after state might be banning gay marriage, but we'd passed gay rights legislation in two more states, New Hampshire and Maine, the President of the United States was speaking out against antigay hate crimes, and 80,000 lesbians and gay men had just converged on Orlando, Florida, for the annual unofficial Gay Day at Disney World. In San Francisco, the 49ers football team was crowding into our bars nightly, attempting to kiss gay butt in order to win votes for a special election in early June that would approve public funds to build a new stadium.

My mind was obsessed with the realization that we were approaching the twentieth anniversary of Anita Bryant's antigay "Save Our Children" campaign in Dade County, Florida.[13] This was one of the seminal politicizing events of my early activist life. It occurred as I was working outside Boston as a closeted gay schoolteacher, spending evenings as a gay activist and writing pseudonymous articles for *Gay Community News,* the only weekly gay newspaper in the nation. Bryant's linkage of homosexuality with child endangerment broke through what remained of my closet door and catapulted me into the political arena. Driving home from work while listening to the radio after a challenging day with sixth graders, I learned that voters had followed Bryant's lead and voted to revoke the civil rights of people like me. I was overcome with hurt and fury. I remember pulling my car over on a busy street, hands trembling as I unsuccessfully tried to avoid bursting into tears.

That event solidified my politicization, buttressed over the next two years by other cities' revoking civil rights for lesbians and gay men (St. Paul, Seattle, Wichita) and then by the murder of Harvey Milk in San Francisco. Is it any wonder men and women of my gay generation appear inordinately utopian and impractical to many younger queers? Those of us out and organizing in the 1970s were championing a cause that was both wildly unpopular and seen as shameful and shocking, even among most liberals and Leftists, and we've seen the world change in our lifetimes.

To this day I feel a special affection for surviving activists from the 1970s. I look back and realize that while our political views may have diverged over the years and many of us have been embroiled in public controversy, I feel linked to these colleagues in ways I rarely feel connected to contemporary cronies in activism. We were participating in the movement at an especially risky time. I remember how lonely it felt being a public queer in the 1970s and how wonderful it was to discover others willing to put themselves on the line for a controversial cause. One gift I received from my years in gay liberation was a profound, almost indiscriminate, love for other queer activists.

It's this deep and abiding affection for queers of all kinds that I bring to my critiques of our lives in community and the cultures we've forged over the past twenty-five years. I also carry with me some hard-earned patience, garnered through countless heartaches and disappointments in our pre-AIDS lesbian and gay organizing. During the 1970s, activists more seasoned than I succeeded in drumming into my head one thing: being a political activist meant laboring in the trenches for the long haul. We might lose in Dade County, but we'd win big just a year later, when we beat back the first statewide antigay effort, the Briggs Initiative in California, which targeted any teacher who supported gay issues. We might be horrified at Harvey Milk's assassination, but we'd be joyous less than a year later when we saw the turnout for the first March on Washington for Lesbian and Gay Rights. Social change wasn't a win-or-lose game at the blackjack table; it was a jig of sorts, steps forward and a few steps back, and none of us should expect the music to stop for a long time.

These twin feelings, the knowledge that all of us concerned with social justice must be in the movement for our lifetimes, along with my long-standing bond with other activists, make me recoil at the current attacks on so-called gay male culture coming from movement colleagues. On the one hand, I value anyone who cares enough about gay people to critique our communities, cultures, and everyday social practices. Even during this time when the mainstream seems obsessed with things gay, few social critics spend time thinking critically about the post-Stonewall identities and cultures forged by queers during the turmoil of the past three decades. While I do not share in what at times feels like a burgeoning consensus in much of the media that gay male culture is sordid, immature, and self-destructive, I do not see these critics as "the enemy." I resist the easy turn that reduces them to self-hating, antisex crusaders, mindlessly targeting our vulnerable sex cultures. At least they care.

On the other hand, I'm struck by the realization that precisely twenty years after Anita Bryant painted a portrait of gay men as sick, sex-crazed, youth-obsessed perverts, who, after turning San Francisco into Sodom by the Bay, were preparing to make Miami into Gomorrah by the 'Glades, gay men themselves are putting forth a portrait of a unitary gay male culture that more than matches her bile. After reading the spate of writing emanating from New York City this season—books by Michelangelo Signorile and Gabriel Rotello, and essays by Larry Kramer—I found myself wondering what's happened to the social worlds of queer men in that metropolis that incites a phalanx of gay white men to reduce our vibrant, multifaceted urban communities to a singular gay culture and then vilify it?[14]

Michael Bronski has critiqued the artificial construct of a singular "gay community":

In recent years—as issues of gay culture and politics have become more a staple of the mainstream press—it is fashionable to declare the existence of a single, cohesive, and unified gay viewpoint. It is not unusual to read in, say *The New York Times*, or *Newsweek*, phrases like "most people in the gay community think . . . " or "is generally believed to have the support of the gay community." Such extravagantly staked claims are patently false. Anyone who has identified with and participated in the "gay community" knows that the very concept of a single-minded and consolidated community is so far from reality as to be, depending upon one's frame of mind, either a myth or a joke.[15]

These overlapping critiques of "gay culture" by Signorile, Rotello, and Kramer make one wonder whether the New York Lesbian and Gay Community Services Center, a beacon of organizing energy filled any night of the week with material evidence that a multitude of gay male (and lesbian, and bisexual, and transgender, and queer . . .) cultures coexist, hasn't become an homogenized mass of twenty-five-year-old muscle boys on ecstasy. If, as these writings suggest, one can collectivize the diverse social worlds that homosexual men inhabit in 1998 as a singular "gay culture," how do New Yorkers as diverse as Paul Rudnick, RuPaul, Moises Agosto, Tom Duane, Antonio Pagan, Martin Duberman, and Harvey Fierstein fit in this tight envelope?

As communities of epicenter gay men emerge from the most intense period of the AIDS epidemic, many are wiping their eyes, surveying the landscape, and offering suggestions for ways of reinventing community and culture. The first part of this chapter will focus largely on Michelangelo Signorile's and Larry Kramer's analyses of "gay male culture" (I discuss Gabriel Rotello's book in the following chapter). I use these men's work to illustrate what occurs when critiques are generated from worldviews locked inside the AIDS state of emergency and epidemiological reports that are scrutinized through the crisis-tinged lenses of 1985. When cultural observers consider the social and sexual practices of contemporary gay men from a vantage point that believes the epidemic is escalating among gay men, they are likely to believe their appropriate role is to exhort men to return to a crisis mind-set.

Next I scrutinize a parallel critique of contemporary "gay community" drafted by therapists, substance abuse counselors, and AIDS prevention workers in San Francisco and published as a centerspread essay in a local gay paper. I argue that, while the language and framing of this piece is steeped in California New Age culture, this manifesto of sorts might best be understood as a West Coast version of the Signorile/Rotello/Kramer analysis. I analyze it in an effort to understand what might be motivating men from both coasts to put forward a unitary concept of gay culture and then describe it narrowly as destructive, sex-obsessed, and intensely self-centered.

Finally, I suggest that the harsh view of gay men illustrated by these essays that has settled over gay communities in the late 1990s can be understood in three critical ways that might not be immediately apparent. First, it can be seen as part of the failure of gay men as a class to come to terms with the AIDS epidemic, a precondition for entering post-AIDS life. Here I consider coming to terms with the AIDS epidemic, not in the way Larry Kramer suggests ("We must stop murdering each other"),[16] but in a manner by which we truly face history and ourselves, and come to understand gay men as neither heroes-without-precedent nor villains-without-comparison, but as ordinary humans confronting a catastrophic event and getting on with their lives.

How do we measure the success or failure of HIV prevention? If we use what appears to be the common standard driving most HIV-education programs, we view each new infection of a gay man as evidence of failure and proclaim there is an expansion of the epidemic. While literally true in terms of aggregate numbers of infected gay men, this kind of evaluation is inappropriate for use with communicable diseases that require long-term, sustained approaches and achievable goals. To mistake the utopian rhetoric that we could end AIDS tomorrow if everyone practiced safe sex 100 percent of the time for appropriate public health strategy is terribly misguided. Instead, I believe the way to assess our prevention efforts is by examining the level of seroprevalance within successive generations of gay men. A realistic aim might be that each successive cohort of gay men in a particular location show a specific decline in level of infection. This means instead of expecting to eliminate AIDS by the year 2000, for example, we aim for gay men who come of age in 2030 in epicenter cities to experience an HIV infection rate of under 20 percent.[17]

Rather than a crisis-driven, drama-queen exaggeration of continuing HIV infection among gay men, coming to terms with the AIDS epidemic means confronting the authentic reality we face: outside New York, San Francisco, and a handful of other cities, gay men in the United States have succeeded for the most part in keeping the rate of seroprevalance to 25 percent or less in almost every city—and below 20 percent in cities such as Boston, Detroit, Baltimore, and Seattle.[18] We are succeeding in bringing about the gradual diminution of HIV among successive cohorts of gay men. Other than hemophiliacs, no HIV-affected population can claim this achievement. Yet our community leadership repeatedly uses statistics from Chelsea and the Castro—statistical outliers in the research on HIV among gay men—to circulate wild claims such as "Fifty percent of all young gay men will be infected before they are forty years old."

Second, I believe this narrow portrayal of gay men has emerged, in part, in response to earlier narratives constructed during the intensity of 1980s AIDS organizing, which produced images of gay men as angels of mercy, valiantly caring for their own and putting aside errant sexual urges once the alarm had been sounded. By adopting a representation of communal response to the epidemic that reduced complex intracommunity dynamics to red-ribbon hype, we unwittingly set the stage for a countervailing image to emerge powerfully just a decade later.

Third, I argue that much of the vocal criticism of muscle boy culture is being put forth in articles, op-ed pieces, and letters to the editor in the gay press by men who are approaching or who have entered middle age. I remind the reader that members of a generation of gay men who were in their twenties and thirties in the 1970s and early 1980s are now in their forties, fifties, and sixties. Many of these men seem intensely focused on gay men in their twenties and thirties. I argue that a generation gap has emerged and a clash is occurring—baby boomers against generation Xers. Rather than address their own misgivings about aging, ageism, and the gay sexual cultures they inhabited in the 1970s and 1980s, some men may be transferring a powder keg of fears, disappointments, guilt, and rage onto young gay men and their emerging post-AIDS cultures.

I do not know or care about the personal lives and erotic tastes of those who intensely criticize the circuit scene. I'm less concerned with the individuals and more with what this trend says about midlife gay men as a collective group. If the authors and energetic letter writers situated themselves firmly in relationship to the circuit culture and illustrated the diversity of identities invented and social practices performed, I would be hesitant to make these criticisms of their analysis. Yet by standing at a distance from the parties, sex clubs, and gyms (as most do) and putting forth analyses that foreground the most extreme members of this gay male subculture and use them to revile an entire tribe of men who populate these sites, these writers replicate an increasingly popular journalistic practice of creating larger-than-life villains out of complex and marginalized populations.

Whether creating cultural bugaboos out of Mexican immigrants or unmarried black mothers or white muscle boys, social critics frequently project a range of cultural anxieties most appropriately attached to a broad population, onto one narrow group. This is a dangerous practice that must be called by its proper name: scapegoating.

SEEING DICK, DICK, AND ONLY DICK: LARRY KRAMER'S "SEX AND SENSIBILITY"

A graphically unassuming commentary by Larry Kramer appeared in the pages of *The Advocate* in May 1997, and set tongues wagging in the coffeehouses I inhabit. Titled "Sex and Sensibility," the piece seems to be a response to three recent events the author found meaningful: (1) the publication of Gabriel Rotello's book *Sexual Ecology: AIDS and the Destiny of Gay Men* (a "terribly important" volume, to Kramer); (2) the appearance of the soon-to-be-published Edmund White novel *The Farewell Symphony* (which Kramer considers "boring" and "irresponsible" because it "parades before the reader every trick [White's] ever sucked, fucked, rimmed, tied up,

pissed on, or been sucked by, fucked by, rimmed by, tied up by . . . ");
(3) the rejection by Yale University's provost of Kramer's offer to
leave the school his apparently substantial estate to endow profes-
sorships in gay studies or fund a gay student center.[19]

These events are worth examining closely and Kramer responds
to each with great alacrity. First he passionately discusses the way
he believes sex is positioned in "gay culture." He reads Rotello's
book as an "undeniable" argument "that we brought AIDS upon
ourselves by a way of living that welcomed it" and faults "almost
every other gay writer—as well as journalists, essayists, poets,
playwrights, painters, photographers, filmmakers" for refusing to
"tell the truth" to gay men who don't want to hear it: "We must
create a new culture that is not confined and centered so tragically
on our obsession with our penises and what we do with them."[20]

Kramer then turns to Edmund White's new novel, which he cites
as an example of the "literature of sex . . . the soft porn of all our
novels and short stories that traffic only or mostly in sex." He
attacks gay writers for what he sees as their limited literary focus:
"Tricks, bushes, S/M, discos, drugs, bathhouses, Fire Island, phone
sex, meat racks." Kramer asks, "Is this all we are capable of writing about or our audience capable of reading?"[21] He wonders why
the scope of gay writing is so narrow and puerile and hungers for a
gay fiction that decenters sex and embraces broader goals:

> Why don't we write about our oppressors and our friends
> and our businesses and our families and our greed and our
> hopes and our crimes and our politics—in other words, our
> real lives? One thing our writers are not teaching us about is
> love. How to love another gay. How to love ourselves. Or
> respect. How to respect each other and ourselves.[22]

The central argument of the first half of the essay is that gay
culture is intensely and narrowly focused on sex, and that this
obsession is responsible for the horror show of AIDS and the continuing toll it takes on our communities:

> After all our history, after all these deaths, we still don't
> have an AIDS literature, and we don't have a gay literature. We
> don't have a gay culture, I don't believe. We have our sexuality,

and we have made a culture out of our sexuality, and that culture has killed us. I want to say this again: We have made sex the cornerstone of gay liberation and gay culture, and it has killed us.[23]

Much of the current wave of criticism of gay male culture has emerged from gay men who have been challenged as inconsistent. After years of enjoying—even exploiting—gay men's sex cultures, as these men approach or settle into midlife, they suddenly announce that they've discovered these circles are "self-centered," "destructive," or "dead ends." Perhaps some of these critics were always on the outside looking in, never committed to what the liberation of the body means, and are only able to articulate their viewpoints during the post-AIDS period.

Yet Larry Kramer, in the late 1990s, may be celebrated for his constancy: he's been haranguing us about our sexual practices since he first entered the queer public sphere in the late 1970s. One can alternately see Kramer as a visionary social critic who predicted the demise of gay culture even before the arrival of the epidemic, or as the original gay man who directed his rage at sexual worlds dominated by the young and pretty. What's striking about this particular piece is not that Kramer tells us anything new about his feelings about our cultures, but that his usual hyperbole takes on exaggerated form.

Kramer as literary critic can be challenged on several counts. He decries the failure of gay writers to produce "great literature," and holds up Tolstoy, Zola, Balzac, Chekhov, or Dostoyevsky as writers unsurpassed in their greatness. By going back to nineteenth century literature to find authors of excellence, Kramer weakens his case. Perhaps, as many have argued, the novel was a nineteenth century form that exhausted itself in the twentieth century.

Perhaps the quality of the writing and the obsession with the self rather than with the self in relation to a broader world is behind Kramer's critique. Kramer seems to want contemporary fiction to match the romance and range of vision of canonical white male writers of a century ago. Yet even these writers treated sex as a part of life in key works driven by passion and desire. In fact, they were as explicit about sex as the cultures of the time allowed. D. H.

Lawrence (a glaring omission from Kramer's list of exceptional novelists given his authorship of the screenplay for *Women in Love*) led the way in incorporating explicit sex and the body into fiction and paid for it dearly by having to respond to numerous lawsuits.[24]

I am not a literary critic, nor do I pretend to value high culture and the literary scene, although I have long been a voracious reader of lesbian and gay fiction. My primary concern here is Kramer's reductionism. This is an ironic charge, I'll admit, considering the thrust of his argument is that other gay male writers are guilty of reductionism in their portrayal of our lives in what he sees as sex-obsessed ways. By simplistically insisting gay literature is entirely focused on sex, and that gay writers do not document the complexities of our lives, Kramer quickly and easily disposes of a panoply of contemporary gay male writers who do not fit his narrow characterization of gay writing. Those whose literary scope goes considerably beyond the erotic are to be understood as no longer "gay writers." The late Paul Monette's *Becoming a Man*, for example, captured precisely the nuanced understanding of the coming-out process that Kramer argues he is seeking, in memoir form, the major literary genre of the late twentieth century. A range of gay men who have written novels, including Stephen McCauley, E. Lynn Harris, Michael Cunningham, Mel Dixon, Carter Wilson, David Leavitt, Doug Sadownick, James Earl Hardy, Lev Raphael, and Bill Mann, have done precisely what Kramer claims he is asking for: they have written about our lives as sons, brothers, friends, uncles, workers, teachers, and fathers, as well as lovers.[25] Edmund White, in all his earlier novels, has done so as well.

Even John Preston, whom Kramer, as well as many others (including Preston), might consider first and foremost a pornographer, produced a body of work that grappled with class, masculinity, geography, family, and other issues implicated in identity.[26] Andrew Holleran, who may as easily have become Kramer's target in this essay as his Lavender Quill compatriot Edmund White, in his latest work, *The Beauty of Men,* has written brilliantly about a gay man's struggles with aging.[27] Yet because sex threads its way through the book, Kramer might again see it as another work about only sex. If sex appears, he sees dick, dick, and only dick.

Michael Bronski offers an alternative way to consider the accusation that gay men are obsessed with sex:

Gay people—and gay men in particular—have always been accused by mainstream culture as well as conservative ideologues of being *obsessed* with sex. And the reality is that it is true. We are obsessed with sex. And it's a good thing. Sexuality and eroticism are extraordinarily powerful forces in all of our lives and gay culture acknowledges and supports that . . . Much of the vitality and social power of gay culture is its preoccupation with sex . . . Mainstream culture is predicated upon repressing or denying sexuality—Freud hypothesizes this in *Civilization and Its Discontents*; Jesse Helms, Newt Gingrich, and their cronies see it as their political mandate—and gay culture, by its insistence on the importance of sexuality, challenges this.[28]

What are we to make of "Sex and Sensibility"? Kramer indicates that his thoughts represent a marginal viewpoint:

Sadly, I feel myself more isolated than ever from my fellow gay writers. But then I always did. The things I believe are things few of my people want to hear, but then they never did. It is disheartening to hope so much for change and to see so little of it.[29]

Yet Kramer's fingering of the supposedly sex-obsessed nature of a toxic gay culture is echoed by other writers such as Andrew Sullivan, John Rechy, Duncan Osborne, Jonathan Capehart, Ian Young, and Dan Perreten, and is increasingly reflected on the editorial pages and in letters to the editor of gay newspapers, as well as in a number of current nonfiction volumes by popular gay male writers.[30] Gay periodicals around the nation are staking out positions in the emerging sex wars, and several have embraced positions that repeatedly moralize about gay male sex and drug use.

This position is best exemplified by *The Advocate,* which appears to be vying for the title of "most moralistic gay media outlet." The publication recently ran the sensationalistic front-page headline: "Sex, drugs, & bathhouses are back . . . A new bio of gay icon Brad Davis reminds us of the dead end we face," in an issue branded with the theme "The Return of Our Bad Habits."[31] A lead article was titled "Men Behaving Badly," and included the outrageous subhead, "The recklessness of the 1970s and early '80s has reappeared on the party circuit, where gay men are indulging in illicit drugs and wild sex with increasing abandon."[32] Kramer clearly found an amenable host publication for his views of gay men's sex. Ironically, Kramer's own piece appeared in an issue of *The Advocate* designated "Special Health Issue," which graphically reduced gay and lesbian health on its cover to two things: AIDS and the gay gene. This is a terribly reductive vision of gay health.[33]

Letters to the editor of *The Advocate* in response to Kramer's essay suggest his message may now be the dominant view in queer communities throughout the nation. A boxed announcement under the headline "Kramer strikes a nerve" appeared in the June 24, 1997 issue, saying:

> Never has *The Advocate* received more mail on one article than we received regarding Larry Kramer's "Sex and Sensibility," which ran in the May 27 issue. Equally impressive: the fact that 75% of respondents agree with Kramer and that so many women were motivated to respond.[34]

The Advocate printed thirteen letters in response to Kramer that together illustrate the challenge of addressing issues of sexuality and culture through polemics. The editorial staff's support for Kramer's views is evident, not only by their choice of heading for this section of the letters pages ("Wake-up call"), but through the content of the three letters they chose to print that challenged Kramer's viewpoint. The remaining ten letters offered great praise for Kramer's bold gesture of bringing the truth to bear on a gay population in deep denial. A man from San Diego wrote:

> It's incredibly painful to have the mirror held up in front of us in this blunt and direct fashion. Bravo to *The Advocate* for having the guts to print a piece so full of truth and political incorrectness at the same time.[35]

A reader from St. Paul echoed this sentiment: "This article is powerful, depressing, motivational, inspirational, and, most of all, undeniable."[36] Another from Memphis wrote:

> I hope, if we're as honest with ourselves as Kramer is about what he has observed in the gay community, that maybe some-

day we'll find our souls and truly become a community, a culture, and a valuable thread in our American tapestry.[37]

Kramer's disapproval of the centrality of sex in gay culture clearly struck a chord in many readers. He urges lesbians "to start getting angry at gay men about all of this," and women responded. A woman from Boston took him up on his call:

> I am one lesbian who has *always* felt infuriated by gay men's inability to look at the world beyond their own cocks. . . . *The Advocate* has let in a breath of sanity and has validated mine. Kramer's statements are not only refreshing, enlightening, and brave, but they also chime loudly as truth. 'Tis rare indeed.[38]

From Alexandria, Virginia, another lesbian writes, "We should be proud of our community's progress and of ourselves and stop glorifying sex in art and literature."[39] A woman in Durham, North Carolina, insists, "Sex can be deadly, and to expect that all we have to do is demand money for a cure and not change behavior is ludicrous and adolescent rationalization."[40]

Kramer's proposition that lesbians should be enraged by gay male sexual practices suggests he believes they hold a single position on issues of sexuality. In a speech given shortly after he wrote this piece, Kramer expanded his discussion of lesbian reactions to gay male sex:

> In my *Advocate* article I suggested that it's time that lesbians started bugging gay men to stop being so promiscuous and to stop thinking only with their cocks. Lesbians have been very polite in letting us get away with something that I know annoys them a lot. . . . Lesbians understand that there's much more to life than sex.[41]

Yet the feminist sex wars of the 1980s made it clear lesbians do not speak in a unitary voice on almost any topic.[42] Starla Muir wrote an angry piece titled "Time to Grow Up, Boys, & Spare Your Brother's Life," in a Seattle gay paper after attending a public forum on the history of gay men's culture and sexuality. Muir chides gay men:

Make no mistake, I am angry at you, not a mindless virus. I'm tired of pretending I'm angry at the disease. *You* are the only ones who can choose to live or die for your dicks. Just as every girl learns she is responsible for getting pregnant, so are you responsible for getting AIDS. Stop screaming about the lack of government response and start screaming about the lack of your own. Government can't stop women from getting pregnant any more than it can stop you from getting AIDS. The choice and its consequences are yours. You've been educated and warned for fifteen years now . . . after losing twenty-three people to AIDS, I'm in no mood to listen to you cry on my shoulder about paying the Piper because you wouldn't control your pecker.[43]

Long-time activist and sex theorist Lisa Duggan, in an article that responds to Kramer, Signorile, and Rotello, recounts the earlier feminist splits and traces the relationship between the current sex panic and a "larger attack on public spaces and democratic public life."[44] As Duggan writes:

There's another troubling little problem for feminists in the discourse of the new gay sexual conservatives. Many of them keep insisting on pointing to a gift for "intimacy" and domestic stability that lesbians are supposed to have, and that gay men might profitably imitate. I feel ill every time I hear it, it sounds so much like something one might hear in church from Pat Robertson—let's all give our thanks to the womenfolk, who know how to keep those home fires burning! (Burn baby burn . . .) I would like to send one message in particular to all gay men who spout this line, as Larry Kramer did in his recent *Advocate* interview—WE DON'T WANT TO DOMESTI-CATE YOU; THAT'S WHY WE'RE LESBIANS![45]

The letters supporting Kramer illustrate many readers' willingness to mistake his highly reduced vision of gay culture for "the truth." Gay men's sex becomes the problem, the engine driving both the continuing AIDS epidemic and societal homophobia. As one man from West Hartford, Connecticut, put it:

For years we have asked the straight world to ignore the sex in homosexuality, while our fiction, art, plays, and films promote it as the essence of our lives.[46]

One must ask, "Who is the *we* here?" This statement highlights the radically different agendas of disparate elements of the gay, lesbian, and bisexual populations. Clearly many queer activists, as well as cultural workers, have long fought to maintain the "sex" in "homosexuality," while more moderate activists advocate for a de-emphasis on sex in the movement. Another letter writer exhibits the current neoliberal view that insists societal respect (as well as civil rights and freedom from harassment and hate violence) is something that marginalized groups must "earn":

It should not take a brain surgeon to realize that our very future depends on how we, as a people, present ourselves. If we do not respect ourselves, how can we expect others to respect us? . . . Respect is not something you can demand; it's something you must earn. It is also something you must prove yourself worthy of.[47]

Equally disconcerting as the supportive letters are the three anti-Kramer letters selected for publication. They suggest that viewpoints opposing Kramer's analysis are held by folks with radical thinking about HIV whom many consider marginal. A doctor from Los Angeles argues AIDS is "a man-made genocide program" that was "seeded into the gay community via hepatitis B vaccine experiments beginning in the late 1970s" and compares Kramer's essay to "blaming Jews and Judaism for provoking the Holocaust."[48] Respected gay activist and longtime AIDS dissident John Lauritsen, from Provincetown, takes on Kramer's insistence that gay writers "tell the truth" about AIDS and gay culture, and writes:

Very well: HIV doesn't do a damn thing. AIDS itself is an infectious disease only to the extent that bouts of VD plus antibiotics are bad for health. The HIV antibody tests are invalidated and meaningless. The leading AIDS treatments are worthless and toxic.[49]

The other letter challenging Kramer compares him to Hitler. Michael Wakefield, a cable access talk show host in New York, writes, "I'm reminded of Hitler's having equally passionate views on what kind of art was appropriate to fulfill another type of political agenda," and insists "Kramer's attitude toward promiscuous gays parallels the genocidal goals of the 'Nazi doctors' who, he says, 'wanted to purify their race'."[50]

While the editors should receive credit for providing space in their publication for alternative views about the genesis of the epidemic and the role of HIV, by selecting only a few critical letters and ensuring that these letters contain views considered heretical by much of their readership, they successfully undercut Kramer's opposition.

At the same time, these letters illustrate a tendency that has become all too commonplace when complex cultural phenomena are discussed through polemics: most of Kramer's opponents write him off as a minority viewpoint, compare him with Hitler, or fail to respond to the intellectual substance of his essay behind the rhetoric. Rather than see oppositional views as offering an opportunity for thoughtful discussion, advocates of any viewpoint denounce, denigrate, and disrespect the opposing voices. While these are tactics that Kramer himself employs, when both sides share an essentially illogical practice, the opportunity for contrary viewpoints to inform each other and shift thinking is lost.

Letters to the editor indicate Kramer might be wrong on at least one of his points. Rather than being more isolated from other gay writers, the convergence of a number of biomedical, social, and political trends (including continuing seroconversions among gay men, the entrenchment of neoconservative political views, an accelerated drive toward assimilation, and the aging of a generation of surviving gay men) has moved Kramer's view of gay men's cultures to center stage for the first time in twenty years. In the late 1990s, Kramer's views about gay men and sex, which he has articulated so powerfully for so long, are being imbibed by legions of gay men and lesbians hungry for his message.

My concern with Kramer's guilt-trippy screeds is not only the profound hatred for gay men that suffuses his analysis and oozes out of his mean-spirited prose, but the ineffectiveness of constructing public health strategy around such harangues. Kramer performs as our community's neighborhood bully as he aggressively strong-arms lesbians to sever their ties to gay men, threatens AIDS organizations who dare lend their names to circuit parties, and attempts to coerce gay male youth into embracing his paranoid visions of apocalypse now and constructing their social worlds to fit his narrow specifications. While such tactics may provide just the encouragement some people need to rise up and assume the roles Kramer has written for them, there is little evidence that a strategy based on guilt, shame, and fear-mongering would prove effective with gay men.

A recently published collection of essays in tribute to Kramer ironically takes as its title W. H. Auden's oft-quoted line, "We Must Love One Another or Die."[51] I am reminded of an exchange I had as a sixth-grade schoolteacher, when I repeatedly witnessed a divorced mother reassuring her ten-year-old son that his father loved him—despite the father's failure to visit the boy or return his phone calls, and the father's emotional abuse. "What you are doing," I cautiously told the mother, "may be telling your son that abuse and disdain may be acts of love. I'm not in your shoes, but I fear such a message encourages a continuing cycle of damage under the guise of fatherhood."

There is a danger in mistaking the abusive treatment Kramer visits on gay men with authentic caring or love. There is nothing loving in Kramer's portrait of gay culture, his analysis of the forces that contribute to its creation, or his choice of words. To confuse vitriol, bullying, and public assaults on colleagues with love runs the risk of creating a no-holds-barred ethos in community discourse and diminishing critiques of gay culture that are authentically loving and respectful, such as the work of Michael Bronski (with whom I often agree) or Daniel Harris (with whom I often disagree).[52]

Resistance to Kramer's perspectives increasingly is emerging from young gay men whom he consistently discusses in condescending ways. In a recent speech, Kramer said of young people:

> These new faces, this new generation—you are awfully complacent. You look great. But I can't hear you. You certainly aren't fighters. . . . What have you done to contribute anything positive to honor the memories of so many of us? How selfish and narcissistic can you be?[53]

In response, twenty-something journalist Wayne Hoffman wrote:

> We young gay men already realize we are more than our
> sexuality. We have style, we have music, we have drama, we
> have politics. While Kramer has been watching the circuit
> queens shake their bubble butts, the rest of us have been writ-
> ing plays, raising families, working elections, battling discrim-
> ination, caring for our loved ones, and struggling to live our
> lives with dignity. We are already full humans, capable of the
> same banalities and extravagances as every other American.
> Why is Kramer the last to know?[54]

Oddly enough, during the same month Kramer proclaimed young
gay people to be "complacent," "selfish," and "narcissistic," *The
Advocate* published a special issue featuring the accomplishments
of queers under the age of thirty. ("They're sexy, they're young,
they're smart, they're gay, they're lesbian. America's future is in
their hands.") Included were a twenty-five-year-old state representative from Vermont, the winner of the men's title in a U.S. figure
skating competition, a United Farm Worker labor organizer in
Washington, a twenty-nine-year-old English professor, a twenty-
seven-year-old physician who serves on the board of the Gay and
Lesbian Medical Association, and a twenty-one-year-old advocate
who single-handedly changed federal policy on harassment in
schools.[55]

MICHELANGELO SIGNORILE: SOUND-BITE SOLUTIONS TO COMPLEX SOCIAL PROBLEMS

If you live in Chelsea in New York City, go to the Chelsea Gym
or David Barton, and hang at bars such as Splash or coffee shops
such as the Big Cup, you might read magazines such as *Next* and
Homo Xtra. Perhaps you style yourself in the image of many of
your white gay male peers, build up a muscular body, shave your
head, and get a tattoo on your shoulder. You may attend the Saint-
at-large White Party in New York in February, Hotlanta in August,
and the Black and Blue Party in October in Montreal. At times you
think of yourself as a circuit boy, deeply involved in defining trendy
gay culture at the end of the century.

Yet gay culture at this point in its trajectory cannot be defined by one narrow population of party-goers, however much a certain sector of the media may embrace the subculture. Men whose identities are rooted in a single subculture, be they circuit boys, bears, men of color, AIDS activists, club kids, trannies, queers, leathermen, or youth, often mistake their special pocket of the gay universe for all of the gay universe, or see it as the leading edge of gay culture. Instead of recognizing the multitude of competing sites in which men enact various queer identities, they make judgments about gay men and gay community based on limited vision.

This is my overarching criticism of Michelangelo Signorile's book *Life Outside: The Signorile Report on Gay Men: Sex, Drugs, Muscles, and the Passages of Life.*[56] Much of what is contained in this 300-page volume offers a vision of gay community that is diverse, comprising various subcultures stretching from rural areas to small towns, suburbs to cities. Yet the frame placed on the book artificially divides the population into an "inside" and "outside," with "inside" representing the "cult of masculinity" currently drawn to muscle-boy cultures and the circuit party scene. Signorile scrutinizes the extremes of this specific gay male subculture, then holds up the entire subculture as destructive to its individual members and to the community-at-large. As an alternative, he offers "life outside," gay men living outside of cities and urban gay men who are integrated into mainstream culture.

I believe it is important to look at all subcultures with a critical eye. I share Signorile's concern about drug abuse, unprotected sex, and the abuses of masculinity, even while I disagree with his analysis and moralistic emphasis on busting out of the circuit scene. If the book initiates a conversation among men who identify with this subculture, something useful might come from it. Circuit boys, however, are not the only gay men who should be discussing abusive masculinities or self-destructive social practices.

This tendency to target gay male subcultures that embrace hypermasculine images and semiotics has long allowed most gay men to avoid reflection on their own relationship to masculinity. In the 1970s, leather culture was targeted in this way, yet often men licking boots or binding another man's wrists had a deeper appreciation for issues of power and equity than those men outside pointing their fingers. Few identify gay politicos and AIDS activists as abusers of power and purveyors of masculinity-run-amok, yet anyone who has spent time in the movement knows the flagrant violations of interpersonal ethics routinely engaged in by activists who have never licked a boot (at least not literally). Recent debates over gay male public sex spaces in New York City certainly suggest gay journalists, activists, and academics might benefit from self-critical exploration of male patterns of discussion and debate.

By positioning circuit culture as the identified problem child of the gay community, the author engages in the game of "good gay/bad gay" that has plagued queers for a very long time. Nothing good comes of it.

This is particularly ironic as Signorile has astutely critiqued the mainstream media for creating a similar representational polarity in its handling of Andrew Cunanan and revealed the double standard used in journalists' handling of gay and straight cultures and relationships.[57] Yet if substance abuse motivates his concern about the circuit, why isn't the alcohol abuse prevalent among other strata of gay men a target of his critique? We can spend years debating circuit boys and ignore the ubiquitous black-tie dinners of gay political groups where we watch respectable board members of gay nonprofits drink themselves into stupors. Wouldn't an even application of this kind of concern for substance abuse among gay men necessitate the sacrificing of advertisements from alcohol companies in glossy gay publications and their sponsorships of AIDS fundraising events?

Despite transparent attempts to qualify his language and offer nods to the greater diversity of the community, Signorile's emphasis in the book and in the promotional interviews that accompanied it is squarely on circuit boys. He takes a population that he acknowledges is primarily white and middle-class and urban and invests it with tremendous powers.[58] The book appears to assume most readers desire to emulate the look and lifestyle of muscle boys, and all of us want to fuck them. This "core" within urban gay life is fingered for everything from luring young gay men into an obsessive quest for muscles to the continuing spread of HIV among gay men.

In a critique of Daniel Harris's recent book *The Rise and Fall of Gay Culture,* Rabbi Denise L. Eger of Los Angeles takes on the issue of mistaking a subculture among gay men for all of gay culture. She argues:

> Harris does not focus on the lesbian community nor on the community of people of color. He does not address how white male gay culture has changed due to its interaction with lesbians and people of color. Instead, his book might be aptly named *The Rise and Fall of White Male Gay Culture.*[59]

Eger's analysis emerges from her perspective as a rabbi of a synagogue serving gay men and lesbians. She argues that the same debates about assimilation versus adherence to traditions occur in Jewish communities and insists that "Jews have also struggled to maintain a balance between complete assimilation . . . and acculturation." Insisting that social critics who "put all of us into an oppressive box" by homogenizing queer cultures do us all a disservice, Eger insists:

> Gay male culture is not just about quips from *Sunset Boulevard* or promiscuous sex. Gay male culture, if truly examined, is still rich with art and humor, courage and caring, verve and vitality. Gay male culture is hardly dead. It is no longer a culture of isolation. Gay men have learned to interact with lesbians and straight folks for the greater good of our community and, especially as we've learned to care for our own, our afflicted loved ones and our children.
>
> Maybe it's time Harris exits the rarefied New York environment to meet the wonderful diversity of gay men that I get to meet each day.[60]

Signorile likewise is misguided in centering, castigating, and blaming circuit boys for the problems he identifies in urban gay cultures. But it would be inadequate to primarily fault the book for simply mistaking a subculture for all of gay culture. The book is also problematic for its homogenization of circuit culture and for failing to understand the complex ways in which diverse masculinities are constructed, negotiated, altered, and reconstructed in this specific site. Researchers once got away with painting any subculture in which men construct gendered identities with a monochromatic color—the "hood" of black urban life, a hockey arena, the weight room in a high school, or a gay leather bar. However, a dozen years of scholarship have created an awareness that a man in any one of these sites is actively engaged in creating identities for himself, and that the identities and meanings he takes from the site may be quite different from those of the man standing next to him.[61]

What's disturbing about Signorile's division of "gay life" into polar worlds is that this tidy segregation does not exist. While certainly gay male cultures exist in gay ghettos as well as outside them, "the scene," as Signorile calls urban circuit life, is hardly composed of men who are separated from mainstream culture. While a small number of men might live primarily within this specific subculture, the majority of men who participate in circuit parties, as well as the majority of men who enjoy any male subculture, such as the bears, the leather scene, the gay literary world, or AIDS activism, have multifaceted lives usually involving jobs in nongay environments, ties to biological families, and residences outside gay-dominated neighborhoods.

The complexity of the lives of the men who participate in this "scene" barely makes a cameo appearance in this book. Perhaps this is because illustrating the messy complications, inconsistencies, and shifting understandings that all of us bring to our social practices makes it harder to stereotype. The book is imbued with a deeply judgmental tone. We see plenty of portraits of men abusing drugs, including steroids, but the large majority of men who are able to use drugs occasionally without proving themselves to be addicts or abusers are less visible. Men who obsess on sex and engage in compulsive practices eschewing safety are the stars of this book, while those who successfully negotiate the complex social and erotic rituals constituting this "scene" are silenced. A portrait is painted in this book that many social scientists would recognize as simplistic, reductionist, and moralistic.[62]

Much of the book mistakes representations of gay men featured in select media published in New York or Los Angeles for the reality of gay men's lives. While there is certainly an active circuit scene in San Francisco, many of us moved here because it offers a wide range of possibilities for gay male identity; friends have made similar claims about New York City. Within five blocks of my apartment in the gay ghetto, various subcultures stake out their own sites. One can be a member of the Metropolitan Community Church, cruise a coffee shop where bears, leathermen, and muscle boys mix, or hang out at a cafe for trendy club kids and literary queens. One can join a gym dominated by midlife gay men who work out hard, another frequented by men under forty who work out hard, or another populated by men of all ages who hardly work out at all. Every night of the week bars are jammed that specialize in black men and their admirers, leather daddies and their boys, young queer kids, and generic "normal" gay guys. Dozens of gay meetings of Alcoholics Anonymous and other twelve-step programs also occur, including meetings focused on men of color, leather folks, men with HIV, and those detoxing from addiction to crystal meth.

My point is this: Gay men in urban spaces have created a wide range of subcultures; they are each complicated and worthy of critical analysis. To place one of them center stage in what one fancies to be the gay male cultural imaginary is to deny and wipe out the work in which all of us have participated as we create post-AIDS identities and cultures. Men who read this book who neither desire twenty-five-year-old, muscle-bound bodies nor eroticize sucking dicks of men who have shaved themselves clean of body hair, might wonder what planet Signorile comes from.

Activist Jim Eigo has criticized Signorile for repeatedly attacking other gay men in his writings and for choosing to focus on "exposés" which "titillate and tsk, tsk, tsk at the same time."[63] Comparing Signorile's recent work to "that favorite pastime of talkshow America: the pathologization of practically everything," he writes:

> Unfortunately, most of the headlines that Mike the columnist has generated in the mainstream media, from the first fury over "outing" to the current one over "barebacking," have occurred when he's pointed his finger and squealed about the conduct of other gay men. The mainstream media are only too happy to parrot Mike: they don't have to dirty their own hands. They are hand-delivered sordid little stories of gay male self-loathing and sexual suicide. And the good ol' boys of the

mainstream appear to enjoy the added spectacle of the ensuing catfight in which all the major combatants are fags.[64]

The tendency to choose extreme examples of errant behavior to pathologize is characteristic of a crisis-driven analysis. Signorile's discussion of "barebacking" reflects this:

> . . . this barebacking thing is devastating and detrimental. This is going to roll back everything we've done in this epidemic. We have a responsibility to each other and to ourselves. Instead of doing anything, our leaders want to coddle each other and feel everyone's pain.[65]

This is not the thoughtful, well-considered analysis of which Signorile has shown himself capable. It's also not an accurate characteristic of community leadership's response to unprotected sex. Rather than address the complexity, Signorile delivers quick sound-bite solutions to vexing social problems. Pointing a finger makes good copy and sells books; it fails to reflect useful processes of self-critique while encouraging the deepening of community divisions.

SELF-ESTEEM VERSUS SOCIAL CHANGE: SAN FRANCISCO'S HEALTH PROFESSIONALS CHECK IN

On a mild June afternoon, as the fog was easing over Twin Peaks, I ambled down the hill from my apartment for tea with friends. As I passed the newsboxes at 18th and Castro, I grabbed the new issue of *Frontiers,* one of the local gay publications. I thumbed through it quickly and chuckled at the cover photo of Quentin Crisp grinning madly, as I crossed Castro Street, heading toward Pasqua, my local coffeehouse of choice.

Since 1992, at least a dozen coffeehouses have opened in the Castro, offering coffee, pastries, and a chance to read the paper, meet with friends, or kill some time. Several of these establishments are part of coffeehouse chains (Peet's, Spinelli's, Pasqua) that have been moving into urban neighborhoods throughout the country since the early 1990s. The proliferation of these businesses had led the Castro Area Planning and Action group to support an eighteen-month moratorium on new coffeehouses in the neighborhood, which the San Francisco Board of Supervisors approved by a six-to-one vote just two months earlier.[66]

While the appearance of a large number of coffeehouses and juice bars in gay ghettos was not triggered by post-AIDS shifts in gay men's communities, queer men have funneled into these spaces in droves and claimed them as primary sites for post-AIDS community building. During weekday mornings and afternoons, many of the Castro coffeehouses teem with gay men. It's not uncommon for visitors from out of town to inquire, "Doesn't anybody work in this city?" Seats may be occupied by men who are telecommuting to work out of their homes, employed in the sex industry, working as writers, retired on disability, or students. Individual coffeehouses and juice bars attract particular types of gay men. They have quickly become an important location for community building and boyfriend hunting for gay men in the Castro.

I frequent Pasqua, selected as the "Best Place to Listen to Tales of Leather and Lace," by the *SF Weekly*, a local paper, in their "Best of San Francisco '97" issue, which described it in this way:

> This Pasqua is the unofficial headquarters for the many self-employed and idle men who make Gay Mecca rock. Adjunct professors, computer geeks, writers, and call boys sip addictive frozen concoctions called Chillinis, talk books, boys, and politics, and trade hugs, weightlifting tips, and tales of sex with priests.[67]

I am one of the writers/graduate students who frequents Pasqua daily. Because I spend most of my time working at home, by two p.m. I frequently feel the urge to turn off the computer, get dressed (finally!), and amble down to the Castro to run errands, visit with friends, and look at men. Pasqua functions for me as the student union of the neighborhood; I see many of the same acquaintances there each day, exchange pleasantries, and read my mail. Occasionally local politicos or gay leaders from out of state stop by. My favorite porn star, Hank Hightower, drops in every few days. Friends pop in and out to talk politics, arrange evening plans, reveal sex stories. While I've never received weightlifting tips at Pasqua, I have enjoyed many hugs and heard more than a few erotic stories involving priests.

Pasqua is an important part of many men's social and sexual lives. As a person who goes to bed nightly at 9:00, I have dreamed for years of a place where gay men could go during the day to socialize and occasionally meet for sexual purposes. This new breed of coffeehouse functions in this way. Most days I spend an hour or two grading papers, editing my writing, meeting with friends, or reading newspapers. Every few weeks I'll give the eye to a handsome man and connect with him for an afternoon romp. Many of these men go on to become part of a friendship circle at Pasqua whose members offer one another referrals to medical providers, advice on boyfriend transgressions, and companionship on weekend shopping trips to Costco or Circuit City.

Pasqua is an ideal post-AIDS setting for me because it unites a group of men across generation, race, and HIV status and allows us to break down many of the rigid barriers that grew up during the most intense years of the epidemic. It is a sexualized space, and the cruising is not always subtle, but the sex does not stand on its own. The projects furthered through the social processes of Pasqua focus on creating and affirming identities, establishing lasting friendships and senses of community, and including humor, warmth, and spirit in with a sexual mix. While some social critics might look at this site and see a group of caffeine-fueled, crotch-sniffing wolves engaged in hypermasculine performances of sexual addiction, others simply would see a group of men of all ages seeking companionship.

The issue of *Frontiers* that I had picked up contained something unusual, a four-page centerspread designed to catch the reader's attention. It sure caught mine. Headlined "Making the Best of It: Could changes in the gay community help more of us live satisfying, healthy lives?," the piece grabbed my interest and I immediately focused my eyes to scrutinize it carefully.[68] The text on the front cover was superimposed on a photograph of what appears to be gay men walking arm and arm in pairs, along a path on a hillside overlooking the Pacific Ocean. The six men pictured are of diverse races and include one older man, perhaps in his fifties or sixties. The photograph portrays a Whitmanesque spirit of homosexuality, a loving brotherhood of comrades, and depicts a multiracial group of gay men in a manner that neither emphasizes nor exploits their sexuality. Its aura is warm and loving in a New Age kind of way. The men seem peaceful, happy, comfortably integrated into the bucolic scene.

I immediately realized what I was reading. For months I'd heard that Dana Van Gorder, the coordinator of lesbian and gay health for San Francisco's Department of Public Health, had been circulating a draft statement about "the community" among health practitioners working with gay men in San Francisco. While I hadn't seen the statement myself, I'd heard various reactions to it, and was eager to read it. As I sat at Pasqua, skimming the four pages of text, I became transfixed. Here, dispersed through the local gay press, was a statement from "a diverse group of over 125 health, mental health, substance abuse, and HIV prevention workers" intended "to offer ideas that increase individual men's awareness about things that may interfere with happiness and health . . . and to stimulate discussion about whether gay culture needs to change so that greater numbers of men will enjoy emotional and physical well-being."[69]

What I read saddened me. Appearing just a month after Michelangelo Signorile's book and while *The Advocate* issue featuring Kramer's provocative essay was still on the stand, this manifesto appeared to me to be a localized version of their viewpoints filtered through the lenses of the self-help, New Age, and mental health movements. Meticulously written to avoid accusations of overstatement and pathologizing the entire gay men's community in San Francisco, the piece nevertheless presents a portrait of a unified gay male culture that is highly sexualized, obsessed with beauty, youth, and muscles, and teeming with abuses of power. How does this portrait fit with the coffeehouse cultures of the Castro?

Many gay men likely picked up this essay, read it, and said to themselves, "Yes! Someone finally said it! I'm glad health care professionals have finally called a spade a spade, and identified the sex-obsessed, beauty-obsessed superficiality of this community."[70] These men may have felt relief, and, after reading the piece, come to understand their own difficult situations in new ways. Instead of feeling that their inability to create a friendship network, find a lover, or get laid is an isolated experience, they can see it now as a mass cultural phenomenon. In many ways, this piece functions to embrace and comfort men who maintain a backlog of anger toward gay community, faulting it for an inability to deliver on their precise social needs.

Again, if this essay helps to stimulate discussion about gay culture, as its authors claim it is intended to do, beneficial things may come from it. As it stands, it functions in three problematic ways, by: (1) denying the presence in San Francisco of many gay male subcultures and creating an artificial, singular gay male culture (or "gay life" or "gay community") that it proceeds to pathologize; (2) failing to appreciate, describe, and value the many life-affirming aspects of various social and sexual worlds gay men have created in San Francisco; (3) offering a vision for community that is inherently middle-class while denigrating the social worlds occupied by working-class, lower middle-class, and poor gay men (for example, encouraging "quality friendships" as a healthy alternative to the seemingly inferior social networks of bars and clubs).

One way to read this piece is as a call to community reconstruction produced by the health industry. This perspective, however, serves to expose a weakness in much of mental health work in the 1990s. It shows the hazards of attempting to understand complex social and cultural phenomena void of political and economic analysis. The cause of most of the problems diagnosed by the 125-plus signatories of this essay is gay men's "low self-esteem." While the piece tokenistically acknowledges that "[t]he source of most gay men's self-esteem problems is homophobia and racism," the authors' continual harping on self-esteem as the root of our problems, rather than homophobia, sexism, and racism, and the failure of the piece to even suggest political activism as an appropriate response, combine to effectively blame gay men for the problems visited upon them by institutionalized sources of oppression. The essay proposes as an answer to societal homophobia and racism only "more services" and "discussion groups" for the victims, rather than the development of political action to mitigate the root causes.

Certainly there are things gay men can do to improve our lives and confront the challenges put in our paths. I am a believer in human agency, the ability of people to effect changes in their lives, even while they must contend with complex and powerful social, cultural, and economic forces. I feel many do a disservice to entire groups of oppressed people by insisting their life conditions cannot be improved absent revolution (or the overthrow of capitalism . . . or the demise of patriarchy . . .). Yet mental health professionals who depoliticize social issues rooted in material economic and political reality, end up participating in destructive, blame-the-victim solutions. A gay man who might get fucked without a condom is encouraged to make sense of his actions and inactions by faulting only himself and his lack of "self-esteem" (a quirky and politically suspect term popularized through the psychobabble of the mid-1970s that I now try to edit out of my own writings and public speaking).

Using concepts and understandings that have attracted huge numbers of gay men to twelve-step programs, the authors tell us,

> Just as we need to help gay men build self-esteem so that the way in which they are received by others has little impact on them, we should encourage gay and bisexual men to renew their commitment to building a community in which caring and integrity mark all dealings with one another regardless of age, race, class, serostatus, or appearance.[71]

Here we find a utopian vision of community that glosses over profound divisions within gay communities. What's problematic here is asking men to commit to building a community that cares for all gay men, without recognizing that we live in a nation where divisions, particularly divisions between races and classes, are in many ways getting wider.[72] This might be acceptable if the essay acknowledged the greater social and economic context; lacking that acknowledgment, this reads as pap from the mouths of the privileged. How can we build a community of caring and integrity without critiquing and working to redirect a nation that is increasingly neither? When immigrants (including gay men) are blamed for all social ills by California's governor, and poor people (including gay men—including gay men with HIV) are kicked off Medicaid and welfare and offered jobs that do not pay a living wage, and the sick (including gay men with HIV and other illnesses) are not afforded adequate health care or treatment-on-demand for addictions, how can our well-intentioned objectives and shiny-faced good deeds build a community of caring?

The authors go on to write:

> The crucial development of an improved ethic of respect, caring, and even responsibility of one gay man for the health and well-being of another is not likely so long as gay men's organizations fail to provide leadership to build a meaningful sense of community and shared destiny among gay men of every race, culture, class, age, and serostatus.[73]

This passage reveals a central problem with this essay. To think that gay community, or gay men's organizations, have the ability to "build a meaningful sense of community and shared destiny among gay men of every race, culture, class, age, and serostatus," is to believe that our organizations have the ability to dupe all of us into thinking something that is not true. Get real! *There is no shared destiny among gay men.* Research by sociologists, anthropologists, cultural studies scholars, political scientists, and public health researchers, as well as popular writings by gay men of color, working-class gay men, and young gay men, have made it abundantly clear that homosexual identity creates a shared destiny primarily among white, middle-class men who have no other sources of oppression.[74] Otherwise, our real-life destinies are not shared. When we are in our seventies and eighties, some gay men will be living in poverty and some will be living in luxury and others already will be dead. When we are sick, some have private health insurance and tremendous access to treatment, and others sit in the emergency room at the nearest public hospital for two days with a knife wound.

The failure to integrate an economic and political analysis is evident throughout the essay. The authors vacillate between insisting the matters of concern are "tough personal problems," and that they are caused by failures in "gay culture." A complex dialectic occurs here that is neither acknowledged nor analyzed by the authors, and primarily individualistic solutions are offered to vexing social problems. For example, the tiny section on socioeconomics is limited to a single paragraph that illustrates the limitations of mental health understandings of the material world:

> A major issue affecting health for many gay and bisexual men is low socioeconomic status, particularly for many men of

color. Poverty contributes to low self-esteem and isolation for many gay and bisexual men, and oftentimes places them in social settings characterized by substance abuse, violence, and victimization. Economic development programs need to be created to help gay men improve their educational and vocational skill levels, and assist them in improving their socioeconomic situations.[75]

Nowhere in this section is there even a hint that unregulated capitalism, a specific economic system, has been put in place that, in late twentieth-century America, mandates that many people (including many gay men) will be unemployed or work in jobs that do not pay a living wage, or that the richest nation on this planet simultaneously produces cultures that uphold wealth as the ultimate indicator of success and relegate increasing numbers of its citizens to poverty. Yet the authors are comfortable portraying poor peoples' communities with simple brush strokes ("characterized by substance abuse, violence, and victimization"), that fail to note the ways people in poverty (including gay men) create cultures and social networks characterized by resilience, determination, and mutual support. Again, the authors buy into neoconservative, culture-of-poverty rhetoric and suggest solutions ("economic development . . . to help gay men improve their educational and vocational skill levels, and assist them in improving their socioeconomic situations.") that blame the victim, suggesting that poor people are poor simply because they lack formal education and job skills.

I am aware some will claim that I am engaging in needless "politically correct" critiques here and that the intent of the authors of this piece was more narrowly focused on improved mental health, not social change. Yet there are models of community mental health that engage closely with social justice work and understand the relationship between mental illness and health, violence and recovery as necessitating political consciousness and action. I think here of the work of Judith Herman and other feminist mental health advocates,[76] as well as Ignacio Martin-Baro's essays in *Writing for a Liberation Psychology*, in which he draws on the work of Paulo Freire and others in examining the consequences of government-initiated terrorism in El Salvador. Martin-Baro highlights the importance of shifting the consciousness of oppressed peoples:

Given the environment of the Social Lie, there arises a need to increase critical consciousness through a process of de-ideologization—to which social psychologists can and should be contributing. What this involves is introducing into the ambiance of the collective consciousness elements and schemata that can help dismantle the dominant ideological discourse and set in motion the dynamics of a process of de-alienation.[77]

He also provides a powerful argument for the linking of mental health work with activism:

If the foundation for a people's mental health lies in the existence of humanizing relationships, of collective ties within which and through which the personal humanity of each individual is acknowledged and in which no one's reality is denied, then the building of a new society, or at least a better and more just society, is not only an economic and political problem: it is also essentially a mental health problem. By the very nature of the object of our professional work, we cannot separate mental health from the social order.[78]

The San Francisco health professionals' limited view of the current economic crisis in this country and the ways social and cultural forces collide with individual lives and wreak havoc might be one reason psychotherapy and other professionalized counseling services are seen as bastions of middle-class indulgence. The growing chasm between the rich and the poor in America has left many people who have both education and job skills (including many gay men) without employment that pays a living wage and without health insurance.[79] The necessary response certainly involves processes of healing, but collective political action to alter the conditions that create poverty and systems of oppression must be central.

WHY IS GAY CULTURE BEING CENSURED AT THIS TIME?

What forces have come together in the late 1990s to create the conditions under which extreme critiques of gay culture appear in

which gay men themselves reduce, simplify, and impugn our varied, complicated, and constantly shifting social worlds? I believe a
number of social, cultural, and structural forces have set the stage
for pathologizing gay men's sexualities and cultures in ways that
deeply resonate as true for large numbers of gay men.

Continuing HIV Infections Among Gay Men

In 1997, we have long crossed an important and usually unidentified line with tremendous significance for gay men. If doctors are
correct that the natural history of HIV causes most people to come
down with infections that give them an AIDS diagnosis roughly ten
years after becoming infected, men diagnosed in 1998 were infected
in 1988, a time when they "should have known better."[80] It has
become increasingly difficult to pretend people with AIDS were
infected "before they knew better." The simplistic understandings
we maintained of safe sex and risk behavior in the 1980s ("Good gay
men practice safe sex 100 percent of the time") allowed us to push
red ribbons as we insisted all people with AIDS—children, hemophiliacs, sodomites—were "innocent victims."

This is no longer possible. I believe increasing evidence that many
gay men occasionally fuck without condoms taps into an immense
pool of sexual shame long lurking just under the surface of gay
men's communities. Because AIDS groups work overtime to keep
the mind-set of the community locked in a state of emergency, gay
men suffer a stark poverty of analysis in attempting to make sense
of continuing HIV infections. Absent a balanced analytical framework from which to consider epidemiological data, men default to
panic, eagerly imbibe damning critiques of gay men's culture, and
rush forward in a stampede of shame-based condemnation. Most of
these same criticisms of gay male culture offered by the health professionals and New York writers could be presented in an even-
handed, even loving manner that would feel less shame-based. The
tone of most of these writings—moralistic, judgmental, disgusted—
suggests profound sexual shame.

The Successful Entrenchment of Neoconservative Strategies Targeting Sex

We are living through a period in which all sex occurring outside of heterosexual marriage is being scrutinized and challenged as contributing to the creation of an enormous social and economic burden on American citizens.[81] While AIDS and sexually-transmitted diseases often appear as the triggering argument in the attacks on sex, recent mass public conversations about welfare, immigration, and health care reform have revealed great concern with the sexual practices of poor people. As Suzanne Pharr writes:

> [The theocratic Right] use inflammatory images and misinformation to dehumanize and demonize lesbians and gay men as sexual predators, just as they have characterized African American men since slavery. Lesbians and gay men become "pedophiles;" African American men become "rapists;" African American women become "whores" and "welfare mothers."[82]

Thus sex is marshaled as a tactic in a broader strategy to effect profound political, economic, and religious changes in American democracy. Michelangelo Signorile and Gabriel Rotello both have expressed concern that they have been unfairly branded by some writers as neoconservatives.[83] Clearly they have histories of gay activism around progressive causes. Yet Jim Eigo, citing the work of Rutgers professor and Sex Panic member Michael Warner, insists, "A range of mainstream gay writers now recapitulate the classic neo-con rhetoric of the last two decades (even as they queer it). Each evokes nostalgia for a lost purity—or for a purity never yet attained.'

The primary neoconservative stance on sex and drug use by teenagers is captured by Nancy Reagan's "Just Say No" campaigns, and emphasizes celibacy, peer pressure, and silencing as primary tactics and considers harm-reduction approaches as tantamount to blasphemy. This seems to parallel the suggestions of some of these authors for dealing with gay men's current sex and drug use with condemnation, stigma, and strict standards. While these writers themselves may not be easily pigeonholed as neoconservative, and their open participation in gay men's cultures clearly distinguishes them from many neoconservatives, their critiques of gay sex cultures often default to solutions to complex social problems that are uncannily similar to strategies embraced by neoconservative social critics.

The Need to Balance the Romanticized Vision of Gay Men's Early AIDS Response of the 1980s with a Demonized Vision of Gay Men in the 1990s

Am I the only one having difficulty placing the representations of gay men's cultures discussed by Kramer, Signorile, and the 125 health workers alongside the earlier narratives of gay men's responses to the AIDS epidemic in the 1980s? While these contemporary writers create a portrait of an uncaring community of men engaged in hedonistic, hypermasculine, self-centered practices, it was just five years ago that writers discussed how "The wildfire of the AIDS epidemic has made gays a community even as it has consumed their lives."[85] Our media featured repeated images of networks of altruistic volunteers caring for their dying brothers, and community members taking care of our own.

We seem to ricochet between exaggerated representations of gay men as a class. We are either seen as drugged out, mindless sex fiends, or selfless Mother Theresas. We are alternately represented unfurling the AIDS Quilt or humping each other on the dance floor. Some might ask if it is possible that gay men actually shift in and out of such characterizations every few years. Instead I suggest that current extreme ways in which gay men are being characterized is, in part, a response to the romanticized vision of gay community that flourished up until the mid-1990s. Rather than continue to falsely depict gay men's cultures in exaggerated ways, an attempt to characterize them in a balanced manner might be more beneficial to community-building.

A Deep Antagonism Baby Boomers Maintain Toward Generation X

For years many have wondered what would happen when the baby boomers grew up. How would they respond to their own children's transgressive actions? Would the generation that got stoned, dropped out, and got laid offer a liberal vision of parenting?

Much of the public representation of Generation X has been created and marketed by baby boomers. A portrait of young people emerged in the early 1990s that depicted Gen Xers as "slackers, cynics, drifters."[86] While each generation of young people in America appears to create distinctive cultures that mark it off from its predecessors, these cultures are not easily reducible to simplistic understandings of motivations and meanings. Yet this is precisely what is imposed on them by their parents' generation.

Much of the hostility directed by gay men of my generation at young gay men must be understood in this context. Larry Kramer begins a speech prepared for San Francisco's gay pride celebration, "Please don't hiss and boo. Please don't throw things. I'm an older man now and older farts deserve respect."[87] Yet in his speech he rails against the "new generations" of queers who "aren't fighters," are "awfully complacent," "selfish," and "narcissistic." Many of Kramer's writings are laced with powerful ageist assumptions (about both young and old people) and profound condescension toward youth. He consistently confuses age with seriousness of purpose and youth with self-centered and pampered attitudes:

> I hope the things that I say don't make me sound like a conservative. I hope, and think, that they make me sound grown-up. I'm tired of our people being told what we must say by a bunch of spoiled children who are feeling deprived because their lollipops might be taken away.[88]

This passage suggests Kramer embraces traditional ageist characterizations of children as brats and grown-ups as sages. Much of the venom currently spewed forth at gay men in their twenties suggests many gay men's profound discomfort with children and youth. They are able to see young gay men in one of three simplistic roles: (1) victims of societal homophobia needing older gays to rescue them; (2) bad boys misbehaving with sex and drugs, prompting their elders to chide them into taking responsibility for their actions; (3) cockteasers flaunting nubile bodies only to frustrate older gay men. Until older gay men forge relationships of equity with young gay men and come to know them as complicated people who are not easily stuffed into these narrow roles, young gay men will continue to need to separate themselves and the gay generation gap will grow wider.

Another way I read much of the contemporary griping that assails the cultures of gay men in their twenties and thirties is as a long, sad, middle-age whine.[89] The majority of the gay men I know who are among the 125 signatories on the San Francisco essay are approaching or well into middle age. What does it mean that some of these men, who may have spent almost twenty years enjoying San Francisco's gay scene, come together in their forties and fifties to begin challenging the "value on youth and physical perfection" supposedly dominating gay male culture? As Dan Savage told me after reading the piece:

> I have felt all along that this sudden harping on the excesses of gay culture—circuit parties, gym bods, etc.—is highly suspicious when it emanates from former participants in that scene who have sadly "aged out" of it, and now can see it clearly for what it is. . . . I say this as someone who doesn't live at the gym, and has never been to a circuit party. But listening to aging gym queens bemoan the emotional and mental paucity of men who won't fuck them anymore is a little ridiculous.[90]

In *Reviving the Tribe,* I argued that many of the gay men of my generation, now in their forties and fifties, who had survived AIDS were walking around with a terrible burden of unacknowledged grief, rage, and terror, and that if they didn't find ways to work through the decimation of the epidemic, they'd turn bitter, decrying their wanton youths, and blaming the "excesses" of the 1970s for the hell they are living.[91] I wonder if part of the energy behind current judgments of circuit boys emerges from the difficult transition some gay men may be making into middle age.[92]

I am left curious about what constitutes "gay male culture" for the authors of the San Francisco essay that insists "Gay culture is also marked by reverence for youth."[93] How does one of the most popular bars in the Castro, Daddy's, which caters to leathermen, a population that has long encouraged a wide range of generations of men to see themselves as sexy, place "youth and physical perfection above most other aspects of a man's personal characteristics?"

Where does San Francisco's booming bear subculture and the Lone Star Saloon with its "bears, bikers, and mayhem" spirit fit within the youth- and beauty-oriented gay culture being critiqued in this essay? How does this gay culture include men in their twenties and thirties who are not identified with either the leather or bear subcultures, yet seek lovers in their forties and fifties? Where is Pasqua in all this?

Dan Savage again cuts right to the heart of the matter. Speaking about the "party scene," he told me:

> Why does this scene get all this disproportionate attention? Because it's where the beautiful boys are. So the critics, as I see it, are playing right into the values they're supposedly criticizing when they spend all their time obsessing about what the lost boys are up to this weekend (circuit parties, pec implants, ecstasy . . .). Don't like the party scene? Don't do the party scene. But don't do it for fifteen years and then it's shallow and demeaning the day after your butt drops.[94]

The essay puts forward an image of gay men in San Francisco that does not hold up under scrutiny. I am alarmed that it is written by health professionals, people who supposedly sit in rooms while gay men pour out their authentic experiences about the social worlds they inhabit. Don't these people realize that large urban areas offer gay men wide playing fields on which we can construct our lives?

Don't like seeing images of pretty boys and smooth-muscle bods? Pick up *Bear Magazine,* published right here in San Francisco. Don't want to hang out at coffeehouses all day being distracted by circuit queens? Fine, avoid Cafe Flore and come to Pasqua, where circuit boys mix comfortably with the leather daddies, computer geeks, and bears. Don't want to dance in a room filled with buff steroid thugs? Fine, don't head to Universe on a Saturday night, and instead walk a few blocks to the Rawhide, where a very diverse country-western crowd enjoys revelry (or go to N'Touch, a bar popular among Asian and Pacific Islander men, or the Litterbox, enjoyed by club kids, or Trannyshack, where genderplay and genderfuck are the rage).[95] Better yet, head to the same building Universe occupies but on a Sunday night, when it is Pleasuredome, a dance scene of thirties, forties, and older gay men.

REDUCING AMERICAN CULTURE
TO LET'S MAKE A DEAL

Casting a critical eye on contemporary life is not the problem. I am not arguing we should unabashedly embrace all aspects of our social worlds and cultural practices and ignore problematic aspects of the subcultures we are producing in the late 1990s. Nor am I saying issues of health, masculinity, addiction, HIV infection, abuses of power, and interpersonal ethics do not merit examination and widespread discussion. Indeed the final sections of *Reviving the Tribe* offer a dozen recommendations intended to "enhance both the ability of individual gay men to reconnect with community and the potential of gay community life to move toward a fuller and more life-affirming state."[96]

Instead, I argue that polemical critiques of gay men's cultures that simplistically paint a rich, varied population with broad brush strokes are not only inaccurate and insulting, but also dangerous. While some cite the perils of Kramer's and Signorile's works as located in the ways such works affirm the political rhetoric of the Christian Coalition, the initial dangers I see are situated firmly within gay male communities.

First, by confusing a narrow gay male subculture with all of gay urban culture, ironically these writers increase the currency of one specific scene. If people did not realize muscle-boy culture was the desirable culture-of-the-moment, after the release of these works, the circuit could only become more central in the cultural imaginary. Second, by failing to consider seriously the relationship societal homophobia and sexism have to the socialization of gay men, the writers suggest limited compensatory strategies while leaving core problems unaddressed. A more useful approach would link political action with individual agency in a lifelong quest to create meaningful lives in the face of continued oppression. Third, because these writers ignore the complex ways cultures are constituted, I fear their solutions would remove much of what many of us value in gay male cultures, what makes them special.

In an essay called "The Impact of AIDS on the Artistic Community," written early in the epidemic, Fran Lebowitz astutely observed:

> The impact of AIDS on the Artistic Community is that when a 36-year-old writer is asked on a network news show about the Impact of AIDS on the Artistic Community particularly in regard to the Well-Known Preponderance of Homosexuals in the Arts she replies that if you removed all of the homosexuals and homosexual influence from what is generally regarded as American culture you would be pretty much left with "Let's Make a Deal."[97]

Without some gay male subcultures probing the boundaries of gender, sexuality, and drugs, I wonder if we'd lose much of what some of us value in many of our gay cultures, much of which superficially seems to have nothing to do with gender, sexuality, or drugs. For example, would the Painted Lady Victorians of San Francisco, which Richard Rodriguez has insightfully linked to gay male aesthetics, emerge from a subdued gay male culture?[98] Would gay male contributions to culture and politics continue? Would cultures that decenter sex, gender, and the body have produced the work of Bill T. Jones, Keith Haring, Allan Bérubé, Robert Mapplethorpe, Harvey Milk, Michel Foucault, Bayard Rustin, Mark Morris, Alvin Ailey? Would a desexed gay culture send forth Versace's fashions, the compositions of Ned Rorem or Lou Harrison, an AIDS Quilt, Tony Kushner's *Angels in America*, Sydney's Gay Mardi Gras, the musicals of Stephen Sondheim, or Armistead Maupin's *Tales of the City?* I do not pretend to have the answer to these questions, but I caution us to consider deeply the risks we take as we consider social engineering as a strategy for HIV prevention.

Finally, and perhaps most dangerous of all, is the powerful affirmation these writings provide to our lifelong socialization that tells us love between men is bad and sex between men is vile. Despite what these writers imagine from their perches in Manhattan or San Francisco, the world has not changed radically enough to produce new generations of queers who believe their desires and passions are good. While they are correct in insisting we do not need a pep rally uncritically cheering on gay men's cultures, neither do we need from our own cultural thinkers a tribunal condemning us as immature, self-centered egomaniacs or self-destructive, diseased pariahs. In the 1970s, we told the antigay crusaders that if they cannot see the diversity and complexity of gay men's cultures, they should not consider themselves experts able to analyze or represent our communities. In the 1990s, we might tell our own critics the same thing: if you cannot see the diversity and complexity, don't fuck with gay culture.

Lisa Capaldini, a lesbian physician in private practice on Castro Street, frames these questions in a useful way. When asked "What is ailing our community?" by a local reporter for the gay press, Capaldini responded:

> I'd like to turn that around and say what is *healthy* about our community. I think in the Western medical model the problem is that we've become too disease-focused. We don't look at how we have managed to overcome adversity. How many communities could survive the various holocausts we've been through, in addition to the personal challenges and tragedies that each of us has faced growing up in a homophobic culture? When I spend time with people from our community, I feel grateful to be living in this struggling, marginalized, alive world. Of course, there are problems with our community, but these problems should be identified and dealt with. They shouldn't necessarily define us."[99]

Like all cultures, our own exhibit strengths and weaknesses, which can bring joy and frustration. Writers determined to critique gay culture have a responsibility to do so with balance, caution, and appreciation of the complex challenges we have survived and the complicated contemporary threats with which we continue to grapple.

Chapter 6

Scapegoating Circuit Boys

Writers concerned about the centrality of sex and drugs in specific gay men's subcultures are not isolated, marginalized voices. In the queer public sphere they represent an increasingly prevalent viewpoint. Their popularity is reflected in letters to the editor of gay papers, cyberspace discussion groups, and sales figures on the books of these authors. The attention given to these writers' ideas in the gay and mainstream media, their participation as keynote speakers at conferences and rallies, and the amount of newsprint devoted to their analyses makes it impossible to pretend they represent a marginal perspective.

Throughout the nation, the quiet consensus that allowed gay men to establish and expand sexual cultures without a great deal of internal community strife has started to rupture. Gay male and lesbian voices check in with concern about the public nature of gay sex cultures, use of drugs at community celebrations, and continuing transmission of HIV among gay men. As same-sex marriage, domestic partners' benefits, and queer parenting attain prominent places on the agendas of many gay organizations, a long-standing difference in political perspective has grown into a wide cultural breach. Queers who structure their social and sexual relations in patterns approximating heterosexual family life and those who do not are increasingly at odds over the organization of communal life and priorities for political action. How wide can the gap get without shattering our illusion of a unified community?

This situation is exacerbated by current shifts in our communal experience and interpretation of the epidemic. While partisans on both sides of current sex debates rhetorically represent AIDS as a continuing crisis, one view supports the deployment of measures

such as state regulation and action, public shaming, and demonization of specific subcultures within gay communities, while the other
encourages libertarian approaches based on the tenets of gay liberation.[1] These various strategies are not simply debated in theoretical
terms; gay men and lesbians now find themselves on opposite sides
of municipal action aimed at regulating, rezoning, and closing public sex spaces. Since 1994, the spaces urban gay men purposefully
have established for sexual liaisons have become highly charged
zones of contention. Cities throughout the nation from Boston to
San Diego, Washington, DC to San Francisco, Cleveland to Austin,
Miami to Minneapolis, have been the setting of increasingly divisive clashes as arms of the state, including public health officials,
police departments, elected officials, and various regulatory boards
and commissions, have targeted gay men's public sex practices for
policing, harassment, and public reprobation.[2]

Those who have been involved in urban gay politics know waves
of entrapment, harassment on code violations, and the accompanying widespread media attention are nothing new. A long history of
police raids on gay bars, attempts to regulate bathhouses out of
existence, and efforts to curtail public sex in parks, beaches, and
restrooms suggests gay male sex spaces have rarely been free from
harassment or secure from attempts at closure. The record indicates
that attacks on sex intensify during periods of social upheaval,
when a range of social and cultural anxieties are projected onto sex
and encourage the state to crack down on anything deemed perver-
sion.[3]

Historian George Chauncey has documented the intensification
of sex panic that occurred after World War II, which targeted homosexuals and linked them to child abuse. Chauncey writes, "As a
result of the press' preoccupation with the issue, the problem of sex
crimes and 'sex deviation' became, to an astonishing extent, a staple of public discourse in the late 1940s and early 1950s."[4] During
this period, a series of gruesome murders of children triggered mass
anxiety surrounding the perils of postwar American life for women
and children. Escalating reports of violence attributed to sexual
deviancy appeared in the nation's newspapers and magazines and
spurred good citizens to demand the state intensify policing efforts.
Chauncey argues that postwar sex panic functioned to reinforce

prewar social and sexual norms that had become increasingly weakened during the war mobilization.[5]

Gayle Rubin describes moral panics as "the 'political moment' of sex, in which diffuse attitudes are channeled into political action and from there into social change."[6] She cites several examples, including the McCarthy-era campaigns against homosexuals and the late 1970s "child pornography panic," and describes the processes and mechanisms that hysterically drive moral panics:

> Sexual activities often function as signifiers for personal and social apprehensions to which they have no intrinsic connection. During a moral panic, such fears attach to some unfortunate sexual activity or population. The media become ablaze with indignation, the public behaves like a rabid mob, the police are activated, and the state enacts new laws and regulations. When the furor has passed, some innocent erotic group has been decimated, and the state has extended its power into new areas of erotic behavior."[7]

Activist and social historian Allan Bérubé has defined a sex panic as "a moral crusade that leads to crackdowns on sexual outsiders."[8] It is distinct from ongoing harassment and vilification of the sexual fringe. It requires ideology, the machinery and power to transform ideology into action, and scapegoated populations, sites, and sexual practices. During a sex panic, a stampede mentality takes hold and alternative viewpoints are silenced. A wide array of free-floating cultural fears are mapped onto specific populations who are then ostracized, victimized, and punished. In recent years, we have seen sexual terrors marshaled to trample upon prostitutes and other sex workers, African-American men, welfare mothers, sex offenders as a class, and men who engage in consensual sex with male teenagers. Gay men have no corner on the market on sex panics.

Currently, debate rages among sectors of gay male communities about whether contemporary spates of police entrapments, closures of commercial sex establishments, encroachments on public sex areas, and vilification of specific gay male subcultures constitute a sex panic. It is important to distinguish between the ongoing waves of harassment and victimization and a full-scale sex panic: while both are destructive to lives and communities, a sex panic alone is characterized by a sustained period of intensified persecution of sexual minorities involving public disgrace, punitive state action, and a powerful cultural dynamic of scapegoating, shaming, and isolation. While communists were harassed and persecuted in this nation during the 1940s, it took the coalescing of a variety of cultural factors in the late 1940s and early 1950s to create the moral panic we have come to know as the McCarthy Period.

I believe we are witnessing the early stages of what may emerge as a full-scale moral panic focused on sexually active gay men who do not organize their sex and relationships following heteronormative models. It is at different stages in different locations. Sex panic looks different in urban, small city, and rural areas and will have different characteristics, contexts, and trajectories. Sex panic has emerged most prominently in New York City, with a sustained period of policing, harassment, and closure of many gay sex spaces and an accompanying discourse in the gay and mainstream media about the need to halt continuing gay male HIV infections.

What we are witnessing in 1998 are several powerful social shifts that could easily and quickly trigger the outbreak of sex panic nationwide. In a postmodern culture, terror and scapegoating may flare suddenly, have widespread ramifications, and cause extensive fallout. At least four factors are contributing to a mounting sex panic:

1. The ascendancy and entrenchment of the Far Right and their development, testing, and successful utilization of sex as a wedge issue that speedily causes divisions within their primary opposition: liberals and leftists.
2. The redistribution and intense concentration of wealth, creating vast economic disparities and making the urban centers of our nation sites of contentious class-based battles over massive corporate landgrabs.
3. A shift in public awareness from the belief that gay men had stopped transmitting HIV to the realization that gay men continue to become infected. This is accompanied by many gay men and lesbians' feelings of embarrassment, shame, and outrage.
4. The relative success of gay rights efforts in which certain victories are offered predicated on the sacrifice of sectors of

our communities or the squelching of certain social, cultural, and sexual processes that seem different from heterosexual social norms.

It is important to recognize that this panic is occurring against a broader cultural backdrop dominated by conservative and neoconservative understandings of sexual morality. These are manifested in efforts to buttress the flagging institution of heterosexual marriage by introducing barriers to divorce and opposing same-sex marriage, limit sex education in public schools and promote abstinence-only programs, and engage in punitive actions against married people who engage in outside sex.[9] Persons convicted of sex crimes may now be released after serving their sentences into a world that legally requires their neighbors be informed of their status as a sexual offender, or they may be held in indefinite incarceration long after they have finished serving their sentences. Many gay men convicted of sex crimes are being identified in their communities as dangerous criminals, simply because they had sex in parks, participated in consensual homosexual activity with another man in a state in which such activities are illegal, or engaged in consensual sex with teenagers.[10]

In this chapter, I provide evidence of the emerging moral panic in the United States.[11] The alarm has initially focused on gay men's sexual spaces, men who participate in circuit parties, and post-AIDS sexual practices such as "bareback" sex. What is unusual about this sex panic is its genesis within gay communities: openly gay and lesbian people, often defining themselves as activists, play a primary role in inciting state action against gay sex. No longer relegated to vociferously defending gay sex spaces by charging homophobia and selected enforcement of regulations, in various parts of the country gay journalists, activists, HIV prevention workers, and public officials have initiated and sometimes demanded crackdowns against gay sex and drug use. Simultaneously, voices within gay communities increasingly encourage the shaming, shunning, and segregation of men who continue to participate in promiscuous sex cultures.

The current moral panic is rooted in the mid-1990s dawning awareness that gay men continue to become infected with HIV and that efforts to prevent AIDS, particularly among gay men under the age of thirty-five, have not fully halted its spread. It is also rooted in the belief that the state should take action to remedy this matter. Rather than grapple with the complex social, cultural, psychological, and economic factors that contribute to continuing AIDS infections, a spirit that some refer to as "prudishness" and others as the "New Puritanism" has emerged.[12] Carmen Vasquez, public policy director of the New York Lesbian and Gay Community Services Center, succinctly characterizes some of the gay men who encourage city officials to regulate or close commercial sex spaces: "The guys are panicked."[13] Gay writers and activists increasingly stereotype and scapegoat one visible population of urban gay men—muscle boys who participate in circuit parties—and accuse them of serving as vectors spreading AIDS throughout the gay community.[14]

Moral panics involve an intense deployment of symbols and representations. At this epidemic moment, we find crusaders investing edifices, architectural designs, even specific structural features of buildings with intense symbolic power.[15] A new spirit of prohibition demands the closure of bathhouses and banning of spaces of privacy. Intense debate may focus on structures as common as a door. Despite statistics that indicate the only U.S. city that fully banned bathhouses during the AIDS years (San Francisco) has the highest rate of infection of gay men in the nation, and research that shows acts of unprotected anal sex are much more likely to occur in private homes than in public sex spaces, a sex panic targeting public sex spaces flares.[16]

Writers, social critics, and a portion of the rank-and-file gay population unleash their fury on the muscular "circuiteers" who attend mass dance parties occurring in urban centers. Portrayed as mindless, drug-abusing Typhoid Marys, Michelangelo Signorile characterized them as middle class and white, and dubbed some of them "Stepford Homos."[17] Despite research showing the infection risk among gay men is greatest among young men of color,[18] his work highlights circuit boys as a core group "that can sustain an epidemic such as HIV for the entirety of a population, keeping seroprevalence high due to multiple-partner unsafe sex . . . "[19]

People in a state of panic commonly blame rather than attempt to understand. The overwhelming feelings that are part of crisis states do not lend themselves to balanced, reasonable consideration of the complex contexts in which contested actions are occurring. As Gayle Rubin observes of earlier wars over sexuality, such battles "are often fought at oblique angles, aimed at phony targets, conducted with misplaced passions, and are highly, intensely symbolic."[20] Those attempting to respond to continuing HIV infections among gay men while locked in the 1980s crisis construct of AIDS are engaging in dangerous actions as they choose strategies, targets, and tactics in the current sex wars.

SEX WAR SCHISMS HIT NEW YORK CITY AND SAN FRANCISCO

It's not surprising that cities hardest hit by AIDS have been sites of the most contentious debates surrounding gay male sex venues during the middle and late 1990s even as men in small-town and rural America continue to face intensive periods of arrests and media exposure. These urban centers were the birthplace of the crisis construct and they are likely to be the last to move beyond it. San Francisco, Los Angeles, and New York City have all experienced intense scrutiny of gay sex cultures by local officials, community activists, and the gay and mainstream press. While such surveillance may have occurred in the past, the current sex panic is spurred by complicated internal community politics. A city-by-city tour of some of the major controversies throughout the United States offers a sense of the range of issues facing advocates who support public sex spaces and the scope of the emerging moral panic.

New York City has been the hub of the most intense debates within gay communities about the politics of regulating and closing establishments men frequent for sexual purposes. The battle over gay male sexual spaces here represents a bizarre clash of intersecting forces highlighted by strong divisions emerging among gay organizers, journalists, and HIV-prevention workers. The election of a mayor seen by some as conservative and hostile to many gay community concerns has added fuel to this fire.

In 1995, one group composed primarily of gay men formed to demand city officials enforce state regulations prohibiting all oral, anal, and vaginal sex acts, with or without condoms, in public spaces. This effort appeared to be triggered by the opening of a new

bathhouse in Manhattan, the first that had opened since the epidemic began. Other gay activist groups immediately formed to
counter this effort and a major battle ensued involving deep ideological and political differences. The mainstream media had a field
day, sending undercover reporters—gay and straight—into gay sex
clubs and running lurid stories on the evening news and in the pages
of daily newspapers.[21]

By 1997, when two books were published by members of the
group demanding enforcement of regulations (Michelangelo Signorile and Gabriel Rotello)[22] some of the opposing groups had been
disbanded while another was launched under the name "Sex Panic!,"
aimed at resisting the closure of sex spaces and offering alternative
viewpoints on gay sexual values, HIV prevention, and the use of
public spaces for sex.[23] Forums and street actions were held, and a
polarized community emerged. One side self-righteously fired off
opinion pieces to the gay press insisting it had been victimized by a
smear campaign branding its members as "neoconservatives," despite
their support for issues such as affirmative action and abortion rights.
Simultaneously, they characterized their opponents as "stuck in
adolescence," and as "the old guard of the gay community," obsessed
with extreme versions of sexual liberation.[24]

The election of Rudolph Giuliani as mayor provides an overarching frame to sex panic in New York. Characterized popularly as a
moralistic conservative hostile to gay community concerns, Giuliani's tenure has seen a marshaling of many arms of government to
restrict, regulate, rezone, and shut down dozens of sex-oriented venues. The gay male activists and journalists who support a regulation-
or-closure policy have been accused of initiating Giuliani's crackdown of gay clubs, theaters, and outdoor sex areas. A flyer put out
in 1997 by Sex Panic! insists "Queer New York is Being Shut
Down!!!" and summarizes the casualties of local regulatory efforts:

Mayor Giuliani has harassed and padlocked:

• Gay and lesbian bars including Cake, Crowbar, Edelweiss,
Rome, Rounds
• Dance clubs, including Limelight, Sound Factory, Tunnel,
Vinyl

- Sex clubs, including He's Gotta Have It, the Vault, Zone DK
- Theaters, including the Adonis, the Capri, David, the Hollywood Twin, King, Naked City, the New David, Prince.

The piers where we have played for years are being torn down, fenced off, and patrolled to keep us from meeting each other.

Giuliani has zoned 85 percent of adult businesses into oblivion, taking Times Square away from us and giving it to Mickey Mouse. Adult bookstores, video stores, strip clubs and even bars with go-go dancers will have to close all over the city.

In the past six months entrapment and arrests of gay men on charges of public lewdness have increased by 40 percent . . .[25]

New York City's only gay newspaper at that time, *LGNY,* has been the paper of record documenting these debates and appears to editorially share many of the views of the regulate-the-sex-clubs-or-shut-them-down activists.[26] They've also printed a number of articles aimed at refuting Sex Panic's central tenet that repressive measures against gay sex venues have burgeoned in New York. These include an article headlined, "Dramatic Drop in City Drive Against Adult Businesses in 1997," by Duncan Osborne, and Gabriel Rotello's writings on "The Myth of the Sex Panic."[27]

The New York Times seems to be taking the lead in whipping up a stampede mentality against sex clubs, circuit parties, and efforts to defend gay men's sexual cultures. The week following a national meeting of organizers seeking to respond to burgeoning attacks on gay men's sex cultures from within and outside gay communities, *The Times*'s Week in Review section appeared with a lead story on the topic. The title reveals the piece's obvious bias: "Gay Culture Weighs Sense and Sexuality."[28]

When letters to the editor appeared one week later, not a single letter represented viewpoints that gay men's sex cultures are worthy of preservation. One gay man expressed his disgust: "My partner and I have virtually nothing in common with the men described in this article. I cringe to think that anyone would think we might behave in those ways."[29] A spokesperson for the Human Rights

Campaign distanced gay political advocacy from gay men's sex
cultures and insist:

> For most gay urbanites, the central features of life are work-
> ing, taking care of their families and building community.
> Many lesbians and gay men are more concerned with winning
> our right to live honestly and to be safe in our homes, at work,
> and in our community.[30]

As if this were not enough, less than a month later, *The Times* ran
Larry Kramer's essay "Gay Culture, Redefined" on the op-ed page,
complete with a graphic of an angel of death with a heart on his
chest and a quotation from Kramer highlighted: "When will we
learn that promiscuity kills?"[31] In the piece, Kramer bullies AIDS
and gay organizations for failing to "speak out and condemn or
even criticize" Sex Panic, a group of New York activists attempting
to counter Kramer's ilk. He incites lesbians (whom he patronizingly
designates as the "other half of our movement") to distance themselves from gay men and, stooping to a new low by doing the dirty
work for neoconservatives, makes a case that gay men's promiscuity "will wind up costing the taxpayer a lot of extra money."[32]

Just one day later, *The Times* printed five letters to the editor
under the headline "Defenders of Promiscuity Set Back AIDS
Fight," none of which opposes Kramer's perspective. This outrageous example of the nation's newspaper of record abrogating any
responsibility for even-handedness and journalistic ethics seems
indicative of the early stages of moral panic. Alternative viewpoints
are made to look ridiculous or entirely muzzled.

Meanwhile, in a move reminiscent of other moral panics, Mayor
Giuliani ran television commercials slamming his opponent Ruth
Messinger for not falling into line and supporting his crackdown on
sex businesses.[33]

While pundits quibble about the scale of closures of sexual sites
in New York City and whether these efforts can be classified as a
full-scale sex panic, Jake Stevens and Christine Quinn of the NYC
Anti-Violence Project present statistical data showing a 62 percent
rise in reported arrests for public lewdness during the first six
months of 1997 compared to the same period of 1996.[34] Is it any

wonder some believe that a full-scale moral panic has hit New York City?

As if to make it clear that the sex-panic impulse may target lesbians and feminists as well as gay men, a women's studies conference on sexuality became the focus of intense media coverage and attacks by conservative public officials during November 1997. The State University of New York at New Paltz sponsored a conference titled "Revolting Behavior: The Challenges of Women's Sexual Freedom," which included discussion of controversial topics such as S/M, lesbianism, HIV/AIDS, and sex toys. Conservatives freaked and, in actions reminiscent of McCarthyism, one trustee publicly called for the university president's resignation, and debates flared in the press and state capitol over whether public universities should be permitted to investigate and discuss these topics. Despite the fact that less than $1,000 was spent to organize the conference, New York Governor George Pataki expressed outrage that public funds were used for the conference and demanded a plan to ensure that such conferences would never take place again on a state university campus.[35]

The sex debates are playing out differently a continent away in San Francisco. Here the controversies initially focused on the city's attempts to enforce regulations that insist sex clubs post guidelines, hire monitors, and ban cubicles (private spaces with doors). These regulations have been informally in place for about a decade, since public health officials and HIV-prevention workers faced up to the continued operation of nonbathhouse public sex venues in the city. A gay member of the Board of Supervisors, working with an advisory group of sex club owners, prevention workers, and public health advocates, attempted to introduce legislation that would simultaneously legalize the sex clubs and formalize the current regulations in 1996. Immediately, a group of "prosex" activists formed Community United for Sexual Privacy to counter the arguments of the original advisory group, oppose the formalization of certain regulations, and demand the removal of restrictions on private spaces. The group swiftly evolved into advocates for the opening of new bathhouses in San Francisco.[36]

The debates in San Francisco have been as fractious as in New York, with the letter-to-the-editor columns in the gay press filled with passionate expressions of diverse viewpoints, reflecting a divided community. Here the controversy has been played out primarily as an internal community debate among queers and the mayor has been shielded from much responsibility for the current sex club policies. Instead "pro-privacy" forces have targeted the Director of Public Health, Sandra Hernandez, a lesbian, as well as the head of the department's AIDS Office, Mitch Katz, a gay man, for promulgating the restrictions in the absence of any research data supporting their rules. An entire cabal of "homocrats," queers working within the city bureaucracy have been fingered for uniting in support of the sex club regulations, including the coordinator of lesbian and gay health, two openly-gay members of the Health Commission, and a lesbian member of the Human Rights Commission.[37]

Thus a particularly ironic case of geographic schizophrenia has emerged. While some gay men in New York City organized to force city officials to implement San Francisco-style monitoring, regulation, and punitive action against sex clubs, in San Francisco gay men's community organizing focused on forcing officials to allow the private spaces and bathhouses currently permitted in New York. Reid Condit, an activist with San Francisco's Community United for Sexual Privacy, pointed out this interesting distinction between New York and San Francisco's current sexual cultures:

> What New York does not have, or has only intermittently between crackdowns, are sex clubs as in San Francisco. While San Francisco seems more enlightened in this respect, its ban on private spaces defies any right to privacy and ignores studies that show less unsafe sex goes on in sex clubs and bathhouses than in private residences and hotel rooms.[38]

More recently, San Francisco newspapers have been filled with coverage of what some have dubbed "The Great Penis Debate." After a few stores on Castro Street featured anatomically correct dolls in their windows or advertisements for gay parties that featured a man with a prominent penis, the heterosexual female editor of a local gay newspaper editorialized against the public appearance of penises in the Castro ("Penis in the Morning: Speak Softly, and Don't Expose Your Big Stick"). News articles, letters to the editor columns, and editorial pages became filled with people checking in with a range of viewpoints about the appropriateness of penises in the neighborhood. Some gay men responded in defense of the neighborhood's sex-positive values; others represented the matter as a free speech issue; still others agreed with the editorial. Because the editor framed the initial editorial with the core question, "What does this say about us as a community?" an entire range of viewpoints on questions of assimilation, community standards, and sex-negativity appeared in response.[39]

What distinguishes the evolving sex panic in gay communities from that of a decade earlier that closed the bathhouses in San Francisco is that current critiques of gay men's sexualities and attacks on sexual spaces are now more likely to be initiated and supported by gay men, lesbians, and their allies than by mainstream journalists and nongay public officials. As activism has propelled increasing numbers of lesbians, gay men, and bisexuals into positions in municipal, county, and state government and the media, an increasingly complicated set of interests influences their public actions and writings. Some of these people feel torn between mainstream values and the liberation values that historically have been embedded in local gay communities. Others hold their authority in a manner that demands queers behave themselves like everyone else in the city or define their professionalism by setting themselves at odds with gay liberation values.

Controversies over gay men's use of commercial sex establishments and public sex spaces in most American cities during the 1980s pitted gay men largely against nongay city officials.[40] Gayle Rubin has argued that San Francisco's experience of bathhouse closures in 1984 can be seen as foreshadowing the current wave of attacks on gay male sexual spaces.[41] In San Francisco, early participation by lesbians, gay men, and bisexuals in the structures of city government and the media had created a level of gay leaders with access to the city's power brokers. The campaign to shut down bathhouses was initiated in large part by these pivotal gay insiders who garnered enough support among the city's lesbian and gay leadership to lead one gay newspaper to publish a list of "traitors" to the community on its editorial pages. While the assaults on bathhouses were supported by a politically ambitious mayor who was judgmental of gay male sexual cultures, they were resisted by a heterosexual public health director who saw closure as bad public health practice. He capitulated only when the mayor, flanked by advocates of closure from within the gay community, forced his hand.[42]

By 1997, the situation in San Francisco had changed in ways that might foreshadow other cities' future debates on commercial sex spaces. Queer public health officials seemed eager to play the lead in initiating and enforcing the privacy regulations. The mayor, who had long touted his early leadership defending sexual civil liberties, appeared to want to avoid a major public controversy over sex, and thus derailed efforts to formalize regulations through a public process, even as he tacitly supported his queer health officials as they did the dirty work. In one short decade, lesbians and gay men had gone from offering behind-the-scenes support for municipal action against sex spaces to leading the campaign for regulation or closure from formal positions within city government.

The current sex panic emerging in gay communities is often informally discussed as a simple case of sexual liberationists versus assimilationists, or queers versus homosexuals. Others have articulated this as a split between responsible gay citizens concerned for the health and well-being of the community and a core group of circuit boys, sex liberationists, and sex club habitués in deep denial about the continuing virulence of the epidemic. Still others see it as a battle between journalists and academics for the role of spokesperson for queer communities. These clean and easy groupings make good journalistic copy and offer a simple way to divide the world into good and evil, yet the contemporary situation is more complex than many accounts have acknowledged.

While the sharply different strategies advocated by diverse interests within gay communities reveal distinct values and understandings of how sexual desires are constituted and how they might appropriately be embodied and enacted, it would be easy—too easy—to narrowly characterize any of the clusters of individuals participating in the current debates. Certainly the tone of the regulation-focused crusaders can lapse into moralism and judgments. Likewise the libertarian rhetoric of the self-identified "sex-positive" defenders of commercial sex spaces can sound naive and romanticized.

Those with historical knowledge of the surveillance and disciplining of sexual dissenters in this century become alarmed when queers themselves appeal to various arms of the state to invoke their powers to police and punish. While San Franciscans, with a liberal mayor, might consider internal community debates over penises as sex panic, they are likely to be able to deter significant city involvement in such actions and avoid a massive crackdown on gay sex. A combination of factors—a conservative mayor, the regulation-focused gay activists' access to mainstream media, the creeping privatization of public spaces—leaves New Yorkers terribly vulnerable to such actions. The circulation of views by gay writers that encourage punitive action against gay men's sex spaces and drug use may provide foundational support for future crackdowns in places outside of New York City and San Francisco. While it is easy for advocates of regulation-or-closure to put their viewpoints forward in the national press and suggest them as a strategy to utilize throughout the nation, most other cities have neither a gay-positive municipal government nor gay-friendly police or health departments. This new climate may prove dangerous in the places where the fractious gay community remains largely outside the city power structure.

EMERGING MORAL PANICS THROUGHOUT THE NATION

Los Angeles may be such a city. A long, unresolved history of tensions between the police department and gay communities makes recent controversies in Los Angeles seem like a throwback to the early 1970s. Since the summer of 1996, Los Angeles has been the site of repeated police action against gay bars, cruise areas, and sex clubs. Cuffs, a Silverlake leather and Levi's bar popular with the after-hours crowd, was a focus of repeated harassment. Joseph Hanania, writing in *OUT*, described an early evening police raid on the bar:

> About 9 p.m. one Saturday night last fall, four Los Angeles police cars swooped down on Cuffs. . . . Charging in with flashlights, the officers immediately turned up the lights in the Silverlake district bar—to find dozens of men stock-still in shock around the small, U-shaped counter.

The cops were citing half a dozen patrons for lewd conduct; they were reportedly caught masturbating. "The [police] wouldn't let us know who was arrested," Dennehy says. "They cited 42 counts of lewd conduct in 45 minutes" when the bar was largely empty.[43]

Cuffs was not the only establishment targeted for harassment. Police have cited staff of gay bars for lewd conduct because they were shirtless. Bars frequented by gay men of color—the Lodge in North Hollywood, Le Barcito in Silverlake, and Club Tempo in Hollywood—have been raided; even discos have been targeted. Public cruising areas in Silverlake, West Hollywood, and Griffith Park have been targeted for stepped-up policing. A gay man who was simply and appropriately using a restroom in Griffith Park was arrested, charged with lewd conduct, and found innocent of all charges a few months later.[44]

By the fall of 1997, the city had succeeded in closing the Vortex, King of Hearts, and Basic Plumbing, three long-standing sex clubs in the city. In November, the Los Angeles City Council, after a series of town meetings accompanied by substantial media coverage, approved a variance that allowed the Barracks, a gay male sex club, to continue operating. Los Angeles Mayor Richard Riordan took the unusual step of vetoing the zoning variance against the entreaties of lesbian city councilor Jackie Goldberg, who showed leadership uncommon to many elected officials by allowing herself to be positioned in the public eye as the primary supporter of the controversial sex club.[45] The club's owners, having exhausted their financial and emotional resources, closed their business immediately following the mayor's veto.[46]

Washington, DC, has been another location where an intense crackdown on gay sex has occurred. A bathhouse opened and was immediately embroiled in controversy sparked by coverage in the gay press and *The Washington Post*. Local gay male leaders of AIDS and gay organizations were the engine driving the media attention. The Green Lantern, a gay bar, had its back room closed and its liquor license suspended. Peep shows were closed in the 9th Street area in 1996, and crackdowns have escalated on strippers and dancers in gay bars throughout the city. Police have raided a neighborhood establishment selling food and periodicals including gay sex magazines, and targeted gay clubs such as Tracks, The Edge, and the Zei Club for inspection, regulation, and punishment for violations. The escalation in harassment of gay bars led representatives of the clubs to form a Gay and Lesbian Business Guild to strategize about a united response. In the suburbs outside of Washington, twenty men were arrested in a vice sweep of an Annapolis, Maryland, video and bookstore. A gay man was arrested and charged with violating Virginia's sodomy law in his own home.[47]

In Boston, conflicts rocked the gay community in 1995, when police arrested thirty-nine men for lewd conduct in the men's restrooms at a Back Bay train station, leading one local gay paper to headline its editorial, "Bathroom sex: A relic of the 1970s." Debates flared over the gay pride parade in 1996 during which a man on stilts repeatedly flashed his genitals at the crowd and a group of Lesbian Avengers simulated sex on a rolling bed.[48] In Austin, Texas, the opening of new bathhouses has ignited contentious debates among gay organizers and AIDS groups, leading one activist to refer to the baths as "HIV-incubation factories."[49] In Miami Beach, police arrested twenty-one men and charged them with lewd and lascivious conduct in a raid on a local gay bar just a few weeks after the Versace murder and suicide of Andrew Cunanan.[50] Richard Mohr, a professor at the University of Illinois, Urbana, has documented a "marked upsurge" in arrests of gay men for "plain air sex," or sex in parks and other so-called public spaces throughout the nation, including Maryland, North Carolina, Missouri, and Nebraska.[51]

In San Antonio, the city council eliminated all funding to the Esperanza Peace and Justice Center, an arts organization with substantial gay and lesbian programming. The center had historically produced high-quality, cutting-edge arts programs including powerful analyses of race and gender and distinctly sex-positive cultural politics.[52] The attack on the San Antonio project is the latest in a long line of attacks on gay, lesbian, and bisexual artists whose work confronts sexuality counter to hetero-hegemonic ways.

Intense sensationalistic media coverage in San Diego focused on the arrest on prostitution charges of the owner of an S/M dungeon space rented out by gay men. Policing of go-go dancers and adult businesses has intensified and lewd conduct arrests have escalated in parks and beaches in the area. The city's long-standing practice of offering first-time offenders the option of pleading guilty to the lesser charge of disturbing the peace has been halted.[53]

Paralleling these debates has been a persistent outcry within gay communities over drug use among gay men. This flared most prominently during August 1996, when a group of gay activists and journalists challenged Gay Men's Health Crisis's sponsorship of The Morning Party, an annual party that draws almost 5,000 gay men to Fire Island. Arguing the prevalent use of drugs such as Ecstasy, cocaine, and Special K among partygoers necessitated a stronger response from the health advocacy organization, crusaders accused the group of promoting drug use and increasing HIV infections among gay men. Larry Kramer was quoted in *The New York Times* about his experiences at the Morning Party two years earlier:

> I was pretty shocked. . . . It was as if AIDS had never happened and I was back in 1974 again. The drugs were rampant and so was the sexuality of it all, the hedonism. I was ashamed of GMHC's affiliation with it.[54]

GMHC leaders refused to withdraw from the event, sending out a letter that stated:

> GMHC helps people address their substance use, not encourage or ignore it. It's a fantasy to think that GMHC's withdrawal from the Morning Party would strike a meaningful blow against alcohol and drug use.[55]

This incident brought out repeated calls for gay and AIDS organizations to distance themselves from such parties and not allow the events to raise money for their groups.[56] Gabriel Rotello wrote:

> You'd think that since intoxication and substance abuse are among the primary reported reasons gay men slip up and get infected, AIDS groups would be deeply concerned that these parties are proliferating. . . . Why is it that in the gay world, where almost half the urban male population is dead or sick from an epidemic closely associated with substance use, there

is still such ambivalence about drugs that AIDS organizations profess to see nothing wrong with raising money from events that glamorize drug use? Why, despite the bitter legacy of AIDS, do we continue assuring ourselves that being gay means we have to be totally nonjudgmental about the very things that have wiped us out?[57]

While the Morning Party in 1996 captured a great deal of media attention and raised the long-simmering debate about drug use among gay men to a fever pitch, other incidents highlight growing community divisions concerning substance use. Community forums sponsored by gay and AIDS organizations in several cities, under titles such as "Ecstasy: What Every User Should Know," "Sex, Drugs, and Rock and Roll," "Ain't No Gay Man High Enough," and "Crystal Use in the Gay Community" have become locations for energetic discussion among starkly divided audiences.[58] The publication of Michelangelo Signorile's book brought out a range of responses to its polemical antidrug message and its characterization of extreme substance use at circuit parties, including some who challenged his views. In *Electric Dreams* (an e-mail magazine), Alan Brown wrote:

> Ultimately, much of Signorile's criticism rings hollow, because it gets lost in the cacophony of guilt and shame that we have slowly and steadfastly learned to ignore. When the sirens fade and the real healing and prevention work begins anew, it will be time to reconcile tough questions from a loving and constructive platform: When does recreational drug use cease being recreational? How can we more effectively disseminate information about drugs—not to promote their use, but to explain their risks and to help prevent abuse? . . . How can we teach young men and women not to go overboard with sex and drugs? How can we preserve and broaden the notion of gay celebration? When can the shame end, and dignity begin?[59]

Community activism in support of the use of marijuana for medicinal purposes has been the focus of whispered, behind-the-scenes criticism by some advocates for a clean and sober gay community, and an editorial in the gay press in support of such marijuana use brought on a letter from one reader that, in Nancy Reagan fashion, stated "Just say no works in the end."[60] In San Francisco, police infiltration and attacks on the group spearheading distribution of marijuana for medicinal purposes have been rumored to be led by openly gay officers.

In the past, when gay men's sex spaces and drug use were increasingly targets of state action, defenders could usually count on a fairly unified community to respond energetically. In the late 1990s, this is no longer the case: communities appear increasingly divided on questions of gay male sex and substance use practices. On the surface, this rift seems caused by different understandings of the role community organizations should play as moral judges of the social practices of its members, and a profoundly different understanding of ways to effect changes in the behaviors of individuals. While this may reveal long-standing differences in values and health strategies, throughout most of the 1970s and 1980s such differences were usually kept within the community. Part of the legacy of increased queer participation in the media and formal governmental structures of urban life is that queers increasingly begin to function as cooperating or catalytic cogs in the machinery regulating queer sex and drug-using practices.

SCAPEGOATING CIRCUIT BOYS

Scapegoating requires two primary tools: (1) a population that can be identified and fingered as bearing primary responsibility for the current problem plaguing society; (2) a theory that explains why the population is a threat.

Gabriel Rotello's 1997 book *Sexual Ecology: AIDS and the Destiny of Gay Men* may be serving as the "science" fueling the moral panic within gay communities over the occasional protests of its author. Utilizing concepts from ecology and the environmental movement, Rotello argues that post-Stonewall gay men have upset the balance of nature by creating cultures that support promiscuity and sexual versatility. To his mind this has made gay men into a sitting target for a host of microbes that might easily invade and saturate the population. Even if a cure or vaccine for AIDS appears,

Rotello argues, other plagues will appear and rapidly take hold through the sexual encounters of gay men.[61]

Rotello's book has been embraced and criticized by many.[62] I share his concern for community and his analysis that cultures that support unprotected anal sex with multiple partners are likely to face many health challenges. I also agree with his belief that we are not prisoners of culture and that gay men can successfully alter the social, cultural, and sexual worlds we inhabit. While I do not share some of my colleagues' beliefs that Rotello is antisex, I do believe his analysis is wrong and his writings are being used to fuel repressive actions that undermine public health.

The polemical features of a book purporting to be objective science, Rotello's inability to acknowledge all science as impure and loaded with biases, and the lack of balance in a book ostensibly about ecology contribute to the book's potential misuse. A forum held by Boston's AIDS Action Committee to discuss the book was somehow granted the title, "Did Gay Sex Cause the AIDS Epidemic?"[63] There is evidence that the book is being put to use by external antigay forces in the evolving sex panic, despite the protests of its author.[64] I was horrified to watch the Sunday morning television news show *This Week* on the morning after President Clinton spoke at a Human Rights Campaign (HRC) dinner in Washington, and hear former Education Secretary William Bennett throw Rotello's book in the face of HRC Executive Director Elizabeth Birch. In a move foreshadowed by Larry Kramer, Bennett then assailed Birch and other gay leaders for refusing to acknowledge and criticize the promiscuity of gay men and hold them responsible for the continuing AIDS epidemic.[65]

Although authors do not control the ways in which our words are used (or misused), we are responsible for carefully considering the political context in which our work appears and doing our best to choose our words carefully. Rotello's discussion of the role of "core groups" in "sexual ecosystems" lays the groundwork for the kind of scapegoating that emerges in moral panics. He defines a core group as "a collection of people who, because of a variety of circumstances, suffer from and transmit STDs at much higher rates than the rest of the population."[66] These people "have significantly higher numbers of partners than those outside," and, Rotello explains, "those partners also have significantly higher numbers of partners *within the core*, creating a kind of biological feedback loop that is primed to magnify disease." This explains how the core group itself becomes saturated with a sexually transmitted disease, but not how a broader population is affected. Rotello solves this dilemma by discussing the "bridging" or linkages that develop and spread the disease "between core group members and those outside."[67]

To his credit, Rotello acknowledges how important it is "to tread carefully around the concept of core groups." He writes:

> To accuse a group of people of contributing to the spread of disease is a powerful way to stigmatize, placing that group in the position of the contaminating Other. . . . In the case of gay men and AIDS, there have been continuous attempts to treat the entire gay male population as a contaminating core, and even within the gay world there has sometimes been a tendency to "blame" the AIDS epidemic on the promiscuous, the denizens of sex clubs, the HIV-positive, and so on.[68]

Yet this is precisely how this book and its marshaling of the core group concept are being deployed both within gay communities and by antigay forces. Michelangelo Signorile makes use of the concept to scapegoat circuit boys. Despite his insistence that "There are in fact many core groups driving the epidemic in the gay population and they are not all white and middle class," Signorile's writings about HIV transmission have almost entirely targeted this narrow subculture.[69] No other gay male "core group" has emerged within popular queer discourse to share the burden of HIV transmission with the circuit boys. Furthermore, Rotello has not protested the increasing representation of circuit boys as "the contaminating other."

This is how scapegoating works. Rotello and Signorile can point to passages and qualifiers in their books to insist they are not engaging in a process of demonization, but the overall understandings that emerge from their work result in the trivialization of complexity, stereotyping of a diverse population, and scapegoating of practices that provide a necessary tool to moral panic. Thus powerful anxieties circulating within social groups are projected onto a single population that is then blown up into larger-than-life demons whose punishment will serve as warning and protection to the broader community. Without a scapegoated population, the fears would continue to circulate until serious confrontation with the true sources of the problem are identified, understood, and remedied.

All writers do not characterize the circuit in this way. Alan Brown is one of the few chroniclers of the circuit scene who examines its sociopolitical dimensions. In an essay on the 1997 Mardi Gras weekend party in Sydney, Brown writes:

> The most beautiful men in the world are gay, and a lot of them love to party. This simple and shocking fact is an essential ingredient in the psychological soufflé that fuels the party phenomenon. The sight of several thousand gorgeous men turning it out on the dance floor is a potent image for participants, critics, and even detached observers of the party world. Notwithstanding the perfectly natural run-of-the-mill insecurity that almost everyone feels when caught in a room full of real and imagined models, the view of a hot dance floor debunks the effeminate gay stereotype and incites a far more threatening notion (among straights, mostly) that a lot of really handsome, strong men were not at all designed for procreation, and that some of these men actually revel in their gayness.[70]

Men who attend circuit parties have been granted the dubious distinction of serving as scapegoats for the current sex panic emerging within gay communities. In retrospect, this might have been predicted. Commonly seen as young, white, muscular, affluent, and hedonistic, they are excised from the daily fabric of their lives and fixed permanently in one of three sites: the circuit event, the gym, or the sex club. They party, dance, and sex. They become men without jobs, families, meaningful friendships, or cultural or political concerns. They inhabit the streets of the gay ghetto, flaunting their bodies, giving off attitude, and making other gay men feel inadequate.[71]

Why has a single, narrow population inhabiting one of many mass sites of collective convergence in gay communities nationwide been targeted in this way? At least three factors contribute to this dynamic. (1) Confronting the complex factors that contribute to significant substance abuse and unsafe sex within many subpopulations of gay men is a daunting process. Projecting the problem onto a single group and labeling them as miscreant bad boys before the general gay population is easier and does not upset the status quo. (2) It is one thing to engage in transgressive sexual and substance using acts. It is another thing entirely to do so without obvious signs of guilt, regret, or embarrassment. (3) To many people, particularly many midlife gay men, boys on the circuit have the audacity to dance and party in the middle of a crisis. How can they celebrate freedom and sexuality in the midst of the epidemic?

One other factor that contributes to the demonization of circuit boys is highlighted in Signorile's book as the "cult of masculinity." Signorile writes that a cult "revolves around an obsessive devotion to a principle, a belief—in this case a rigidly defined physical ideal of 'masculinity'—that followers see as a source of control over their present lives as well as their future happiness."[72] He then takes extreme examples of circuit queens obsessed with muscles, drugs, and sex and uses them to denigrate an entire population. This allows him to mistake culture for cult. Following his example, any gay subculture that has obsessive adherents might be disrespectfully tagged as cultish and have the complex meanings of its participants simplistically reduced and discounted. It's almost as if we are all encouraged to say, "The social worlds I occupy are cultures; those I dislike, fear, or feel cut out of, are cults."

The iconography of hypermasculinity embraced on the circuit includes features that have been considered problematic among activist gays for many years. I recently saw a billboard for Titan Video's *Naked Escape*, a gay male porn movie, displayed on a bus station in my neighborhood. The advertisement featured two butch muscle men, complete with tattoos and relatively hairy chests. Someone had scrawled over the advertisement in thick black marker, "How about less straight-acting, less self-hating, more self-loving, more queen-acting?"[73]

Circuit boys are purported to ape a specific form of masculinity resonant with macho values of fierce independence, profound arrogance, and unquenchable desire for bigger muscles and ever more intense sex. Because many gay men grew up victimized by other boys and men and mocked as sissies, a profound distrust of conventional masculinities pervades community life.[74] When gender is played with as a parody, it is acceptable. When a muscular man with traditional manly appearance talks and moves like a queen, it is almost acceptable. But when a gay man fits traditional masculine conventions entirely, he is likely to be seen by some as self-hating, antigay, or less authentically queer.[75]

In an article titled "Circuit Queen for a Day," Peter McQuaid visits the White Party in Palm Springs, and describes the men:

> At least half these so-called circuit gods aren't intrinsically beautiful. They're tan; they have good haircuts; they have nice clothes; and, most intrinsic to the equation, fabulous bodies. Big or small, they've clearly put in a lot of gym time, just said no to sundaes, and perhaps yes to nandrolone and testosterone cypionate.[76]

Yet many circuiteers talk and move like queens. Once immersed in party culture, it becomes clear that a variety of masculinities are performed and negotiated within the circuit. Only a cursory glance allows for a superficial impression that circuit boys as a group conform to narrow hegemonic masculinity. How much easier it is to identify patriarchal abuses in men with muscles than to do so in queer academic circles or amid gay male journalists or drag queens! Yet populations of gay men who embody traditional masculinities—leathermen, bears, the gym crowd, and circuit boys—have served as routes of entry into gay community for many working-class men.[77] One friend, raised in a working-class Irish family in Massachusetts, recently told me that, if he hadn't discovered Chaps, a Boston bar populated in the 1970s and early 1980s by clones of the period, he would never have come out of the closet. When he visited other gay bars, he saw men with whom he could neither identify nor to whom he felt attracted.

I find it ironic that critics become transfixed by the muscles of men on the circuit and ridicule these men's participation in gym culture. One other subcultural category of which I am a member, middle-aged Jewish men, is repeatedly visited with warnings about diet and exercise and the fear of heart disease that have plagued our kind for years. This group is chided for becoming overweight and not exercising while the gay men on the circuit are criticized for being lean and muscular and spending too much time at the gym. Signorile provides extreme examples of circuit men obsessed with their pecs, addicted to a life of steroids, and never satisfied with their size. But there is no evidence that these men are typical of those who participate in life on the circuit. Few contemporary observers appear happy to find a population of men in their late twenties, thirties, and forties committed to being physically fit.

Yet another source of the scapegoating of circuit boys may rest in gay men's long-standing tendency to be hypercritical of ourselves and our community. Sometimes this has emerged from an intense need for things from community that could never be fulfilled, and at other times from the societal homophobia that is bred into us throughout our youth. These intense judgments of gay male cultures take several forms, as is clear from letters to the editor in the gay press. One man wrote to *OUT:*

> Let's face the simple truth about the rise in steroid use. It's not that gay men want to look like the Nazi image of a manly man, or because they hate womyn: the simple fact is pure and unadulterated narcissism. What a sad commentary on those parts of the community that can only accept a physical facade that leaves the inner person empty and wanting.[78]

A young gay man from Cleveland wrote to *The Advocate:*

> I'm 28 years old and have never experienced a gay world without the threat of AIDS. Leave it to self-indulgent, irresponsible queers to behave in a way that brought on this epidemic to begin with. Do me a favor: Cut off the protease inhibitors, put them out of our misery, and serve the cocktail to some deserving soul.[79]

Disgust for other gay men has appeared throughout the post-Stonewall period, targeting at different times the gay hippies, early gay libbers, effeminate gay men, leathermen, drag queens, and Castro/Christopher Street clones. Any group of gay men who identify themselves in opposition to the broader community is likely to become a target for broad communal enmity.

This is increasingly prevalent as many people within gay and lesbian communities assimilate into mainstream culture and distance themselves from the seedier types. A letter to the editor in *The New York Times*, in response to its coverage of Andrew Cunanan and the murder of Gianni Versace, illustrates this dynamic:

> It's important for the public to know that Andrew P. Cunanan represented the seedier side of gay life, not the norm. I am a forty-three-year-old gay man who has been in a loving, monogamous relationship for twenty-one years. We lead an everyday life like any married couple. Neither of us has ever partied in South Beach, been to a bath house or taken illegal drugs. Mr. Cunanan had as much in common with ordinary, decent gay Americans as a man from Mars.[80]

In a moral panic triggered by continuing HIV infections among gay men, the circuit crowd seems currently positioned as the scapegoat. Seen as a uniform group of affluent white men suffering neither race nor class oppression, their position of relative privilege only positions them more visibly as a target. This is especially likely to occur in the absence of a deep understanding of the subculture that could be gained from rich, ethnographic study. While some of the writers who scapegoat circuit culture acknowledge attending parties and fly-in weekends, none have engaged in systematic empirical research seeking to probe the meanings of the social practices of the circuit.

Yet research on this subculture does exist. A detailed study by Lynette Lewis and Michael Ross, titled *A Select Body: The Gay Dance Party Subculture and the HIV/AIDS Pandemic*,[81] was published in 1995 and focuses on parties in Sydney, Australia. The book offers insightful analyses of the relationship between homophobia, HIV/AIDS, and the historical role of community rituals of dance. By allowing a cross-section of dance party habitués to speak for themselves, the authors succeed in presenting a rich portrait of a complicated social structure and avoid glossing over problematic features or simplistically reducing complex phenomena.

The qualitative methods utilized in the study allow for a nuanced understanding of the meanings that emerge from circuit sites:

> The respondents suggested that many gay men sought validation of their identity within the context of the dance parties

because of the dominant culture's rigid opposition to their radical transformations of social prescriptions related to sex, death and drugs. . . . Many gay men have been continuously reminded of the need for self-control in one of the most important areas of their lives: their sexuality. For many of the respondents it was like walking on a tight-rope, particularly if they had used psychoactive substances that removed them from their everyday responsibilities and awareness of safe-sex guidelines.[82]

Rarely have American gay writers discussed relationships between mass circuit events and gay identities, nor have they elucidated the relationship between the self-control demanded of gay men and the need to let go of control. Instead we default to discussions of "personal responsibility" and insist that, whatever "extenuating circumstances" exist, adults bear ultimate responsibility for their actions. The approach of these Australian authors doesn't seek to blame or absolve from blame; rather they seek to uncover the diverse social and cultural forces out of which emerges the circuit scene.

The authors include in their analysis a cross-cultural look at how many populations have made use of dance rituals to shift beyond the crisis state:

A culture in crisis often develops rites or social structures in an effort to re-empower itself, particularly when the established paradigm fails to contain or subjugate the life-threatening crisis, such as the current medico-scientific paradigm and the HIV/AIDS pandemic. The dance party milieu is a social structure where gay men may derive positive reinforcement for their identity, meet potential partners and ventilate their accumulated stress and anxiety over HIV/AIDS-related issues. . . . The greater the loss of control among a subculture in crisis (such as the increased risk of HIV infection among party patrons) the higher the drug consumption. Although the drugs the party patrons use (such as Ecstasy) are relatively new compounds, the optimism they endow is ancient. The consumption of intoxicants is perennial and universal for the transformation of perception and emotion, particularly among a culture facing a life-threatening crisis.[83]

Perhaps most useful to the current debates about unprotected sex and drug use by American gay men are the authors' suggestions for interventions that might assist dance party patrons with safer sex and drug use:

> First, the patrons should be taught the technique of cognitively "pre-programming" their memory by keeping a "little corner in [their] mind very straight," following their use of psychoactive substances within the context of the dance party institution. Second, they need to learn how to negotiate safer-sexual guidelines with a potential sexual partner in an open and honest manner . . . rather than relying on flawed symbols, such as the "straighter-than-straight" identity symbol. Third, the dance party and recovery party venues should openly reinforce safer-sexual behavior by reminding their patrons about the importance of safe-sexual and drug-related behaviour via a wide range of context-related media.[84]

Rather than scapegoat the subculture, these scholars have approached their research with the intent of understanding the complexity of the party scene and grasping the diverse meanings that gay men forge through participation. Drug use, unsafe sex, masculinities, and gay identity are scrutinized deeply in this book. This allows the authors to provide no easy answers and no simple solutions; instead, they take a long-term approach to issues of health and safety.

My discussion of the circuit is not intended to deny issues within the cultures of circuit parties and muscle boy gyms that merit concern. I share the belief that leaders within circuit culture (producers, writers, deejays) ought to assist partygoers with developing a critical awareness of sexual practices, masculinities, interpersonal relations, and the use of substances, including drugs, alcohol, and steroids. While I have seen no evidence that indicates most circuiteers who use substances are unable to do so without becoming addicts or damaging themselves, this is one of several gay male cultures that

exhibit an amount of prominent drug use that merits continuing
critical examination and significant public education.

My previous book, *Reviving the Tribe*, has been embraced by
many men who participate in circuit events. Men who attended the
Saint-at-Large White Party in New York City in February 1997
report "a white banner unfurled onstage at one of the party's peaks,"
proclaiming "Revive the Tribe."[85] An article by Christian Hart,
PhD, titled "The Circuit: Drugged-Out Party Boys, or Neo-Tribal
Spirituality," which appeared in *Circuit Noize*, the quarterly publication of the circuit scene, quotes from the book and uses my
analysis of celebration and dance as key elements of community
regeneration to argue that the parties "have become at once an escape
from the plague and a way of meeting the needs of those who require
our care."[86] I am glad circuiteers find my work useful, but nowhere
do I argue that the events need to be effective AIDS fundraisers to
justify their existence. At the same time, attacks on AIDS organizations' sponsorship of these events seem misguided to me.

I do not believe, however, that wholesale scapegoating that
comes from a place of crisis and panic assists members of any
subculture in developing critical consciousness. Instead, subcultures develop oppositional stances and social processes that lead to
isolation and alienation; a dangerous, polarizing dynamic emerges.
This sets in motion the precise processes by which the isolated and
scapegoated group is pathologized, blamed, and eventually punished for crimes that are not of their making.

A similar dynamic has emerged that scapegoats one particular
sexual practice, now known as "barebacking" or "raw sex." Prior
to 1996, this practice was known simply as "unprotected anal sex."
Few men talked publicly about their own participation in such
activity. Then a series of articles appeared, often of a confessional
nature, that placed into the public sphere gay men's accounts of
fucking without condoms.[87] Stephen Gendin wrote a controversial
piece in *POZ* titled "Riding Bareback" which began:

A year and a half ago at a conference, I heard a talk by a
really cute positive guy on the fun of unsafe sex with other
positive guys. He was beautiful, the subject was exciting, and I

soon ended up getting fucked by him without a condom. When he came inside me, I was in heaven, just overjoyed.[88]

While Gendin discusses issues of reinfection, multidrug-resistant viruses, and exposure to other sexually transmitted diseases, letters to the editor in response to the piece expressed outrage at his article. One writer described the piece as "selfish, specious musings," accusing him of "preaching" a kind of "kamikaze sex code."[89] Another wrote that he felt "disgusted and saddened," by Gendin's article, and insisted "Unless you're on a suicide mission, protection is absolutely necessary."[90] The author of an article in a San Francisco gay paper chided him, "Mr. Gendin, I would like to suggest that you conduct your sex life as if your life depends on it. BECAUSE IT DOES."[91]

Within a short period of time, unprotected anal sex was discussed as an erotically charged, premeditated act, and accounts began appearing of HIV-positive men who were gleefully fucking one another without condoms at invitation-only parties. Next, orgies supposedly became popular, for men of both antibody statuses to enjoy "raw" sex together. "Barebacking" became a subject of widespread debate, took on heightened erotic charge and cultural cachet, and was increasingly cited as the cause of the continuing epidemic among gay men.[92]

Instead of seeing everyday, run-of-the-mill unprotected anal sex as the primary activity resulting in HIV transmission among gay men (certainly transmission occurs through the sharing of needles, anal sex where condoms fail, and, occasionally, oral sex), people see the barebacking parties and men who cruise the Internet seeking raw sex as *the* culprits transmitting HIV. We reduce our judgments toward other incidents of unprotected anal sex, and reserve our strongest condemnation for those that occur within barebacking parties. Like circuit boys, the group most frequently linked to this practice, barebacking becomes a convenient screen onto which gay men are asked to project all our anxious, confused, and angry feelings and let them loose in self-righteous expressions of shock and horror. This is precisely how scapegoating works.

A POST-AIDS PERSPECTIVE
ON CONTINUING INFECTIONS

Some of us are not panicking about continuing HIV infections among gay men. We do not experience them as a crisis or believe they are evidence that something is terribly wrong in gay male cultures. They do not make us feel shame or embarrassment about gay men as a class or diminish our achievements of the past fifteen years in responding to HIV/AIDS. We do not believe they indicate the ethics of sexual liberation are misguided. This does not mean we are unconcerned about gay men's health or do not believe there are problematic aspects of the various subcultures comprising gay communities throughout the nation.

By considering gay men's sex thoughtfully and without knee-jerk condemnation, many of us are accused of encouraging or romanticizing unprotected anal sex. Anyone who fails to fall into line and spout the hollow rhetoric of the new gay moralizers is seen as an advocate for HIV transmission. In an especially malicious attack on Sex Panic, an informal network of people working to provide understandings of gay men's sex cultures different from the Kramer/Signorile/Rotello representation, Log Cabin Republicans Executive Director Richard Tafel wrote,

> These men pretend that the gay community hasn't been decimated by AIDS, using the language of freedom and individual rights to justify sexual behavior that can be deadly. . . . Fulfilling their own need for victim status, they imagine themselves under assault for being gay, with thoughtless unsafe sex complete with HIV infection as the ultimate liberation. Their callous selfishness has the potential to guide another generation of gay young men toward potentially deadly choices.[93]

I am involved in Sex Panic and was an organizer of a conference Tafel refers to throughout his essay. This is a gross mischaracterization of our work, yet I can understand Tafel's inability to understand our work and our analysis of HIV and gay men's sex. He is yet another impassioned voice repeating the safe-sex mantra and ordering us back into the state-of-emergency mind-set. In an appalling action reminiscent of the McCarthy Period, Tafel and his group called on "every gay and lesbian organization in the country" to join in denouncing the group which "romanticizes sexual behavior that could lead to death." The wholesale condemnation of a small group of activists whom he either does not know or willfully mischaracterizes is a frightening move. If a full-scale moral panic hits, I would be surprised if Republican gay men—particularly those from a libertarian tradition who are among the gay men most staunchly supporting sexual liberation values—aren't included among the victims.

The crisis construct that underlies much of the panic over sex and drugs in gay communities must be understood in its historical context. The narrative that has taken hold in the mind of America claims gay men in the mid-1980s made dramatic changes in their sexual practices in response to the hazards of AIDS. Once the alarms were sounded, men called the party to a close, stopped much of their promiscuous sex, and focused on taking care of their sick friends and building community health organizations. Safe sex education is credited fully with bringing down the rate of newly infected men in the mid-1980s.

The narrative goes on to explain that gay men behaved themselves throughout the 1980s but, as the epidemic proved tenacious, began to "relapse" into unsafe practices as the 1990s dawned. Thus a "second wave" of gay AIDS cases emerged prominently on the scene, composed predominantly of young gay men who somehow had not been successfully reached with effective safe sex messages.

In *Reviving the Tribe*, I critique this narrative and insist this is a romanticized, sociologically and historically unsound explanation that, while satisfying many gay men's need to appear as the epidemic version of the teacher's pet, would come full-circle and cause tremendous damage.[94] Instead, I argue the mid-1980s was a conflicted sexual wasteland, brought on by the shock of the epidemic on our communal psyche and body politic, and triggered most intensely by men's personal experiences with deaths and the arrival of mass HIV testing in 1985. Men did not simply stop having unprotected anal sex and begin using condoms; they ceased most of their sexual activity and entered an era that included long periods of celibacy, intense binges of sexual release, and withdrawal into supposedly monogamous relationships. Infections fell off for two primary reasons in addition to the advent of safe sex education: (1) men had much less sex; (2) a large portion of the men who enjoyed getting fucked had already been infected.

I do not subscribe to the view that a second wave of gay AIDS has emerged in the 1990s. Instead, infections occurred throughout the late 1980s, albeit at a reduced rate due to the saturation of the gay male population that occurred earlier in the decade, and the infections of the new decade should have been anticipated as younger men entered gay communal life.

A number of studies have been brandished to claim that 50 percent of the gay men currently aged eighteen to thirty will be infected by the time they turn forty.[95] Yet the data from these studies have been used in questionable ways (I have been guilty of this myself in earlier writings). For example, Richard Elovitch, Director of HIV Prevention at Gay Men's Health Crisis, recently published an open letter to the gay community titled "Four Percent and Counting . . . " in which he writes:

> It is intolerable that a generation of young gay men now growing up are becoming infected with HIV at a rate of up to 4 percent a year. That may sound low to you, but at that rate, one half of the gay men who are now eighteen years old will be infected by the time they turn thirty.[96]

Elovich and others take data from studies that have found a single year in which 2 percent or 4 percent of this cohort seroconvert in San Francisco and New York City, and simply multiplied by twelve years (the number of years between eighteen and thirty) to conclude that 50 percent will be infected by the time they turn thirty. This is an improper use of the data for a number of reasons: these studies do not indicate whether this level of seroconversion is typical or unusual, so extrapolating to 4 percent (the highest figure in any study I could find) *every year for twelve years* seems wrong; such conclusions do not factor into the analysis the saturation of a population and that many gay men do not practice anal intercourse; these studies are limited to New York and San Francisco and the data have not been replicated at this same level in other cities. While "Four Percent and Counting" certainly is an attention-grabbing title for the piece, misusing the data in a manner intended to stir up feelings of continuing crisis mars an otherwise thoughtful piece about new directions for gay men's AIDS prevention. Can't prevention leaders find options other than the crisis construct to use in generating interest and involvement by gay men? Is it possible to be satisfied with the gradual diminution of HIV rates in successive gay male generational cohorts? Or is total elimination the only goal that will satisfy us?

It feels difficult to balance a sense of sadness that *any* gay men continue to become infected in the 1990s with the reality that plagues do not end suddenly and swiftly. I continue to believe that displacing the utopian vision of prevention is critically important to the well-being of gay men. As I wrote three years ago:

> If 80 percent of the at-risk population of epicenter city gay men from the early 1980s have been infected, and one-third of the following generation of at-risk queer men are expected to be infected by the time they are thirty (and many additional men might be expected to be infected before reaching the age of fifty), it is a suitable objective to aim to bring the rate of infection under 30 percent within three gay generations (approximately the year 2030)?[97]

If we created this narrative of gay heroism in the 1980s, fabricating politically useful explanations for the decline in new infections in order to win public sympathy and gain funding for AIDS services, we should not be surprised that it has come around to confront us just a few years later. If a vaccine or cure had appeared, perhaps a rethinking of the epidemiology of the 1980s would not have been necessary. Without such assistance, the heroic narrative of the first decade of AIDS couldn't help but be transfigured into a demonic narrative in the second decade.

Many people, clinging to the "Best Little Boy" story of gay communities in the 1980s, cannot fit gay men's contemporary sex and drug-use practices alongside that rapidly fading narrative. Those who have resisted romanticizing gay men's response during the early years of the epidemic and avoided seeing gay men as the superheroes we became through the lenses of the media, are more likely to consider current patterns of drug use and sexual activity without shock, horror, or blame for any particular subcultures. This is one post-AIDS perspective on continuing gay male HIV infections: we are neither untouched, wracked with horror, nor filled with shame when we hear of incidents of unprotected anal sex that occur between partners of different antibody statuses. Instead, we see our aim as diligently and gradually reducing the level of HIV infection over a period of decades. We are in this work for the long haul and bring a balanced perspective to our review of epidemiological data.

Part of this post-AIDS perspective involves a commitment to supporting both the health of the community and the continuing diverse ways gay men construct their sexual identities and practices. While some would consider these as paradoxical or contradictory aims, I see them as interrelated. Thus it is critically important for people committed to the continuing centrality of desires, bodies, and masculinities in gay community life to create a broad and sex-positive gay agenda of health and wellness. Our concerns would not be fixated solely or primarily on deterring HIV infection but would be concerned about health—including sexual health—more broadly. This has long been an important part of the project of gay liberation. As Douglas Crimp has written:

> We demanded the fundamental right to experience sexual pleasure as an ethical human ideal in and of itself. This was part of the wider movement for sexual liberation that fought for the rights of all people to enjoy consensual sex, regardless of their relation to the institution of marriage or the propagating of the species. We thus took part in the ongoing radical historical shift from understanding sex as serving the purpose of procreation to understanding sex as fulfilling the human need for pleasure.[98]

One of the unfortunate legacies of allowing a limited understanding of gay men's health to dominate the community agenda for almost two decades, and allowing AIDS to be a catchall metaphor for gay men's health, is that our valuing of sex and attention to sexual health have been greatly narrowed.[99] Once the state-of-emergency communal mind-set has arisen, unprotected anal sex becomes an issue of debate solely around HIV transmission. Men who are already HIV positive are cautioned to continue using condoms primarily to avoid "reinfection," a concept whose possibility continues to be debated among medical researchers.[100] Other health concerns such as hepatitis, gonorrhea, syphilis, and other sexually transmitted diseases rarely appear prominently on the community agenda.

Historically, gay men have been willing to take many risks to fulfill their desires for specific sexual acts with other men. Men have risked loss of jobs, loss of families, and loss of life. This should tell us something. For many, sex is about much more than the simple pleasure invoked by a touch of the mouth, a finger up the butt, a squeeze of the nipple, or the taste of testicles. As Ilan Meyer has aptly observed, "Gay sex is also about identity."[101] While identities are mutable, and shift and change daily, many gay men also believe our identities as sexual beings are worth preserving. We have spent most of the past two decades attempting to balance concerns about sexual health with the enactment of desires. We are unwilling to sacrifice either, though at times we are willing to creatively modify both.

Those of us defending gay male sex cultures are not indifferent to HIV-prevention efforts. Many of us are leaders in both areas. We know that effective prevention is built on sexual empowerment and believe that decades of public health research show that tactics of guilt, fear, and repression exacerbate public health crises rather than deter them.[102] It is precisely because many people have become frustrated with HIV prevention and feel at a loss to chart new directions for our work that the time is ripe for an escalation of support for coercive measures to stop gay men's sex.

Those standing up for sexual freedom are neither lost in a romanticized vision of the golden age of the 1970s, nor dick-hungry men who are selfishly seeking more power and more privilege, as our critics have claimed. We have been condescendingly characterized as immature children who haven't grown up and who need to get with the times, put our pricks back in our pants, and apply our energies to the real challenges facing our communities, like gays in the military and gay marriage. Yet even a cursory look at the histories of our movement will show that sexual liberation has been inextricably bound with gay liberation, the women's movement, and the emancipation of youth.[103] Among the most effective ways of oppressing a people is through the colonization of their bodies, the stigmatizing of their desires, and the repression of their erotic energies.[104] Continuing work on sexual liberation is crucial to social justice efforts.

Those taking action to monitor, de-track, and resist the emerging sex panic find ourselves increasingly at odds with mainstream gay efforts to present a sanitized vision of our people and replace butch/ femme dykes with Heather and her two mommies, and kinky gay men with domestic partner wedding cakes. Can we not advocate for a pluralistic queer culture in which we affirm everyone's right to self-determination in the ways they organize their sexual relations and construct their kinship patterns?

Individuals dubious about sex panic and mainstream gay groups which are frightened to support these issues should remember that when moral panics flare, history has shown, in Lillian Hellman's words, it's "scoundrel time" and there are limited roles from which social actors can choose.[105] There are the scoundrels who blow the whistle, point the finger, name the names. There are the resistors who take the risk, go out on a limb, take the fall, and get trampled in the mindless stampede. And there are the vast masses who find themselves locked in silence by confusion, misgivings, self-protection, ambivalence, and fear. When the panic is over and attention has shifted to other issues, when we all shake our heads and say, "How did we ever let it get to that stage?," these people are complicit in the destruction. There is no neutral here. Hence, regardless of perspective, all should:

1. Stand up firmly against any efforts that mobilize arms of the state to restrict the right of sexual and reproductive self-determination. Do not invite the police, public health officials, or the media to monitor and close down gay sex spaces due to continuing HIV infections.
2. Refuse to cast off any section of our community in order to gain privileges and social acceptance. Demand a continuing commitment to a pluralistic vision of community. Resist scapegoating subcultures you do not know and understand.
3. Try to understand the historic role sex cultures have played in the formation of queer identities and communities and resist seeing them simply as an unfortunate by-product of antigay oppression. Are our sex cultures evidence of our historic

stigmatization, abuse, and reprobation? Or, to borrow James Baldwin's language about a different matter, can they be understood as "cultural patterns coming into existence by means of brutal necessity," and can they be seen as strategies for survival?[106]

Perhaps the real trouble with gay men's sex cultures is that they alone give testimony to the fact that gay men as a class have not completely assimilated into that vast melting pot of America.

Contrary to the rantings of the Larry Kramers of the world, we are aware that our entire identities are not focused on our erotic desires and our cultures are focused—not solely on sex but also on spirituality, love, genderplay, and political action. Contrary to the exaggerated claims of Michelangelo Signorile, we do not see any identifiable group standing out as the cause of continuing infections among gay men, and we will not participate in demonizing individuals, groups, or specific spaces. Contrary to the views of Gabriel Rotello, we believe that we are already making progress in bringing down the level of infection among gay men, and we are not panicked by the realization that, absent a vaccine, this is likely to take many decades.

A VISIT TO LEATHER BUDDIES

I wasn't sure I wanted to go out on a rainy November night. My lover was out of town and I was getting fidgety at home until a friend called and reminded me that "Leather Buddies," the once-a-month sex party for leather pigs, was occurring that evening. Weighing the attractiveness of a warm bed and good book against the stormy weather and good sexual encounter, I immediately went to my closet and pulled together an outfit with sufficient leather to allow me to pass muster with the dress code and get me past the front door into the South of Market sex club. I was going out on the town!

To my delight, the place was jumping when I arrived at 10 o'clock. I checked my coat, stripped off my shirt, and entered the sex rooms in leather vest, arm and wrist bands, black 501 jeans, and my tall black boots, acquired at a clothing store for police officers.

As I walked slowly through the club, allowing my eyes time to adjust to the dimness, I came across various friends and acquaintances: a buff boy from the gym who was unusually friendly, a hot daddy who, on closer inspection, turned out to be a famous dermatologist active in gay political causes, and my friend Vince who treats sex club attendance like twelve-step meetings and refuses to divulge who he's sighted during his frequent visits South of Market. I found a spot to stand and cruise next to the entrance to one of the club's specialty rooms, and nestled in.

I watched men come and go from the mazes where they lure one another into small cupboard-type spaces, or the sling room always filled with eager voyeurs, or the glory-hole area where countless opportunities present themselves if one seeks to suck or be sucked in that fashion. The music was good, the men looked even better, and I was miraculously perky for being up so late. Somehow I found my mind drifting off—not to the erotically charged fantasies the club aims to create but to a previous day's argument I'd had at Pasqua about promiscuity's place in gay culture. I thought about all the critiques of gay men's sex cultures I'd been reading over the past few months and wondered what relevance they had to the events unfolding all around me.

Are these the men Larry Kramer finds obsessed with sex? Are their lives focused so entirely on erotic pleasures that they make no contributions to the world? Vince walked by and jokingly grabbed at my butt. Here is a man who works energetically all week for his company and travels to Southern California regularly to visit his aged mother and numerous brothers, sisters, and the accompanying nieces and nephews. Is Vince the kind of guy Kramer would consider to be stuck in a cycle of superficial encounters and meaningless sex? Does Vince's muscular butt and penchant for fisting keep him trapped in a sex club–focused life that leaves him without authentic friendship and love, constantly moving from one man to another, unable to find the partner he is seeking? Or is he simply one of the many gay men who have designed lives for themselves that do not privilege coupledom over friendships, and who considers his kinky sex as just one of his many interests, including motorcycle riding, deep-sea fishing, and volunteering for AIDS organizations?

I thought about Michelangelo Signorile's critique of circuit culture. There were a number of muscle-bound hunks in their late twenties and early thirties walking by, who bore the signs of circuit clones: tattoos in all the right places, bodies shaved smooth, and sideburns but no facial hair. Are these men trapped in a culture that offers them limited options and forces them to continuously repeat cycles of drug use and sexual frenzy? Matt, the buff boy from my gym, leaned into the wall next to me and made idle chatter. Is he one of the souls lost on the circuit scene, I wondered? I knew he went dancing Saturday nights at Club Universe, because he had once explained that was why I would never see him at the gym on Sunday mornings. He certainly had the look and attitude I had become familiar with from my few visits to circuit parties, and I knew he did the drugs. How did this fit together with his life as a corporate attorney, avid cyclist, and president of the board of a local nature conservancy? I had once talked to him about being HIV negative, but I wondered whether he had become infected since that chat, another soul lost in the dissolute gay world of sex and drugs.

As I was chatting with Matt, the dermatologist walked past and gave me a friendly wink. What is he doing in here? I tried to remember if he was one of the health care workers who had signed the manifesto about creating a better gay culture. He had been a longtime volunteer at the San Francisco AIDS Foundation. Was he on the list of signatories? As my mind tried to remember who had signed the list, a tall, lean man passed by and gave me the kind of look that says, "Follow me." I disengaged myself from my chatter with Matt and made a beeline for the door to the patio which I had seen this man pass through. I walked past the smokers, lounging around and conversing, and headed toward the small outdoor maze where men commonly have sex.

He was exiting as I entered. I caught his eye and tried to project interest yet still look disinterested enough to maintain his interest. He whipped around and followed me into one of the dark corners. "I've had my eye on you for a while," he said in a deep voice with the hint of a New York accent. Pressing me against the wall, he started deep kissing me as his arms wrapped around my body.

I immediately realized who he was. Two weeks earlier I had cruised this tall, lean, and hairy man one Saturday morning at the gym. He had at least two things I wanted: a bald head and a short goatee getting peppered with gray. I had caught him eyeing me a few times, but he seemed intent on sticking to his workout, so I didn't get to talk with him or exchange names and phone numbers. I thought to myself that he must be an out-of-town visitor. If I had seen this one before, I would have remembered!

We made out while our hands roamed over each other's torsos. I reached under his tank top and felt his hairy chest and stomach as his hand came up and squeezed my tit. He was alternately kissing me hard on the mouth and then licking his way through my beard. I felt incredibly excited as this tall, strapping wolf was devouring me. His aggressive ardor both excited and frightened me. Where was all of this going to lead?

Just then I felt another hand on me, this one unsnapping the buttons of my jeans. I opened my eyes, looked down, and saw the smiling face of the dermatologist as he yanked out my dick and took me into his mouth. While I have enjoyed group sex on many occasions, I am ultimately a one-on-one sort of guy and often find myself shooing away interlopers who intrude on my encounters in sex clubs. I'm the type of guy who goes to sex clubs to meet men and bring them back to the privacy of my home. As I felt him swallow my dick, bobbing up and down on the shaft and licking my balls, my friend from the gym had moved on from my face and was now licking my neck and chest. I sank back against the wall and eased my body and spirit into their ministrations.

Once again my mind tripped off into the sex debates currently raging in the community. Was this safe or unsafe sex I was having? My gym pal was simply licking my body. What was the risk there? The dermatologist was blowing me. Unless I have some kind of disease of which I'm unaware, or he has the clap in his throat, this is a safe sort of act. Would Gabriel Rotello believe our little orgy was fated to culminate in ecological disaster? Would the Log Cabin Republicans condemn this act? Suddenly I remembered an article I had read in a local gay paper. Wasn't the dermatologist a Republican?

I didn't have time to answer the questions reeling through my brain. The guy from the gym had shifted me so that my shoulder leaned against the wall. He yanked my open jeans down to my knees and crouched behind me, bringing my butt to his face. He kissed my ass cheek and I felt his face moving toward my butthole. Immediately my mind raced in all directions: Is rimming allowed at this club these days? Did the rules that I initialed on entering the club say anything at all about anal/oral contact? What were my own concerns about health and safety in regard to rimming? I wasn't concerned about HIV but did fear parasites. Was Leather Buddies a place where I should allow myself to be rimmed?

I immediately turned my body in a way that indicated my reluctance to be rimmed. I placed my hand on the back of my buddy's neck and pushed his face to my balls. "Lick my nuts!" I heard myself say, as his tongue flicked out over my balls and began licking my legs as well. I noticed a small crowd had gathered watching the three of us carrying on and I simultaneously loved and hated the attention. The dermatologist was a great cocksucker, but it was difficult to maneuver in the tight space and he and my gym pal repeatedly jostled against each other. Other hands reached out to touch my chest. I looked up to see an attractive Asian man whom I had noticed earlier, smiling sternly as he twisted my nipples.

This was all too much. Excitement was racing through my body and I felt my legs tremble as an orgasm approached. "I'm going to come!" I heard myself say. Immediately the dermatologist pulled his mouth off of my dick and began jerking me off manually. The gym man still nuzzled my nuts, and my chest was hurting from the firm twists the Asian man was giving them, but hurting in a good way. As my body began to shudder, I felt myself cry out. My dick jerked in a series of spasms and the semen shot all over the dermatologist's hands and my gym pal's bald head. As my body stopped quaking, the Asian man brought his lips to mine and kissed me deeply. For a moment, my mind went blank.

As we pulled ourselves together a moment later, wiped sperm and saliva from various bodies, and readjusted our clothes, the questions filtered through my brain once again, finding no easy answers. Is this encounter a healthy part of my life? What effect does this degree of sexual freedom have on our communal cultures? Is it possible to maintain gay subcultures that treasure promiscuity without causing plagues to constantly cycle through the community?

Chapter 7

A Framework
for Low-Risk Promiscuity

In March 1997, I was invited to present a keynote address at the National HIV Prevention Summit sponsored by the Centers for Disease Control and Prevention (CDC) in Atlanta. I was simultaneously surprised and flattered by this invitation: surprised because in my earlier writings I had critically challenged the reigning paradigm of HIV prevention for gay men supported by the CDC, and flattered because I hoped the alternative ways of working with gay men's sex that I suggested would be seriously considered by policymakers. Jumping at this opportunity, I broke a promise I had with myself to turn down engagements that would cause me to desert my students and skip classes at Berkeley. I was eager to speak with folks from the CDC.

The primary participants in the conference were leaders of CDC-funded HIV-prevention community planning groups convened at local, state, and national levels throughout the nation. Over 700 prevention leaders were expected to attend the three-day conference at the Atlanta Hilton. Organizers informed me the conference was aimed at gaining grassroots support for a consensus statement developed by the National Institutes of Health titled "Interventions to Prevent HIV-Risk Behaviors."[1] I requested a copy of this statement because I thought I might use it as a starting point for my talk, elucidating the document's strengths and weaknesses regarding gay men.

When the document arrived and I scanned it, I was stunned. The statement, though developed through a lengthy and rigorous process, gave scant attention to gay men, the principal at-risk population in the United States. It offered little new thinking that might strengthen our collective work. For example, Section 2 poses the questions, "What Individual-, Group-, or Community-Based Methods of Intervention Reduce Behavioral Risks? What Are the Benefits and Risks of These Procedures?," but only a single paragraph focuses on "men who have sex with men":

> Considerable research has focused on risk reduction in men who have sex with men. Descriptive studies and non-randomized studies with control groups show positive effects, as do randomized studies. The studies with random assignment to groups have clustered in two areas: individual interventions delivered in small group settings and programs aimed at changing community norms (e.g., using peer leaders in community settings to deliver programs). These intervention programs focus on information, skills building, self-management, problem solving, and psychological factors such as self-efficacy and intentions. Studies with clearly defined interventions, retention of samples to allow follow-up periods as long as 18 months, and reasonable sample sizes show substantial effects for intervention over minimal intervention or control conditions. More intensive interventions (e.g., more sessions) boost efficacy.[2]

This draft of the document seemed to be saying simply that programs attempting to shift community norms by placing gay men in counseling, support group, and peer leadership settings have greater effects when significant effort is made. I was struck by the narrow ways the document's authors considered HIV prevention for gay men and the limited scope of activities they consider worthwhile prevention. If this document had been drafted a decade ago, before the "new thinking" emerged from Walt Odets, Ralph Bolton, Cindy Patton, Simon Rosser, Michael Wright, Michael Ross, and a dozen other prevention theorists, researchers, and writers in Western Europe and Australia/New Zealand, it might be excused. As a statement about gay male prevention in 1997 it seemed embarrassingly narrow and woefully inadequate.

The full limitation of the government's brain trust of prevention experts is evident late in the document, in section 4, titled "How Can Risk-Reduction Procedures Be Implemented Effectively?" The limitations of what passes for HIV prevention in the mind of the CDC are clearly displayed:

> Based on current research, a number of interventions have been evaluated and are ready to be implemented within communities. Interventions at the *individual level* include the following:
>
> • Community outreach, needle exchange activities, and treatment programs for substance-abusing populations
> • Cognitive-behavioral small group, face-to-face counseling, and skills-building (proper condom use) programs for men who have sex with men.
> • Cognitive-behavioral small group, face-to-face counseling, and skills building (i.e., negotiation, refusal) programs for women that pay special attention to gender-specific concerns (e.g., child care, transportation, and relationships with significant others)
> • Condom distribution and testing and treatment for STDs for sex workers
> • Cognitive-behavioral psychoeducational skills-building groups for youth and adolescents in various settings.
>
> At the *family* or *dyad level* interventions include counseling for couples (including HIV sero-discordant couples) in both the United States and other countries. Within the *community,* interventions include changing community norms through community outreach and opinion leaders for men who have sex with men.[3]

As I scanned this document, I realized my hands were holding evidence of precisely what needs to change in the ways we think about HIV prevention work with gay men. Since the start of the epidemic, prevention efforts have focused almost exclusively on interventions on the individual level designed and championed by the public health establishment. Our energies and resources have been directed to cognitive-behavioral work that, at best, is simply one piece of the work necessary to bring about the needed changes.

Efforts at the community level which sociologists, anthropologists, social theorists, cultural studies scholars, and many grassroots prevention workers have argued should have been prioritized as the short-term crisis was transformed into a multigenerational plague, remain sorely undertheorized, underresourced, and misunderstood.[4] If "changing community norms" is understood primarily as buttressing community outreach and influencing opinion leaders, a decade's worth of social science efforts to educate the prevention establishment about meaningful community-level interventions have gone unheard.

I thought carefully about what I was going to say to the prevention wonks gathered by the CDC. I had twenty minutes in which to make my presentation—thus I had to choose my words carefully and plan my talk strategically. What I said to the CDC provides my encapsulated analysis of the history of gay male HIV prevention in the United States and suggests directions for the future.

WHAT THE CENTERS FOR DISEASE CONTROL HAVE YET TO UNDERSTAND . . .

In the 1980s, prevention work with gay men was pulled together quickly and chaotically by a socially isolated, politically maligned population with most of its members deeply closeted in their work lives and invisible in their communities of origin. In five short years, gay men rapidly moved through denial to shock to terror to action. Gay men in hard-hit cities developed an understanding of AIDS as crisis. This captured our experiences as we searched our stomachs for purple spots, watched our sex lives shift from places of pleasure and comfort to sites of fear and dread, and opened our weekly gay papers to dozens of obituaries of handsome men with whom we'd danced, tricked, and built community.

Our prevention focus was aimed at keeping men safe from what seemed like a lethal syndrome about which we knew little. We aimed to get information out as rapidly as it became available, design interventions to get men to use condoms all the time, and change community norms about sexual practices, drug use, and involvement in community life.

It is easy to look back at this time critically without acknowledging the miracles of the period: programs were developed even before funds became available; a diverse population wracked by internal bickering and racism managed to keep working together, and, despite a powerful antigay, antisex backlash from the Theocratic Right, gay men did not go back in the closet, but came out in a spirit of service to develop care and prevention programs for our many communities.

Some important lessons were learned from our work of the 1980s:

- Prevention efforts must take seriously the differences within the populations we call "gay men." What works for affluent white gay men may not work for gay men who are first-generation Central American refugees. What works for educated, middle-class, African-American gay men may not work for African-American gay men living in poverty. What works for forty-year-olds may not work for twenty-year-olds, or for sixty-year-olds.
- A population with a long history of victimization by government, medicine, scientific research, and the media will not easily and quickly see these sectors as trustworthy partners in prevention. Our communities must have ownership of prevention in word as well as deed. We must lead it.
- Sex is a core part of most gay male identities and cultures and telling men not to have sex will not work. Programs that judge men with multiple partners or a taste for kinky sex will rapidly lose the confidence of much of the community.

There are lessons that were not learned from the 1980s, but need to be, as demonstrated by the consensus statement drafted by leading "experts" in 1997:

- Context is everything. By designing urban prevention programs for gay men on cognitive-behavioral models, prevention leaders are responding to an experience of crisis that dominated epicenter gay communities in the 1980s and is now outdated. The context shifted by the 1990s, making these models less appropriate. Prevention for gay men in epicenter cities has rarely acknowledged these shifts and has failed to embrace sociocultural models enjoying great success throughout most of the West.

- There are several different gay male AIDS epidemics. Programs for gay men rarely take seriously the different geographic, generational, and economic class-based gay epidemics.
- People will take matters into their own hands if they are treated with disrespect, disgust, or deception. Our work in earlier years told gay men they must use condoms every time, trivializing their authentic desires and treating as unimportant the meanings many find in being fucked and receiving another man's semen inside. Our efforts overlooked the central position of specific sex acts in many men's identities and treated anal sex with abhorrence and queer bodies as sites to be colonized. While claiming to "empower" we used methods of manipulation, policing, subtle guilt-tripping, and outright shaming. This has created the community we inhabit today: cities populated by increasing numbers of gay men who distrust, disbelieve, and do not practice the rigid guidelines set forth by our own organizations.

As the second decade of AIDS draws to a close, we need to take a deep breath and reexamine the theoretical foundations of our prevention work. We might take a serious look at whether our methods are respectful, honest, and appropriate to the changing context of various gay AIDS epidemics. The crisis-driven behavior-change cognitive approaches so popular among public health traditionalists may no longer be effective in the approaching third decade of the epidemic. Prevention for gay men is at a turbulent crossroads. We can continue fine-tuning traditional interventions focused on providing individual gay men with information, motivation, and skills. Or we can acknowledge the complexity of sexuality and trust and support gay men truly to manage their own risk.

When we hear that men are fucking without condoms, these days discussed as engaging in "raw" sex, or "barebacking," why are we shocked? When friends confess they swallow semen, why does it seem staggering to some of us? We can either pathologize men or understand them as doing their best to develop strategies to reduce risk while continuing practices that offer core meaning to their identities and work to support them in their efforts. While both perspectives characterize some gay men, the former viewpoint has been dominant in prevention and functions as a catchall explanation for all men's unprotected sex. Pathologizing leads some public health planners to ask, "How can we use peer pressure to intervene in both public and private sex acts?" An alternative viewpoint might lead us instead to ask, "What can community offer to gay men that is affirming and life-sustaining?"

The NIH consensus statement might be improved by a greatly expanded notion of prevention tackling the social and cultural questions that ultimately determine infection rates. For example, how can we analyze shifts in the epidemic thoughtfully and carefully? Too often gay men buy into the simplistic and misguided analyses of tabloid journalists. I wonder if upswings in unprotected sex in some areas may be attributed, not to hearing discussions about protease inhibitors or reading articles about "The End of AIDS" and deciding to keep the condom in the wallet, but to the insistence by prevention groups that we remain locked in a state of crisis when our authentic everyday experience of AIDS directs us otherwise.

How do we lift the imprint of AIDS off gay identities? The merging of "gay" with "AIDS" is said to lead many young gay men to believe infection is inevitable. Finding ways to separate AIDS from gay identity seems critically important. Perhaps circuit parties, which are celebratory and build spirit, can be seen as valuable sites where gay masculinities are performed, experimented with, and transformed, without a dominant focus on AIDS. How can we support gay men to have greater authority and responsibility for their sex? These are tough questions we must be asking as post-AIDS cultures emerge in the late 1990s. As we abandon crisis-based prevention efforts, what kind of programs will take their place?

MAKING ROOM FOR MONOGAMY

In a speech titled "Learning from Each Other or Monogamy: Pleasures and Pitfalls," presented at the 1997 National Lesbian and Gay Health Conference, *Village Voice* writer Mark Schoofs said:

Our culture has erected a false sexual hierarchy. It reserves the bottom rung for anonymous sex. On the rungs right above that perch the various species of promiscuity: casual sex, where at least you exchange names and conversation, fuck buddies, sex with friends, and sex outside a primary relationship. On the top rung, all smug and sure of itself, sits monogamy. Of course, monogamy can be wonderful—I've been in a very happy monogamous relationship for a year and a half—but monogamy is not necessarily superior. What's right for one person might be wrong for another. There is no hierarchy.[5]

Gayle Rubin has diagrammed a "sexual value system" which functions to "rationalize the well-being of the sexually privileged and the adversity of the sexual rabble":

> According to this system, sexuality that is "good," "normal" and "natural" should ideally be heterosexual, marital, monogamous, reproductive, and non-commercial. It should be coupled, relational, within the same generation, and occur at home. It should not involve pornography, fetish objects, sex toys of any sort, or roles other than male or female. Any sex that violates these rules is "bad," "abnormal," or "unnatural." Bad sex may be homosexual, unmarried, promiscuous, non-procreative, or commercial. It may be masturbatory or take place at orgies, may be casual, may cross generational lines, and may take place in "public," or at least in the bushes or the baths. It may involve the use of pornography, fetish objects, sex toys, or unusual roles.[6]

This sexual hierarchy or value system currently is at center stage in the gay male sex wars of the late 1990s. Post-AIDS prevention workers see the politics inscribed in this system, struggle against the tendency of crisis-driven communities to default to judgmental approaches, and appreciate, even exult in, sexual variation. Gay men maintain a wide range of relationships with our community sexual cultures. Some men opt for authentic monogamy, long-term relationships in which sexual activity is focused solely on one's lover. Others embrace "postmodern monogamy," Michelangelo Signorile's term for couples who strive for exclusivity and aim for "bonding, commitment, and closeness," but occasionally and discreetly trick out on each other.[7] Still others participate in serial monogamy, various levels of activity with multiple partners, or enjoy unabashed promiscuity.

Prevention workers might commit themselves to creating projects that respect individual men's decisions regarding how they situate themselves in relation to sex and gay male sex cultures. The job is not to judge or moralize, but support, affirm, and assist. The tasks at hand are to provide the information and resources needed for men to make their own sexual choices and manage their own risk, and work with the overseers of community institutions, including public sex venues, to help them critically consider their sites' relationships to gay men's health.

AIDS education too often has given lip service to respecting gay men's diverse sexual strategies while failing to fully value men's varied options. Men who identify as monogamous may be viewed with suspicion, considered by some within gay communities as "less gay," sex-negative, or secretly screwing around on the side. Promiscuous men may be derided as mindless, immature sex addicts, oblivious to the risks of casual sex and incapable of authentic commitment. We judge all who construct their erotic lives differently from the way we construct our own at any given moment.

A recent thesis completed by Daniel Geer, while a social work graduate student at San Francisco State University, surveyed San Francisco gay men about the way they organized their sex.[8] Geer argues that, while monogamy became popular among male couples during the first decade of AIDS, in the 1990s, "as men realize that safe sex works," increasing numbers of men have entered nonmonogamous relationships. The majority of the respondents had been monogamous at some time in the past, but most for a period limited to less than one year. Among his interesting findings, Geer corroborates Signorile's analysis of "postmodern monogamy" by discovering that, "of the men who identified as monogamous, 37 percent reported having sex outside the relationship."[9]

Geer's small study suggests gay men, even those in a sexually liberal city such as San Francisco, choose to construct their sexual relationships utilizing different definitions, values, and boundaries. Along with other studies, it provides evidence that most urban gay men do not live for long periods of time in relationships in which they have no sexual partners other than their lovers.[10] Despite this, many men continue to consider monogamy a worthy goal.

While some sexual liberationists might consider claims by gay men that they aim for exclusivity in their erotic lives to be dubious, prevention efforts should take as a starting point some men's honest desire for monogamous partnerships. Since the early days of prevention we have tailored workshops and programs to fit the needs of specific subcultures of gay men. In large cities, it is possible to find targeted prevention campaigns for gay men of various races, antibody statuses, ages, and sexual proclivities. Yet rarely have programs been planned thoughtfully around men's relationship to monogamy, promiscuity, and the other ways we conceptualize and structure our sex and relationships. Nor do we find many projects tailored to assist men in enhancing their abilities to negotiate within sexualized gay sites such as parks, tearooms, sex clubs, and bathhouses.

Those who would consider modeling all gay male cultures on a romanticized version of heterosexual marriage might consider instead a more limited project carving out social space for male couples. They might start by creating organizations, publications, and social networks of gay male couples seeking to socialize with other gay couples and by supporting already-established efforts. Groups that currently exist in the San Francisco area include San Francisco Bay Area Couples, and Bayshore Couples, centered south of the city. These groups are not limited to monogamous couples, but focus more broadly on providing "a social, educational, and humanitarian forum for gay and lesbian couples, to promote the validity of same-gender relationships, and to endorse the gay and lesbian couple as socially responsible units."[11]

Recently, the back page of a San Francisco gay paper was filled with a full-page advertisement for a new dating service:

Single? Personal Introductions for Lesbians and Gay Men:
If you've completed your education and are on track with your career, your thoughts may move to companionship, romance, and love. You aren't alone. At Quality Partners we work with attractive and successful lesbians and gay men who lead healthy and happy lives that they hope to share with someone special.

Mo • nog • a • my (mo nog am me)
state of being romantically and passionately involved
with one person
Quality Partners
For Selective Gay Men and Lesbians Seeking Long-Term
Committed Relationships

Bonds Limited is another San Francisco gay and lesbian organization committed to "building stable relationship foundations in our community" and aims to help those seeking "loving, stable, monogamous life partners." A seven-step process of recruitment, screening, selection, and matching provides clients with "meeting opportunities" with like-minded individuals. This group's mission is to:

- Bring together loving, stable, carefully screened same-gender partners committed to long-term monogamous relationships.
- Serve the needs of both women and men equally, while honoring their differences.
- Contribute to the well-being of our clients, community and culture.
- Protect the confidentiality of our clients.
- Profit by adding value to the lives of those who employ us.[12]

I am curious whether substantial numbers of urban gay men flock to such organizations, but informal conversations with men in certain parts of the nation (particularly the South and the Midwest, and men in suburban and rural areas) lead me to believe significant numbers of men might embrace such an option. A monogamous gay male subculture might be prudent to guard against thinking itself superior to other subcultures, and men committed to monogamy might work to avoid smugness. Post-AIDS gay communities will aim to allow room for men of different priorities and values and neither exalt nor trash those whose views differ. There is room for both monogamous gay couples and sex pigs in the same big tent of gay community.

JUST SAY YES

If creating monogamous subcultures among gay men feels like a daunting challenge, prevention groups are likely to have a far greater problem creating what Jim Eigo calls "a framework for low-risk promiscuity."[13] While safer sex campaigns of the 1980s and 1990s were ostensibly designed for urban gay cultures that offer gay men many different opportunities for sexual contact, only a few of these programs currently are implemented with full respect for the diverse choices men make about their sexual practices. This becomes clear when one considers how few U.S. prevention groups have seriously embraced "negotiated safety," an Australian program with counterpart efforts throughout Canada and Western Europe, aimed at "gay men who want to consider not using condoms in their relationship."[14] Despite being heavily discussed in the gay press and at AIDS conferences since 1993, and widespread evidence that many gay men are not using condoms during some of their anal sex activities, most AIDS prevention groups have yet to embrace such a program.[15]

Yet in post-AIDS worlds negotiated safety is precisely what prevention groups should be intent on, not only for gay men in primary relationships, but as a foundational concept informing all work with gay men. A brochure published by the AIDS Council of New South Wales titled "Talk, Test, Test, Trust . . . Together" states:

> Using condoms remains the safest way of having anal sex, but . . . if you are in a gay relationship and you want to fuck without condoms, then there are 4 steps to take together: (1) Talk about it; (2) Both get tested; (3) Get tested again; (4) Trust each other to tell.[16]

The last point, "Trust each other to tell," seems to me to lie at the heart of the concept of negotiated safety:

> Reach a clear agreement about sex inside and outside the relationship. Possible agreements include: (a) no condoms together; (b) no anal sex outside the relationship; (c) all anal sex outside the relationship is with a condom; or (d) no sex outside the relationship. Recognize that people don't always stick to agreements, and that accidents can happen. If a slip-up occurs, it doesn't mean the end of the relationship. It does mean you will both have to go back to using condoms again.

> Don't punish each other for telling the truth. Agree to start the TALK TEST TEST TRUST process again. . . . together.

Additional information for couples who are of different antibody statuses, as well as couples who are both positive ("the choice to fuck without condoms is up to you . . . "), appears on the brochure, as does a warning that sounds like something one's mother would say: " . . . but remember, unless you follow these four steps use a condom every time."

Negotiated safety within male couples provides new ways of working with gay men's sex that might be used to generate a framework for low-risk promiscuity. A number of useful concepts are employed here that should serve as building blocks in creating post-AIDS prevention efforts. (1) Fucking without condoms is not automatically pathologized. Instead it is discussed in a manner that is reasonable, thoughtful, and not highly charged. (2) Conscious agreements can be reached (with oneself or with a lover) about the levels of sexual risk one is willing to take. The utilization of critical decision-making skills based on previously agreed-upon limitations encourages men to be active participants in sexual strategizing. (3) Dialogue is emphasized as a critical tool in sexual negotiations. Why should we limit our talking only to our lovers? Sex club contacts, tricks, fuck buddies, and long-term affairs might also include intimate conversation around issues of safety, not in the way prevention groups have encouraged, but as part of the sexual scene-setting stage preceding action. While differing levels of trust may be appropriate with one-time tricks than with long-term fuckbuddies, in a post-crisis period, it is unlikely men will maintain the rigid practice of assuming "all men lie" that has dominated prevention in the past.

Negotiated safety might be considered broadly by gay men considering adopting harm reduction strategies in their sex lives. Rather than limit its application to HIV transmission, harm reduction approaches to other health-related matters might be considered: hepatitis and other sexually transmitted diseases, substance use, hate-violence, heart disease, cancer. Gay men using negotiated safety as a central strategy would be encouraged to view each sexual encounter with a lover or a buddy in the Jacuzzi at the gym as meriting reflection, analysis, and occasional dialogue linked to a range of sexual health matters.

A framework for low-risk promiscuity may be utilized not only with men as they become masters of their health, but also with those who shape environments in which gay men are creating new identities and evolving relationships to their bodies, emotions, and spiritualities. Unlike some of my colleagues on what has been simplistically categorized as the prosex side of the sex war debates, I believe community organizations have a role to play in working with owners of sex clubs, producers of circuit parties, and managers of gay bars and other queer social spaces. Yet the objective of this task should not be to become arms of the state and order sex clubs to unhinge doors on private spaces or demand event producers put up signs dramatizing the dangers of drug use.

After being hounded in *The New York Times* op-ed pages by Michelangelo Signorile about potential drug use at the 1997 Morning Party, Gay Men's Health Crisis (GMHC) responded by inviting federal law enforcement officials—the same people who regularly entrap gay men in nearby cruising areas—to patrol this Fire Island fund-raising event undercover and wearing GMHC identification badges. These plainclothes narcs secretly policed the event and made arrests for drug use.[17] As Matt Foreman, then executive director of New York's Anti-Violence Project, wrote:

> How sickly ironic, then, that GMHC would welcome this force and its tactics into the Morning Party. How utterly disgusting that GMHC played an integral and helpful role in having nearly two dozen persons facing federal drug charges. (These aren't mere "tickets"; at a minimum, the victims will carry a drug arrest and conviction on their records forever.) At this point, the use of the word gay in GMHC's name borders on sacrilege. There are plenty of organizations in the struggle against AIDS that deserve our support. GMHC is not one of them.[18]

When I encourage AIDS groups to work with the producers of events and the owners of establishments for gay men, this is *not* what I am suggesting. Instead the primary mission might be focused on initiating noncoercive, reflective dialogue about gay men's health issues with those who shape queer environments.

Mark Schoofs has discussed sex as a "survival strategy" for some gay men:

> In my own life, I've enjoyed splendid casual and anonymous liaisons, as well as fantastic sex in long-term relationships. In all these forms, sex can be play and recreation in the best sense, rejuvenating and sustaining to us. A friend of mine, who is single, says that if he doesn't have sex for a few months, he begins to feel anxious and irritable; at those times he goes to a bathhouse, after which he feels much more calm and refreshed. I recently interviewed a seventy-five-year-old gay Jewish Holocaust hero. This man led an underground resistance group in Berlin and saved about 100 Jews from Hitler's ovens. An elf-like man, he is an outrageous flirt, and he had sex right and left through the war with many, many different men. But for this Holocaust hero, sex was not just a frivolous pastime. It was a survival strategy. He told me that one reason he was able to be so strong and so brave was *because* he had lots of sex and love. For this hero, for my friend who goes to bathhouses when he wants the touch of another human being, for myself, and for many people, sex is a source of emotional energy and power.
>
> I would even go a step further. I don't think AIDS is anywhere near as horrible as Hitler's Holocaust, but the epidemic is terrible and dangerous. For some of us, sex is part of our survival strategy.[19]

Many gay men consider sex to be an activity of central value to our identities and lives. We may see it as a survival strategy that makes living satisfying and worthwhile. This does not mean we are obsessed with sex or have no interests or activities besides sex. It means we value the enactment of our desires and will not always give them up in a grand gesture of sacrifice to the epidemic. We may understand that, in the value system of middle-class America, a long life and safety are supposed to be motivation enough to throw a cold blanket over our smoldering desires, but many gay men will not give up meaningful sexual acts uncritically or forever.

When I talk at gay town hall meetings about the various reasons some gay men have unprotected anal sex, some men believe I am endorsing or encouraging men's fucking without condoms. We have become so steeped in fifteen years of safe-sex rhetoric that anyone who attempts to offer more nuanced understandings of sex is seen as a heretic. A rigidity has set in, and we are given a choice of either falling into line and espousing superficial and simplistic perspectives on buttfucking, or being seen as outlaws inciting men to infect themselves. More than once I've been confronted by angry gay men demanding to know which side I was on.

Because I maintain a lifelong commitment to gay liberation, I see the survival of openly gay men as an important priority. Too many threats against our people ensure too few of us will live to our seventies, eighties, and longer. While I neither romanticize old age nor pity those who die young, I believe it can be a radical act for gay men to enjoy lengthy lifespans. My career as a gay organizer has been focused on creating spaces for queers to heal the wounds of a hostile culture and emerge powerfully as social change activists. I do not want gay men to die early deaths.

However, I hold this commitment alongside other priorities, including support for a wide range of ways gay men organize their sex lives and social relationships. This makes it difficult for me, easily and quickly, to judge acts of unprotected sex as bad or wrong. When a man in Atlanta recently asked me if unprotected anal sex was ever okay, I had to answer that I believed it was. He was horrified. It made no difference that I cited examples I consider easy to defend (two HIV-positive men, or two HIV-negative long-term lovers). To this enraged, red-faced man, I was irresponsibly encouraging unsafe practices and should be banned from the queer public sphere.

I believe sexual health is important and that two HIV-positive men or two HIV-negative men should incorporate into their decision-making processes about anal sex an awareness of sexually transmitted diseases besides HIV/AIDS. This might encourage them to use condoms despite similar HIV antibody statuses. For many men, however, an important part of anal sex *is* semen exchange—receiving another man's semen in the butt or ejaculating one's semen into another man—and the use of a condom alters the meaning of the act in a way that is not always acceptable. I will not judge these men harshly. I also understand that, despite what many prevention leaders seem to think, for most men, sex is not primarily a rational activity, created through conscious decision-making processes.

RATIONING RIMMING

Perhaps my reluctance to judge comes from my own sex. Anal sex is not a source of conflict for me because I have not gotten fucked in fifteen years and I enjoy using condoms when I screw guys. My primary act of sexual risk is rimming, at the top of my hit parade of carnal knowledge. While rimming is not going to give me HIV, it could easily expose me to all kinds of microscopic critters that could mess up my health for a long time. I feel fortunate to have gotten through twenty-five years as an avid rimmer and never acquired parasites. I've supported friends who have been unable to rid themselves of intestinal parasites acquired through rimming, despite slurping up Flagyl for more than a year. This is not something I am eager to endure.

In a societal value system of sexual acts, having one's tongue on a butthole would not be categorized as one of the more acceptable activities. My lover makes faces of disgust when he hears I've rimmed a guy, and another friend wrinkles her nose and cries, "Gross me out!" Yet having my face in a guy's hairy butt drives me wild and makes me happy. And resting my own beefy butt on a man's face, feeling his goatee against my cheeks as his tongue licks up and down my crack, can bring me to a quick and intense orgasm.

So how do I place my concerns about health alongside my penchant for rimming? I've tried several types of barriers but they don't work for me: the whole point of rimming a guy is to put my pink little tongue in contact with his dark hairy hole. Have I retired rimming to the junk heap of forbidden sex acts? Is it now an activity I imagine in my fantasies as I jerk on my dick, but would never perform in real life? No way! It's too important to me—too pleasurable and too meaningful. So what's a guy to do?

I've made rimming into a special treat I allow myself to enjoy on special occasions. I do not save the activity for my birthday and

Valentine's Day (Lord knows, my lover won't let me put my tongue anywhere near his butthole!); instead I allow myself to rim four times a year and get rimmed four times a year. Yep, I ration rimming. This makes me choose the buttholes I tongue with some discretion, and encourages me to think twice before sinking my face into just any beefy butt.

One December, I faced an incredible dilemma. I'd picked up a short, squat, muscular Italian guy at the gym and lured him home for an early morning assignation. It was clear when I climbed into his pickup truck and he put his hairy paw on my knee and started feeling up my thigh that he was eager to take control. "I like big boys like you," he said through a leer. I immediately became incredibly excited. His thick forearms, near-black goatee, and balding head made me quiver. My dick was poking out of my gym shorts.

When we got to my home and sat on the couch, he immediately jumped on top, reached under my tank top, and started feeling me up. As I felt his hand slide down to my butt and squeeze my cheek, I realized I'd better say something soon if I hoped to quell his determination to fuck me but avoid alienating him from other possibilities. After explaining to him that I was not up for getting fucked, he whipped out his dick to show me that, while it was quite thick, it was not very long. I countered that my disinterest in getting porked had nothing to do with his great-looking cock; I simply didn't enjoy the act and this was nonnegotiable. He immediately climbed off me and peeled down his sweatpants. "If you won't let me fuck you, then we'll have to do my next favorite thing," he insisted as he exposed his butt, beautifully framed by his jockstrap. I thought he might be inviting me to penetrate him. Instead he started maneuvering his crack toward my face.

Wow! My mouth immediately started drooling and I delightfully envisioned being smothered by his great butt. Suddenly I remembered I'd already used all four of my rimming opportunities for the year. The last one was just a few weeks before with Darrell, a handsome black man who'd picked me up at the Gauntlet in Los Angeles. I ultimately felt I'd wasted one of my rim opportunities on him because no sooner had I licked his butt up and down than he spread his legs, grabbed my dick, and started prepping me to fuck him. It counted as a rim job, because the tongue-butthole contact thing had occurred. Yet I felt just a bit robbed because the rimming had been immediately eclipsed by a randy fuck scene.

So here it was, early December, and I'd used up my allotment of rimming for the year. And here was Phil, maneuvering himself so he could shimmy down and rest on my face. I had to think quickly. I didn't want to alienate him by turning him down twice, but I had my rules and I had to follow them. What's a rimdog to do?

I came up with a quick solution in my head, just before I settled myself back on the couch and eased my face up to his butt. In a move that came to me from my years as a schoolteacher where students would grab an extra snack one day in exchange for a snack from the following week, I simply borrowed against my four rim jobs for the next year. I'd get the enjoyment of licking Phil's butt, and sacrifice one of next year's snacks.

That's exactly what I did. I had a great time rimming Phil—our tastes clearly coincided in this area as he loved being rimmed—and then I suffered through 1996, knowing I was only allowed to rim three times. My distress was alleviated somewhat by my new pal Phil. He returned for a repeat rim job, which made me quite happy.

SHIFTING FROM AIDS PREVENTION TO GAY MEN'S HEALTH

AIDS work in the early 1980s was initiated within the context of a nascent lesbian and gay health movement. The earliest meetings about "gay cancer" were convened at the annual National Lesbian and Gay Health Conference, and local groups of gay health professionals in cities throughout the nation, often gay male doctors, nurses, and social workers, took the lead in confronting the mysterious new syndrome manifesting itself among gay men. The massive AIDS organizations upon which many gay men with HIV and AIDS depend these days commonly were started in gay male sexually transmitted disease clinics. AIDS Project Los Angeles began as a phone line in the Los Angeles Gay and Lesbian Community Services Center health clinic. Boston's AIDS Action Committee was initially a unit within the Fenway Community Health Center. Whitman Walker Clinic in Washington, DC, was a general gay health center with a large sexually transmitted disease program that transformed itself into an AIDS center over the past fifteen years.

During the mid- and late 1980s, AIDS work was removed from its original position embedded in the gay health field, as it began to produce its own freestanding system. This was understandable because nongay populations were also deeply affected by the epidemic. Yet ties between gay health and AIDS were never cleanly severed. The mammoth New York City AIDS organization serving multiple populations retains its original name, "Gay Men's Health Crisis" and the annual National Lesbian and Gay Health Conference continues to meet alongside the National AIDS Forum. We spun through cycles of de-gaying AIDS and re-gaying AIDS and debates sparked back and forth, which never found resolution.[20] Although all parties acknowledged that AIDS work with gay men of all races and classes had to be culturally sensitive to community needs and values, it was never clear whether the work was best situated in gay-identified organizations such as community centers or in AIDS-identified organizations.

In 1997, prevention planners might revisit these questions with an eye to shifting the ways we conceptualize our work and the frameworks from which we operate. If exposure to HIV no longer occupies the central, overarching position in gay men's consciousness that it did throughout the 1980s, our work must respond accordingly. We have long known that a range of other health issues, from substance abuse to mental health to hepatitis and other sexually transmitted diseases, are linked to HIV transmission and some organizations worked diligently to incorporate such concerns into their efforts. Yet in an era when some believe more gay men are contracting HIV through sharing needles than having unprotected sex, and where repeated bouts of gonorrhea might prove destructive to HIV-infected men, a holistic approach to gay men's health might be merited.

Lawrence Mass, MD, has argued persuasively that our discussions of oral sex often focus narrowly on questions of HIV transmission and ignore other sexually transmitted diseases:

To date, safer sex guidelines have been negligent in qualifying that not only is there risk, however low, of HIV infection from unprotected oral sex, but there is also the longstanding risk of a whole host of other STD's, and that risk extends to both partners. The other risk needs to be much more clearly and consistently spelled-out in "oral sex is safer sex" materials.[21]

Likewise, discussion of popper usage in gay men's communities has frequently focused on the limited question of whether popper use increases one's risk for Kaposi's sarcoma or other HIV-related opportunistic infections, while skirting a range of other health risks associated with the drugs. Hank Wilson of ACT UP Golden Gate produced a synopsis of studies that focus on poppers and unsafe sex and seroconversion, as well as their relationship to more generalized immunosuppression.[22] Because poppers have returned as a ubiquitous feature of many urban gay dance parties and sex clubs, intensive community-based education about their risk should be initiated.

There is another important reason why gay male HIV prevention might best be situated in a more general gay men's health project rather than a broader AIDS organization: the primary gay populations experiencing significant new infections are young gay men and gay men of color.[23] While efforts have been made, especially in large urban centers, to create population-specific programs to best serve these communities, rarely have leaders of mainstream AIDS organizations responded to the broader health needs of these two groups. A metropolis might have an excellent HIV prevention program for Chicano men who have sex with men, while resources to assist these men with other pressing health concerns are nonexistent. A well-funded HIV-prevention campaign for gay male youth means little when housing programs targeted for street youth are underresourced and substance abuse treatment programs have waiting lists of five months.

HIV-prevention work that emerges from a holistic understanding of gay men's health is likely, in the long run, to prove more effective than isolated, crisis-driven models. Transforming gay-focused AIDS prevention projects into gay health programs is one way to encourage this shift. Ironically, much of the pre-AIDS work on gay men's health issues was interrupted as attention shifted to the plague. For years, the agenda of the National Lesbian and Gay Health Conference was overwhelmingly dominated by HIV/AIDS and offered few workshops on non-AIDS gay men's health issues and fewer still on topics concerned with lesbian health. In 1997, the conference programming began to return to a broader range of priorities, reflecting post-AIDS prevention thinking.[24]

AIDS prevention efforts targeting gay men should be reconceptualized, restructured, and reinvented as multi-issue gay men's health programs that include strong components concerned with substance use, basic needs (food, housing, and clothing), and sexual health (broadly defined). They would no longer take as their central mission limiting the spread of HIV, but instead aim to improve the health and lives of gay men. AIDS should be seen as one of many challenges to gay men's health and our work should no longer position HIV prevention as the overarching focus. AIDS should join a list including suicide, substance abuse, hate crimes, other STDs, cancer, domestic violence, heart disease, and poverty as important threats to gay men's lives.[25]

Some may consider this recommendation outrageous; some may believe I am trying to wipe AIDS off the agenda of our communities. This is not my intent. I believe post-AIDS identities and cultures currently being produced by gay men make ineffective intensive prevention work narrowly focused on HIV/AIDS. Men who have integrated contemporary realities of HIV disease into their understandings of the worlds they inhabit may best take in helpful information about transmission in a richer context including other health concerns.

Any attempt to broaden the agenda beyond narrow AIDS work as conceptualized in the mid-1980s will raise hackles and move some people to issue extreme statements. As one gay man wrote in a letter to *The Village Voice*:

> A couple of years ago, in the throes of Clintonmania, there was finally a palpable sigh of relief: finally the AIDS crisis was over (sort of). Marriage and the military became hot issues. By changing priorities, gay leaders implicitly granted permission to HIV-negative men to start throwing away their condoms. Fifty years from now, "queer" historians might rate this as a moral betrayal of monstrous proportions.[26]

I do not expect AIDS prevention groups to embrace this shift into broader health work easily or without rancor. Gay-focused prevention programs situated in large mega-AIDS groups may find it especially difficult to imagine themselves spun off or transformed into a gay men's health program. One factor might serve as an effective impetus to change: money. For a long time prevention has been the unwanted stepchild of many large AIDS groups, glaring jealously at the large resources channeled toward direct services, treatment, and housing for people with HIV/AIDS. It is common for prevention departments to be funded at a small percentage of what is assigned to direct services departments. If private donations to AIDS groups continue to drop and if government funding also declines, AIDS groups are going to be forced to make hard decisions.

Yet there is evidence in some urban centers indicating that funding for gay health programs may be rising.[27] This presents an especially ironic situation, as throughout most of the past twenty years, funding for non-AIDS gay male services has been minimal or nonexistent. Grant writers seeking funding for gay youth services commonly have had to argue that because queer youth are at great risk for HIV, funds should flow to youth-oriented social programs or beds in youth shelters. If public concern about gay youth continues to rise, it might be possible in some areas to mobilize private giving, including donations from nongay sources, in a manner that parallels AIDS fund-raising during the 1980s.[28] Washington, DC's Whitman-Walker Clinic, which is a primary organizer of that city's gay pride celebration, plans to turn the event into a "mini-AIDS Walk" intended to fund non-HIV-oriented lesbian and gay health programs.[29] Tapping into growing concern about drug abuse also might provide opportunities for expanded resource development.

To discuss funding for gay men's health programs without noting the profound imbalance of resources directed at lesbian health services would be unethical. Mixed lesbian and gay community centers and health centers rarely distribute resources equitably between genders and this is becoming increasingly problematic for women's health advocates who have grown sick of gay men giving obligatory speeches thanking dykes for caring for their brothers with AIDS but failing to translate that gratitude into active support for

lesbian health services. As gay men consider reconceptualizing
their HIV prevention work amid a broader framework of gay men's
health concerns, we might also reexamine our commitment to co-
gender community life and the redistribution of funding in an equitable manner.

Forces are converging that support the reinvention of HIV education for gay men as a broader campaign to improve the health and
lives of all gay men. The Massachusetts Department of Public Health
has grabbed a place in the vanguard of this shift by initiating a broad
effort addressing the health concerns of the gay, lesbian, bisexual,
and transgender community. They have undertaken studies and
needs assessments and engaged in media-based educational programs, mass media advertising, and the initiation of new health
services for this population.[30] Their understanding of the health
needs of gay men is comprehensive and broadly based. Health
promotion planners would be wise to follow Massachusetts' lead and
ensure gay male health programs are not conceptualized around the
needs of the visible white, middle-class gay male population. Large
urban centers, in fact, might reproduce the pattern of population-
specific projects that have flourished during the AIDS era. Separate
programs or groups might be developed under names such as "Queer
Youth Health Project," "Men of Color Health Resources," or "Gay
Men of African Descent Health Center."

Signs of change in prevention programs are already visible and
there is evidence some organizations are rethinking HIV prevention
as they shift paradigms, reinvent themselves for a postcrisis era, and
terminate narrowly conceived programs in order to launch broader
gay men's health initiatives. Gay Men's Health Crisis in New York
City has initiated a major shift in its prevention programs, launch-
ing "Beyond 2000," an "effort to mobilize the gay community
around prevention."[31] The new program aims to recruit 2,000 men
of all serostatuses as volunteers and peer educators who will "help
uninfected gay men stay uninfected through the year 2000, and
beyond." Among the strategies employed are "helping gay men talk
openly about their sex practices and relationships," "complicating
gay men's thinking about risk categories and safer sex," and "using
oral histories as an intervention and a way of learning more about
gay men's lives."[32]

At the core of Beyond 2000 is a commitment to harm reduction:

> We are trying to help gay men think through the values they attach to their specific sexual practices and relationships, the attendant risks and the formation of realistic and individualized risk reduction strategies. . . . A harm reduction approach allows individuals who participate in our programs to honestly identify and talk about their desires, sexual practices and relationships. This approach also allows prevention professionals to move beyond the "one-size-fits-all" model in order to help individuals shape their thinking, clarify their decision-making and develop effective communication skills. In the process, the HIV Prevention Department is seeking to transform conventional condom or "latex education" into a more holistic, meaningful and credible "sex education."[33]

Richard Elovich directs the program and, in many people's minds, is the force behind GMHC's pronounced shift towards harm reduction, which builds on his earlier work in substance use counseling and needle exchange. Elovitch has explained:

> Harm reduction means not judging, but helping people to be more conscious of the kinds of choices they're making. Our counselors frequently hear gay men say, "It just happened." And then what we want to say is "Okay, how did it happen . . . walk me through it." And that's the beginning of counseling.[34]

Harm reduction strategies are not free from controversy. Gay Men's Health Crisis has been criticized for the way its harm reduction philosophy is being used with gay men's health. Duncan Osborne, writing in *LGNY*, has argued:

> Harm reduction techniques applied to injection drug users—distributing clean needles, safer sex education, and information on avoiding needle sharing—have a proven effectiveness in reducing the transmission of HIV. . . . There is no evidence that harm reduction reduces unsafe sex among users of K, X, crystal, or ecstasy. There is only some evidence that these drugs promote unsafe sex, though it is implicit in the

GMHC harm reduction philosophy that they can. In some European countries where harm reduction for injection drug users was once in vogue, advocates are now questioning the philosophy. While it did reduce HIV transmission, it did not reduce the population of users.[35]

GMHC's increasing focus on harm reduction also is reflected in Proyecto P.A.P.I. (Poder, Apoyo, Prevención e Identidad, or Power, Support, Prevention, and Identity), a program aimed at helping HIV-negative Latino gay and bisexual men remain uninfected. Daniel Castellanos, the program's manager explained:

> Each participant has to decide by himself what's "the best" for himself given that he's the only one who owns full information about his life. The relationships we engage in, the kinds of sex we have and like, where we have it and with whom, and what these sexual practices mean for us, are some of the issues that are not addressed in slogans like "Keep it up" or "Use a condom every time . . . " Change has to happen from inside and not from norms imposed from outside. We facilitate the process by which people become more conscious of the flexible choices they are making around condom use. Since we started the program with a discussion group a year and a half ago, we have seen many of these Latino gay and bisexual men become more comfortable when talking about their sexual lives and their Latino identity. Their ability to talk and discuss within different settings about HIV risks in their own lives has helped them to make informed and flexible decisions about the sex they want to have. *This process has come from deep inside because the decision making process is done within and incorporates his expertise about behavior and risks.*[36]

While remaining situated within an AIDS organization, the organizers of Proyecto P.A.P.I. realized that discussing cultural isolation, employment opportunities, immigration status, masculinity, and gay identity, as well as a broad range of related health issues, is essential if they hope to create an effective program.

As Gay Men's Health Crisis shifted paradigms, an hour south of New York City an organization was undergoing a more radical post-AIDS transformation. Philadelphia's SafeGuards Project, long one of the nation's most innovative prevention programs, expanded its mission from addressing primarily HIV prevention, to a "broader and more comprehensive mission of promoting the over-all good health and well-being of gay and bisexual men."[37] While HIV prevention continues as part of the group's work, other neglected issues such as testicular cancer, smoking, hepatitis, and health concerns related to aging are now included in the mix. The group took these steps because:

> . . . our own participants have told us that they have many other health issues that urgently need to be addressed. They have told us that we need to build communities as a way of addressing health issues, including, but certainly not limited to, HIV prevention. . . . Gay men, both HIV positive, HIV negative, and uncertain, have recognized *already* that there are a number of big issues that we've put on hold while we dealt with a crisis for more than fifteen years. These men realize that the future of our communities *depend* upon addressing these issues *now*.[38]

New programs have been initiated by the reinvented SafeGuards, including seminars for men over forty focused on health issues, support groups for people with poor responses to new HIV treatments, and discussions of "substance use and misuse." New workshops have been developed on hepatitis and other sexually transmitted diseases, and a mentoring program has been established for men in their twenties. The project has also considered developing programs on eating disorders and body image, issues facing mixed HIV-status couples, and antigay violence. Leaders of the program have articulated their rationale for making these changes:

> The SafeGuards' change in mission is a recognition that HIV prevention does not equal gay men's health. It is a recognition that our communities need to plan for a future that struggles with a broad range of community work. . . . Our change in mission also recognizes that community health work

is *dynamic*—that it must change to reflect the realities of the communities it serves. At SafeGuards, we have made the change because we believe in what we've heard from the men we serve. These men, of all serostatuses, races, classes, and ages, have urged us to create a health project that promotes our health—not only a metaphor of our health.[39]

Chris Bartlett, Heshie Zinman, and other prevention leaders in the SafeGuards brain trust have identified the ways HIV/AIDS has functioned as a catchall metaphor for gay men's health:

> In essence, in HIV prevention as in care services, AIDS became a metaphor for gay men's health. Urgency led to focus, and a clear and penetrating focus on HIV meant that other health issues fell squarely into peripheral vision.[40]

More than anything else, preventing the continuing confusion of HIV/AIDS with all of gay men's health must be the hallmark of post-AIDS prevention programs. It can be reasonably argued that substance abuse, hate crimes and domestic violence, and hepatitis and other non-AIDS sexually transmitted diseases pose as great a threat to gay men living outside epicenter cities as HIV/AIDS. In the changing epidemic moment, gay men's HIV-prevention programs that rigidly cling to narrow missions may not only fail to limit HIV transmission and improve gay men's health, they may ensure their own demise.

SECTION III:
HIV WORK BEYOND THE PROTEASE MOMENT

I became a victim of the very songs I sing.

—Candi Staton, "Victim"

Things can only get better.
They can only get better if we see it through.

—D:Ream, "Things Can Only Get Better"

Chapter 8

Closing Down Prevention Programs

AIDS prevention groups that do not radically reinvent themselves by closely examining their foundational assumptions and the paradigms out of which they operate will find themselves increasingly marginalized or openly criticized by gay men for being vestiges of Jurassic times. These prevention programs may find themselves out of business in the next few years.

The title of this chapter is intentionally provocative. I believe many—not all—current prevention programs targeting gay men are best understood as relics of the past. They do not speak to the current epidemic context within which most gay men find themselves. Not only do they fail to make positive contributions to the task at hand, but, in some cases, they function in harmful ways. Programs are needed that educate new generations of gay men about HIV and communicate changes in the epidemic to the gay rank and file. Yet I believe there are a number of very important questions about the designs of these programs that should be asked at this time: Are prevention programs for gay men best situated in AIDS organizations or in more broadly conceived gay health promotion projects? What are the goals of such programs and what kinds of objectives would be reasonable to adopt? What should be done to transform crisis-driven programs that remain stuck in the event of AIDS of the 1980s?

I do not mean to suggest everything must be scrapped or that all lessons learned through the first two decades of prevention work should be scuttled. Indeed, prevention workers might return to their roots as gay community advocates who insisted that effective prevention work be situated within a cultural context and take as its starting point the social worlds gay men occupy. This would

241

encourage a fresh look at many of the basic messages still served up by education campaigns. If our mid-1980s work with gay men was embedded in communities that were rapidly cycling through states of terror and grief, is it appropriate to assume that the expectations we maintained at that time would be suitable to a period when gay men are not particularly overwhelmed by sadness or panic-stricken?

It was one thing to expect gay men to practice safe sex 100 percent of the time in the context of 1985, when many expected this sacrifice of sexual pleasure and meaning to last only another year or two. It is quite another thing to maintain similar expectations in 1998, when becoming infected does not promise a swift and ugly death, and we have been asking men to forgo such activities for almost twenty years.

This raises an issue prevention leaders seem unable to confront, which ultimately may make or break prevention organizations in the coming years. In epicenter cities since 1995, while many remain infected with HIV, significantly fewer gay men are sick and dying than in the early 1990s.[1] We expect men either not to notice this shift in the material reality of their lives, or to allow it to have no effect on their worldviews and the ways they organize their erotic lives. Since 1996, we've known many men who have made remarkable recoveries thanks to combination therapies, yet we also expect this knowledge to remain compartmentalized, separated from the information men factor into social and sexual strategies. We read about the so-called "morning-after pill" (which is *many* pills, not a single one, taken over a *lengthy* period of time, not simply on a single morning) and notice that media coverage always includes doctors bemoaning the powerful effect they fear any discussion of postexposure treatments might have on efforts to halt transmission.[2] All our efforts to improve the possibilities of what happens when one is infected with HIV—the result of grassroots community-based perseverance of the past dozen years—are expected to have zero effect on prevention.

The worlds we occupy as gay men in the late 1990s have changed radically in the past few years, but our prevention work has not kept pace. If we can no longer count on a foundation of terror to serve as the impetus motivating gay men to alter their sexual practices (some convincingly argue fear was never an effective impetus for self-protection)[3] we must rethink our strategies and develop new tactics more appropriate to the contemporary climate. Prevention efforts must be radically reinvented at this time.

In considering such a radical rethinking of prevention, I am aware many may feel frustrated because I am not able to direct prevention workers methodically through the step-by-step reconceptualization and restructuring of their work. This is because the transformations I suggest in this chapter must occur within specific contextual arrangements that vary greatly. In some large urban centers, for example, it might be best for HIV prevention for gay African-American men to be situated in black neighborhood health centers rather than mainstream AIDS organizations. In others, it might best be placed within a local organization of black gay men; in still others it might best remain in a mainstream organization. Likewise, in small towns and cities, where various projects focused on distinct populations share office space, I am suggesting that—on a project-by-project basis—stakeholders reconsider and reenvision their work.

I am aware that the systemic changes advocated in this chapter have enormous implications and may seem daunting to folks working in the trenches of prevention. What I am attempting to do here is motivate fresh thinking which will prioritize new events of HIV and the emerging needs of gay men over the weight of bureaucracies and fear-based investments in rigidity and permanence.

TACKLING BIG-PICTURE BARRIERS TO HEALTH

Moving beyond mind-sets dominated by crisis-driven, stop-AIDS-now thinking, prevention workers who remake themselves as gay health advocates will discover many new opportunities to reconceptualize their work. Since HIV prevention for gay men began, most efforts have been rooted in the belief that fully halting the epidemic among gay men within a short time span is a reasonable goal. While this has provided a righteous cause to champion, it has encouraged the deployment of methods more suitable to short-term objectives than to complex, big-picture health challenges. The everyday life of most prevention groups is chaotic and high-pressured; a community of crisis emerges and feeds on drama, panic, and intense interpersonal interactions. Little time is devoted to long-range planning or thoughtful analysis of complex phenomena.

Prevention workers' time is spent planning social marketing campaigns, sitting in excessive numbers of meetings, and organizing public events. Few organizations are structured to encourage systematic and planned group discussion of research data and their implications for education programs. On a recent visit to a major prevention project targeting gay men, I perused the books on the single shelf of their AIDS education library. A staff member commented that the organization's staff hadn't read the books (including works by Gary Dowsett, Walt Odets, Andrew Sullivan, Cindy Patton, Gabriel Rotello, and Urvashi Vaid, among others). "We don't have time to read books," he said casually. "We've got too much work to grab a few moments to sit and read."

This is not a challenge faced only by prevention groups. Contemporary organizational life is structured in ways that limit thoughtful, unhurried consideration of issues. This is as true of law firms as AIDS organizations. Yet organizations determined to make significant changes in business-as-usual with their interventions will not succeed unless organizational processes are reconceived to provide time and space needed for well-considered reflection and analysis. Rather than seeing such discussions as either a luxury or a wasteful exercise, gay men's health groups might understand them as essential to their work. Mindlessly churning out health services or educational interventions often results in reproducing the very problems programs aim to ameliorate.

Understanding the social, economic, and cultural forces that converge on our bodies and contribute to the health or illness of gay men is necessary for successful health promotion. Yet rarely do health care workers see their work as related to larger efforts addressing the sociopolitical issues of the time. Few gay political and health care organizations understood the impact welfare reform would have for gay men with AIDS, even though many people with AIDS are unemployed, homeless, and living in poverty. Fewer still understood the powerful effects it might have on the quality of life of all poor gay men, regardless of HIV status. Many are not accustomed to making linkages between health care, identity, and politics, and training programs for doctors, public health workers, and health educators usually do not adequately address the interrelationship between wellness and political matters.

Although AIDS has allowed some to make a leap and understand how homophobia in Congress translates into a lack of appropriate AIDS education for gay male teens, few are able to link non-AIDS-specific political issues such as the restructuring of the health care system, limits on immigrant rights, and Internet censorship to gay men's health or HIV care and prevention. A community beset by many health challenges somehow fails to place universal health care access at the top of its agenda.

If we abandon the state-of-emergency mind-set and understand HIV as a challenge that will be with us for our lifetimes, even as the landscape of prevention, services, and treatments changes, we may be better able to understand the need for long-term planning that addresses big-picture issues related to HIV prevention. Gabriel Rotello and I disagree on some important things, but we appear to share an interest in understanding how specific sexual acts, such as getting fucked, become central foci of the desires of large numbers of gay men.[4] If erotic desires are not hard-wired into us, it may be possible to learn how specific acts come to hold a central position in the sexual imaginary of a population and create strategies for decentering them. While Rotello recommends incentives, inducements, and a reward system to shift gay cultures, I wonder whether such tactics do not actually bring out a rebellious streak in many gay men and make them determined to enjoy precisely what they are being urged to give up.[5]

Alex Carballo-Dieguez, PhD, has studied the relationship between societal taboos and transgressive acts and argued "homosexual men in Latin America developed survival strategies based mainly on transgression." Carballo-Dieguez writes:

> Transgression is doing what one was told not to do. Where a rule was laid down forbidding men from living their sexuality openly, homosexuals found ways to circumvent that prohibition. . . . Among homosexuals, transgressions range from the maintenance of another man's gaze to signal a personal interest, to overt defiance of prohibitions by gathering in known cruising areas or holding gay parties while bribing the infil-

trated police. Transgression is present at a more intimate sexual level, as violation of cultural taboos with its ensuing pleasures.[6]

Carballo-Dieguez's analysis of the paradox of transgression suggests gay men as a class may develop cultural coping mechanisms that might complicate prevention work. Does telling men to use a condom every time they fuck actually increase some men's desires to fuck without condoms? We do not have answers to this and other questions that seem critical to charting directions for gay men's health promotion in the years ahead. We lack the answers for a few reasons: (1) our focus has been on education under emergency conditions and this leaves little room for long-range thinking; (2) theorizing about prevention uses narrow approaches and ignores disciplines that offer new and valuable thinking; (3) few of us are probing the deeper issues that ultimately determine the effectiveness of our work.

SAVE-OUR-SEX ACTIVISM

Post-AIDS gay health efforts must find a way to energize activism. For too long, advocacy work has focused narrowly on treatments for HIV-infected people. Not only has research on issues related to HIV prevention and education been underfunded and kept isolated from core issues related to gay men's sexual cultures and broader health status, but community activists who have so successfully influenced the processes of developing and testing treatments have failed to target broader health issues, including sexual health maintenance. As Thomas Coates and Michael Shriver have written:

> Though successful at creating pressure for HIV therapies and treatments, gay men have yet to mount a groundswell of activism for prevention. Perhaps this is because drugs and doctors are "normal," what we grew up with, what we find comfort and cure within. The discussion has turned to one's right to access the new treatments. What about the right to be protected from HIV in the first place?[7]

This failure in activism is not solely the result of comfort with drugs and doctors but about the shame and vulnerability gay men feel in asserting our right to community sexual self-determination. This has created significant gaps in our knowledge base about gay men's health. For example, while we now know that having someone ejaculate in one's mouth can result in HIV transmission (although transmission occurs much less easily through oral sex than anal sex) and that pre-cum may contain HIV, we lack much of the information necessary for prevention workers to better support gay men making decisions about cocksucking. Developing activism focused on HIV prevention and non-HIV health issues seems urgent if many gay men remain sexually active with many partners and may likely face a range of health concerns.

When word reached me in 1995 that "prevention activism" was sweeping New York City, I was initially heartened that people were finally motivated to make demands in this area. I had long been disturbed that gay men were willing to become street activists when it involved extending our lives (treatment issues) or easing our deaths (funding for services), but not when it involved saving our sex. I became quickly disheartened when prevention activism in New York swiftly defaulted to encouraging state regulation or closure of sex spaces.[8]

There is an entire sex-positive agenda of activism around gay men's health begging for a mass movement to coalesce:

- **Condom access and availability:** Absent societal proscriptions about anal sex, condom distribution practices would be an essential part of sexually transmitted disease prevention. Seventeen years into the epidemic, few public health departments have seen fit to make condoms widely available in places where men meet to have sex, and many gay establishments do not make them freely available.[9] We should demand universal access to low-cost condoms.
- **Condom research and development:** Two decades into an epidemic in which anal sex is a common mode of transmission, the Food and Drug Administration has not approved a single condom for anal sex usage.[10] When the history of this period of the epidemic is written, this failure will be one of the clearest indictments of the federal government under both Republican and Democratic presidents. Nor is the develop-

ment and testing of anal microbicides central to most activists' agenda.[11] The failure of many HIV-prevention groups to assist gay men in gaining access to the "female condom," proven popular among many gay men during limited distribution attempts, may reveal sex-negative strains in community activism.[12]

- **HIV vaccine development:** While reports have appeared in the press which alternately argue that a vaccine against HIV will never be developed *and* that such a vaccine is just around the corner, no movement has coalesced effectively to demand increasing governmental efforts to make this a priority. Absent such a movement, research on vaccines will be granted limited funding and take place without an appropriate sense of urgency.[13]

- **Sodomy law repeal:** All Americans of conscience should be enraged that prohibitions against sex acts between consenting adults remain on the books in almost half the states. That gay men are targets of the enforcement of most of these archaic laws should incite a radical movement to demand change. A decade ago, the National Gay and Lesbian Task Force made this a visible priority for its work; some organization again ought to place this at the top of its agenda. Sexual prohibition's effects on gay men's identities, legal status, and collective mental health are staggering.[14]

- **Funding for gay men's health:** If post-AIDS prevention work best occurs embedded in a broader project for gay men's health, educating public and private funding sources about the need for this shift is important. Skills, tactics, and even the chants we've used to pressure officials to fund AIDS treatment and services must be transformed to demand funding for research, treatment, services, and prevention surrounding a wide range of gay men's health needs. Gay male health advocates might learn from leaders of the lesbian health movement who, after years of organizing, are now seeing some federal attention directed at their health issues.

As prevention projects undergo metamorphoses in post-AIDS gay communities, they must become self-reflective communities engaged in ongoing study and critical analysis. Such a transformation poses formidable challenges. The simple formation of a weekly study group where teams of workers collectively discuss a research study, for example, will quickly be undermined if the culture of the organization remains crisis driven and the value placed on reflective practice is not permitted to permeate the organization. We hunger for models of health education that solidly rest upon a foundation of thoughtful, critical analysis.

MINDFUL STRATEGIES FOR COMMUNITY BUILDING: SEATTLE'S GAY CITY HEALTH PROJECT

Community building is the most important part of the work of gay health organizations in the post-AIDS era. While this is the dominant theme of *Reviving the Tribe,* the issue merits inclusion here because I have become aware that it is extraordinarily difficult for groups to make the transition from a mind-set of disaster relief to a model of community building. The cultures of most AIDS organizations seem to work against effective long-term community building, yet this is precisely what is demanded in the wake of the destruction of the past two decades.

Many neighborhoods in urban centers throughout the United States have nonprofit and for-profit development corporations charged with long-term planning. These corporations take a strategic approach to development, gathering a great deal of data, filtering it through a participatory community process, and initiating a multiyear (sometimes multidecade) plan for the transformation of the neighborhood. Such groups consider future shifts in demographics, emerging needs of the local population, and innovative ways to generate and balance new housing, neighborhood services, and commercial establishments. Community development is neither an easy nor a speedy process and controversy often arises every step of the way. Yet over a lengthy period, a competent planning process can strengthen the local community and provide for a healthier and more secure future.[15]

Community development is sorely needed by gay men throughout the United States but, because we are a geographically dispersed population and rarely dominate specific neighborhoods, we are usually not central to current processes. Yet the aim of community development efforts to ensure a stronger future for the community through a meticulous process of research, planning, and project initiation has great relevance for contemporary gay communities.[16] Democratically organized processes of planning that welcome mass participation and create blueprints for the future may be especially useful today.

Networks of gay men throughout the nation—in urban, suburban, small-town, and rural areas—who are interested in forging community might form community development groups to investigate and evaluate their current conditions, and begin a process of identifying future needs and prioritizing options. Perhaps a small-city alliance of diverse gay men may decide to initiate formation of a community center that includes gay men, lesbians, bisexuals, and transgendered people. A rural group might identify the need to form support groups for queer youth. An urban black gay men's community might prioritize population-specific health care programs. The possibilities are endless, and a thoughtful, planned process involving the assessment of the strengths and weaknesses of local communities (more than one "gay community" is likely to exist in any specific location) and the prioritization of projects might draw new energy from local gay men.

No one should enter community development efforts thinking they will be quick, easy, and without conflict. Because such processes grapple with fundamental issues close to the hearts of most constituents, they tend to be contentious; participants bring passionate feelings to the issues and, in a diverse community, priorities are likely to differ. Yet the work of negotiation and compromise, if entered into with open eyes and good faith, has the potential to unify a community and bond participants closely together. During the post-AIDS era, this bonding is what many of us are seeking.

Community building by post-AIDS prevention groups also involves the creation of programs that draw men into a collective working relationship over time and promote an ongoing spirit of fellowship and friendship. As masses of men exit the state of emergency, it becomes increasingly clear that the bonds of community have become frayed and need restoration. The intensity of life in the epidemic during the 1980s and early 1990s, particularly in large urban centers, frequently resulted in profound alienation and fragmentation within gay male communities. Not only have surviving men lost lovers, friends, and entire social networks, but the stresses of social upheaval divides men from one another in countless ways. At the height of the epidemic, it sometimes seemed as if we needed one another more than ever, but found it impossible to connect as lovers, friends, and comrades.

Assisting gay men in restoring these linkages is crucial to revival of gay community life in the United States. Some prevention groups perform this function, albeit in limited ways, by offering support and discussion groups, community forums, town meetings, and social activities. Yet because these groups usually maintain narrow missions focused on reducing HIV transmission, the scope of the programming is limited. Groups are formed to discuss what it means to be an HIV-negative gay man and forums are held on the impact of combination therapies on people with HIV. A picnic is organized to afford gay men with AIDS the chance to meet peers, and a town meeting is called that focuses on continuing HIV transmission among young gay men.

These kinds of programs continue to have a place in our work but, in a post-AIDS era, must take a back seat to a broader program of community building. Prevention groups might deploy the earlier tactics—support groups, forums, town meetings—but feature topics not explicitly related to AIDS: male friendships, dating in the 1990s, cross-race relationships, the widening generation gap, class differences within gay communities, sexual pleasures and meanings, and the many forms of spirituality embraced by queer men.

These discussions must be allowed to take place without an obsessive emphasis on AIDS or HIV transmission. In fact, conversations about dating that acknowledge antibody status as an issue, but as one issue among many, accurately situate the topic in a place of balance in our current cultures. New kinds of programming might be considered, focused on storytelling, dance and art therapy, creative movement and drama, activities that encourage men to tap into a range of creative energies.

What would a program focused on community development look like? The work of Gay City Health Project in Seattle offers one window onto post-AIDS community-building efforts. Founded in 1995 by a group of gay men critical of existing HIV-prevention efforts, the organization wisely chose a name that was not specifically AIDS-related in order to embrace a broad agenda determined to support and develop the gay city in Seattle. The organization's brochure opens with a statement proclaiming "Gay City is a Vision":

> Imagine no more poignant memorial services. No more "twenty something and HIV-positive" support groups. No more AIDS protests, no more AIDS fund-raisers. *And no more fucking red ribbons.*
>
> Imagine a future of equality, diversity, community. Imagine a time when gay men count gray hairs, not T-cells. Imagine a world where we're raised to love ourselves as healthy, whole and beautiful. *Imagine.*
>
> Imagine a place where holding hands is not an act of courage. And having sex is not against the law. Imagine no more fear, no more grief. Imagine no more new HIV infections.[17]

The organization aims to develop gay community in Seattle and energetic staff and volunteers organize community forums that are creatively promoted and well produced. Staff function as community organizers and activists, rather than as professionals standing above or aloof from their peers. Hundreds of gay men turn out for these town hall meetings. The group also hosts smaller events aimed at bringing men into community: discussion groups, special events, seminars, noncompetitive ball games, even summer camp. Topics focused upon by Gay City have included dating, local community history, political activism, and the creation of a local gay community center—not your usual fare for more narrowly-conceived prevention programs.

When I visited Seattle, Gay City arranged for me to lead an informal afternoon conversation with leathermen focused on community-building. We expected twenty or thirty men to attend and, thanks to the staff's impressive promotional efforts, over 100 appeared, forcing us to relocate to a larger venue. What impressed me most about our dialogue probing generational shifts in the leather scene, sexual decision making in an S/M context, and power relations between men was the openness of the participants to new thinking. These men, like many throughout the nation, eagerly participate in community when afforded the opportunity.

BUILDING COMMUNITY THROUGH INFORMAL STRUCTURES: ATLANTA'S SECOND SUNDAY

Efforts to build community should never ignore what John Peterson, an associate professor of psychology at George State University, calls "naturally occurring self-help mechanisms" in communities of gay men and men who have sex with men throughout the nation.[18] Networks of friends, neighbors, and social acquaintances have proven invaluable to efforts to care for people with HIV, yet are frequently overlooked by community planners who prioritize formal organizations and institutions. In my own experience, commercial establishments in my neighborhood have served as sites for men to build connections and a spirit of community.

Two particular establishments have been meaningful to my own search for community in the Castro. The Cove Cafe, a small restaurant featuring down-home American food, has been my home-away-from-home throughout the decade I've lived in San Francisco. It is a place I see old friends and make new ones; it functions in a manner similar to the bar on the television show *Cheers* and creates links between people. The restaurant's walls are covered with over 400 framed, glossy photographs of past and present patrons, including many who have died. I visit the Cove to enjoy the food, exchange casual conversation with the staff, and nurture my ties to a broader community.

Gyms may be spaces for body building, but gay gyms have long served as primary sites for community building. For ten years, I have been part of the 6 a.m. workout crew at Market Street Gym, which opened the month I moved to the city. From its creation, the gym distinguished itself from Muscle System, a gay gym located on the next block, by attracting a younger crowd (gay men in their twenties, while Muscle System was popular among gay men in their thirties), welcoming both men and women, and affecting an ultrahip image. I joined this gym, despite feeling like one of its older members (at the time, approaching thirty-five), because the men at Muscle System both attracted and intimidated me. In those days, Market Street Gym was as much as I could handle.

The gym has been one of my major windows into the cultures of young gay men. I've observed their semiotics and aesthetics, listened to their music and gym banter, observed their flirtations and dalliances. I've watched these men as they buffed up, shaved their bodies, pierced their nipples (and occasionally their noses, navels, or cocks), and aged from the mid-twenties to mid-thirties. Some of these men I've seen at 6 a.m. every morning for years, but have never seen them outside the gym. A few have become friends; more commonly they've become social acquaintances, men with whom I chat at the grocery store, greet on the street, or dance at various clubs.

The gym has served me as a supportive site as I've gone through the ups and downs of life. To find safety in a space commonly depicted as intensely competitive seems ironic to me, yet my gym cronies have been quietly supportive of me as I've held community leadership positions, endured media scrutiny, and published controversial books. They've watched me lose and gain and lose weight, develop muscles and change my image, try out a goatee and shave my back, shoulders, and upper arms. The 6 a.m. crowd these days is largely made up of men (and a few women) in their mid-thirties and forties, and we've collectively contended with the joys and trials of aging in the gay ghetto.

Market Street Gym, the Cove Cafe, Pasqua, and similar commercial establishments are valued places where gay men are creating new identities and building community. I make this statement fully aware of the creeping privatization that has swallowed up public spaces, and the ways commodification and the commercialization of our social worlds presents both barriers to and opportunities for social change. While gay men continue to forge community through political and social service organizations, nonprofit cultural groups, and formalized social networks, increasingly many of our lives and identities seem inextricably bound up with the places where we dance, dine, drink coffee, and work out. The gay men with whom I enjoy tea are as central to my life as my political colleagues, twelve-step friends, and HIV prevention cohorts.

While community organizers committed to gay men's wellness might continue to make efforts to limit privatization and increase the development of new public spaces, they should not fail to direct efforts toward all the sites in which gay men currently are creating new identities. At best, gay health advocates see these venues as either problematic or as potential walls on which to hang posters promoting safer sex or fund-raising events. More useful ideas might emerge through discussions with staff and patrons of the establishments.

Much of the community-building work among gay men during the past two decades has occurred outside organizations that maintain overtly political or health advocacy agendas. Gay men have established a wide range of social groups including bowling leagues and sports teams, choruses and bands, ethnicity, neighborhood, and race-based discussion groups, motorcycle gangs, fetish-focused networks, and hobby-oriented clubs ranging from square dancers to stamp collectors to bird watchers. Health advocates diminish their effectiveness when they do not understand the potential of these groups to nurture men and improve the overall health of communities.

Much of the energy that was directed toward establishing AIDS organizations in the mid-1980s is being directed into social organizations that constitute the infrastructure of community life for increasing numbers of men in the post-AIDS period. Although some may minimize the value of these groups, wishing resources were diverted into overtly political and health-advocacy groups, groups such as community centers, ethnicity- and race-based discussion groups, and even sports or musical groups, may serve as valuable points of entry for gay men who may be initially hesitant with political involvement but later go on to participate more fully in such activities. They are also valuable in their own right.

Black gay men throughout the United States are one population currently experiencing mass community building, often through social organizations and informal networks. A circuit of black lesbian and gay events has emerged over the past few years, drawing thousands to Washington, DC, on Memorial Day weekend for Black Gay Pride festivities, Los Angeles for July 4th At The Beach Party, and to Atlanta over Labor Day for In The Life Atlanta parties. As one local participant in the Atlanta event enthusiastically told me:

> Over Labor Day you see a *lot* of brothers and sisters that you've never seen before just walking down the street, in the parks downtown, attending parties all weekend. The clubs are *packed*, with lines going around the corner.[19]

One group enjoying great popularity in Atlanta is Second Sunday, a support organization "created to assist the collective growth of gay, bisexual and transgendered men of African descent through educational, social, spiritual and cultural activities."[20] The group meets on the second Sunday of the month and focuses discussion on a specific topic. Anywhere from 100 to 200 men come together for conversation, socializing, and a potluck supper.

The genesis of Second Sunday exemplifies many men's need to come together for bonding and sharing of mutual concerns and interests. Three Atlantans visiting Washington, DC, in 1992 attended a rap group for black gay men, and were determined to start a similar program in their own city. The first discussions were held in men's homes and attracted no more than ten or twenty men who were involved in either the local black community or the black gay and lesbian community. From the start, an attempt was made to create a safe, nonjudgmental space that felt homey and relaxed.

By 1994, people "were packing into people's homes and you'd have forty guys packed into a guy's living room . . . there were people sitting on the floor, standing in the kitchen, sprawled out in the corners."[21] The group next moved to more public spaces, a local church, and then a municipal building. The informal processes of the founding members were replaced by elected officers, organizational bylaws, and task-oriented committees. In addition to the monthly discussion group, Second Sunday sponsored house party fundraisers, picnics, and a retreat. Currently the group has a membership of 300 men and a mailing list of 400 to 500 people.[22]

Craig Washington, one of Second Sunday's cochairs, told me that the group is focused on "community building, not AIDS prevention," though he believes the two are related:

I think the most powerful thing about Second Sunday is not even what we're talking about that day, but that we're here together, 150 strong. It's the fact that there is so much potential out of the group for establishing linkages. This can be about having a network of folks in terms of their job skills and professional affiliations, so you know there's a brother you can go to if you need a printing job, for example. That's part of community-building. People think that's just economic, and economic is part of it, but there are also the intangible support mechanisms.[23]

John Peterson, the associate professor at Georgia State University and a participant in Second Sundays, also sees community building as the primary function of the group:

It is very clear to me that the men who are coming [to Second Sunday] are not coming with primary interest in HIV risk and prevention. They are coming with many needs that have to do with their experience in a subculture of the African-American community, as men who have sex with men, most of whom, to my knowledge, identify as gay . . .

No matter how pressing the epidemic has become, Second Sunday can never become an AIDS organization. To address AIDS in the African-American men who have sex with men community, you cannot simply address HIV prevention or risk. In the cultural context of this population you have to address the issues that involve sexuality and identity for this population as much as you address HIV risk. Community development is the really difficult issue. Dual identity has just as much importance as HIV risk. Men come to us with multiple issues.[24]

Groups such as Second Sunday may be experiencing widespread success during this post-AIDS period because, in the face of AIDS' impact on gay communities throughout the nation, men feel deeply that community rebuilding is in order. Second Sunday provides a focus for men's efforts to reinvent identity and recreate social networks, as they continue to struggle with HIV/AIDS and tackle broad issues of cultural development.

QUEER PROMISE KEEPERS:
DESIGNING OUR OWN MASS RITUALS

Throughout America there seems to be a hunger for mass rituals that unite diverse people, counter the fragmentation and alienation that accompany postmodern life, and create meaning beyond self-centered urges for money, career, and achievement. People seek not only one-on-one relationships, small friendship networks, and intimate social groups, but also connection to much larger groups, symbolic communities that allow us to feel tied to some mass movement outside ourselves. A late twentieth-century quest for connection seems aimed at countering forces in our culture that leave us divided and isolated.[25]

This longing is reflected in the success of Right-wing networks of Promise Keepers that pack stadiums full of men promising to fulfill their "God-given" roles as husband, father, and breadwinner. Joe Conason, Alfred Ross, and Lee Cokorinos described a Promise Keepers rally in *The Nation:*

> Very early on a Friday morning in July, hundreds of men walked toward Three Rivers Stadium through the still-dark streets of Pittsburgh. Mostly white and of varying ages, they looked like ordinary sports fans, except that their baseball caps and T-shirts didn't bear Pirates or Steelers logos but were adorned instead with pictures of Jesus and catchy slogans like "His Pain, Your Gain" and "Christ: The Real Thing." Many were accompanied by their sons, but none by wives, girlfriends or daughters. As they entered the stadium and filled the bleachers, the first arrivals began to clap, sing and engage in warm-up cheers. . . . For two full days, the stadium echoed with chanting as a throng of almost 50,000 from Pennsylvania and surrounding states joined in a stirring, brilliantly produced spectacle combining elements of religious revival, rock concert and football rally. Gazing down from their seats at an enormous, stage-like altar on the field, they listened raptly as professional evangelists, sports figures and Christian musicians bombarded them with preaching and music about the worthlessness, sinfulness and possible redemption of the American male. By sunset on the last day, in what appeared to

be a spontaneous outpouring of emotion, nearly every one of these men threw his arms around the friends or strangers standing next to him. Weeping with cathartic joy, they bowed before the altar's huge video screens, hands raised in supplication, swearing to become better husbands and fathers and to "take back the nation" for Christ.[26]

While criticized from the Left as "antigay and antiwoman," and dubbed "the return-to-male-supremacy Promise Keepers," this burgeoning wing of the evangelical movement may be tapping into powerful social needs that social change groups would be wise not to ignore.[27] Kerry Lobel, executive director of the National Gay and Lesbian Task Force, knows this:

> There's a real need for some to feel more connected to family and community. The rhetoric of Promise Keepers fills that need. However, the reality is that the organization scapegoats women and gay people, blaming them for the collapse of family and community.[28]

I do not intend to say that the political underpinnings of the Promise Keepers are worth emulating, or that the identical forces that draw men to their rallies are operating among most gay communities. Yet I believe current configurations of masculinities leave most men of all races and sexual identities longing to heal wounds engendered by male socialization and hungry to connect with other men through mass cultural processes.

This powerful urge may resonate at various places where gay men gather en masse: the San Diego Gay Rodeo, summer retreats for black gay men, twelve-step round-ups, bear expositions, weekend workshops for men with AIDS, circuit parties, and rural new age gatherings. I feel it regularly at the Sunday beerbust at the San Francisco Eagle, my local leather bar; I've experienced similar feelings at community forums organized by prevention groups where men gather to discuss the relative safety and risk of oral sex, the relationship between HIV-positive and HIV-negative men, and the impact of protease inhibitors on prevention work.

Organizing mass rallies around fundamentalist religious practices or reactionary political beliefs is quite different from aiming for similar effects to emerge from gay male communities composed of men of different religions, politics, and cultures. The success of the Promise Keepers is grounded in a comfort level with authoritarianism and militaristic practices that is not shared by many gay men. Yet I believe creating our own form of Promise Keepers, situated within the political and cultural milieu of gay male communities, merits exploration.

If we can come together to affirm our identities as leathermen, Asian gay men, circuiteers, or gay Harvard alumni, and if we can spend time engaged in dancing, cruising, and social banter, it might be possible to join together to affirm broader identities as gay men committed to reinvigorating identities and cultures. Judging from events such as the Hotlanta raft race weekend, Hellfire Inferno, the MCC International Convention, In the Life Atlanta, and gatherings of Billies, the talent clearly exists to create our own "brilliantly-produced spectacles" that do not share the Promise Keepers' underlying aim of affirming male supremacy.

A community without rituals is vulnerable to fragmentation and discord. The primary rituals shared by gay men—coming out and attending Gay Pride marches—do not function to provide meanings that draw us together in the 1990s. Because coming out often occurs in isolation, and Gay Pride marches in many urban centers have become aimless, depoliticized celebrations with little clarity of focus, gay men as a class currently could be considered a population without mass rituals symbolically linking our various subgroups.

This is an urgent and daunting challenge for those concerned about building gay male community. Can we envision stadiums or auditoriums full of gay men united behind specific themes, sharing in song and chants, and inspired by unifying speeches? Would it be possible to take on the formally articulated objective of the Promise Keepers, reconciliation among racial groups and between men and their wives and children, and adapt it to our own cultural contexts and political values? Could this be achieved without lapsing into authoritarianism and superficiality? What could these mass-produced events contribute to restoring the health and well-being of gay male communities?

At this particular juncture in our history, gay men may be simultaneously attracted to and repulsed by such ritualistic events. Some of us are perpetual outsiders and will never feel comfortable in large group situations, let alone in stadiums filled with thousands of gay men. Yet my memories of being in Yankee Stadium for the closing ceremonies of the Gay Games in 1994, while it was jam-packed with gay men, lesbians, and supporters, make me believe such extraordinary convergences are both possible and valuable. Thoughtfully planned and carefully produced events focused on injecting into gay male cultural life themes such as promoting caring in our social, sexual, and political lives, combating racism, and healing rifts between generations of gay men can assist us in jump-starting processes of community building. While not the sole answer to the complex and shifting needs facing gay male communities or the issues that divide us, mass rituals can provide one useful arena in which to tackle tough issues facing our communal life.

ABANDONING THE ROLE
OF MORAL JUDGE OF THE COMMUNITY

Few prevention groups believe they assume a role of moral judge in their work. After all, they pass out condoms, use vernacular terms such as "fucking" and "blow jobs," and don't bat an eye when men casually mention fisting and watersports. Since the early days of the epidemic, educators of gay men have expressed a commitment to supporting diverse values and avoiding admonishment and moralizing. We have tried to offer nonjudgmental information and support to men whose sexual practices we do not share and whose sexual values seem different from our own.

Sometimes, however, judgments and moralizing sneak into the work, even into good efforts by organizations that aim to avoid preaching and finger wagging. Once again, Gay City's brochure provides a text for review. A few pages after the vision statement is a page that reads:

> Gay City Is In CRISIS
> 50,000
> Gay and bi men live in the Seattle area.
> 10,000
> of us are HIV-positive.

2000
of us have died of AIDS so far.
2000 more
of us will get infected with HIV in the next 5 years.
The government is not giving us HIV.
The Christian Right is not giving us HIV.
We are giving HIV to each other.
It's up to us to save our tribe.[29]

This statement reeks of moralistic judgment and Larry Kramer-style guilt-tripping. Not only is Gay City a dozen years late in attempting to shake Seattle area men awake to their belief that they are in crisis, but the drama-queen statement "We are giving HIV to each other" is gross simplification of a complex matter. Turn the page, and Gay City's "Call to Action" appears, stating:

Somewhere along the way, a lot of us started slipping back into unsafe sex. And a new generation of risk takers came of age. Today, an alarming *40 percent of us are fucking without condoms*. There are a thousand reasons why and no simple solutions.

This section raises difficult questions. If Gay City realizes "there are a thousand reasons" why gay men fuck without protection and there are "no simple solutions" to what they clearly conceptualize as a problem, why represent gay men engaging in an act that has transcended centuries and cultures as "slipping back" or regressing? Why reduce buttfucking to "unsafe sex"? Why simplistically characterize young gay men attempting to create meaningful erotic lives amid the threats of their contemporary social worlds as "a new generation of risk-takers"?

The answer can be found on the next page, where the organization's mission appears:

Our MISSION is to dramatically reduce the number of new HIV infections in Seattle-area gay and bi men by the year 2000. Gay City is committed to building community, promoting communication and nurturing a culture where gay men see their lives as worth living.

With one glaring exception, this is a wonderful mission statement and succinctly captures the key elements of community-wide health revival: expansive communication, affirming cultures, and building community. Yet burdening these nurturing objectives with the goal of *dramatically cutting new HIV infections* infuses a powerful dose of crisis-driven determination into the mix. By taking as its central aim the drastic reduction in unprotected sex, founders of Gay City may have ultimately undermined their loftier, more life-giving goals. Perhaps government grants demand prevention groups maintain a primary focus on reducing infections, but short of coercive measures such as quarantine, closure of sex spaces, and the elimination of gay bars and meeting places, no one truly knows how to effect such a reduction (particularly a "dramatic" one) in a short period of time.

It may be appropriate for some gay groups to keep HIV prevention in a prominent position in their mission statements and in their organizational work. Yet I believe maintaining a narrow focus on reducing infections, as opposed to placing this aim in a context of general overall health promotion, triggers a single-mindedness that easily shifts into moralizing and subtle coercion. This may lead prevention programs to take on a traditional schoolmarm role, wagging their fingers, and chiding the bad boys to stop the mischief. By not making behavior change the criteria for success or failure of a project, staff members would be granted the breathing space and creative freedom to experiment freely with new ideas.

Some have argued that there is a distinction between "being moral and being 'moralistic.'"[30] While I agree the terms are distinct, they frequently are defined from vantage points that do not acknowledge bias. Gabriel Rotello attempts to make a case that things are immoral when they are harmful, "especially in a way that is almost certain to destroy human life." He continues:

> In the same way, individual sexual behaviors that traditional moralists might consider "always wrong" can still be considered perfectly moral so long as they don't produce widespread harm. But those behaviors must be considered immoral when they do. Harm is the key—ecological harm. The principle will come to be employed more and more as the earth gets increas-

ingly crowded and its ecosystems increasingly strained. It does not seem regressive to put it to use in the service of gay survival as well.[31]

Yet Rotello does not fully grasp that "harm" is a relative term, socially constructed, and not universal. Instead he essentializes the concept, ignoring, for example, many Americans' belief that same-sex relations are "harmful" because families may be divided and wracked by pain, gays may be discriminated against, and gay men are a population at risk for HIV/AIDS. Does that make one's choice to live as a homosexual immoral? Although his argument has surface appeal, it exemplifies how easy it is to confuse moralism and morality.

Post-AIDS prevention programs relinquish moralizing and judgmentalism because they do not operate under the emergency conditions Gay City believes it is facing. Once organizations step beyond the crisis construct and accept the epidemic as a long-term challenge against which we need to develop long-haul tactics, they are freed from the pressure to condemn every incident of unprotected sex or feel personally responsible for every new infection. They know that moralizing is not sound public health strategy with gay men.

What does this look like? AIDS prevention projects provide gay men with information, support, counseling, and advice, and assist in the regeneration of our communities by allowing each gay man to find his own way forward. Incidents of unprotected sex are neither shameful embarrassments nor red badges of courage, and men who become infected with HIV are seen neither as condemned to an early death nor as hot studs who made the "ultimate sacrifice." Post-AIDS prevention work takes much of the charge out of these matters and inserts gay men again into the fabric of a complex culture. We neither romanticize nor demonize specific sex acts. Our work is about supplying current information, assisting men in acquiring appropriate social and sexual skills, and supporting men as we collectively create lives that are worth living. We do our best at these aims and trust, over the long haul, that HIV-infection rates will decline. We do the education work and prevention will follow.

Chapter 9

The Final Days of AIDS Inc.

In October 1996, I traveled to Washington, DC, to experience the mass display of the Names Project's AIDS Memorial Quilt. I made the trip because I had to, even though I live three short blocks from the Quilt offices in the Castro and walk past their storefront almost every day. I am one of the gay men whose history and identity are deeply sewn into the Quilt's panels. Displays of the Quilt serve as a catalyst for release of grief that accumulates inside me. When I first heard the announcement of the "final display of the AIDS Quilt in its entirety," (yet again), I immediately blocked off the dates on my calendar. I had to be there.

The trip took on unexpected urgency because of the recent losses I'd suffered when Frank and Dick died during the preceding summer. Dick had insisted no formal service be held and, because I was not close to any of his surviving friends, I mourned him in isolation. Frank's funeral felt like a big deal to me, one of those small, serene gatherings that his Shanti volunteer organized in a bucolic park in West Hollywood. The feelings of grief I held for him, however, were greater than any single event could release. I saw my visit to Washington for the Quilt display as a chance, once again, to make good use of that huge communal ritual.

During the months that led up to that October weekend, I found it difficult to get any of my East Coast friends to commit to joining me at the Quilt. For many of them, it seemed, the Quilt had outlived its purposes and seemed archaic, a vestige of the past.[1] Some were caught in judgments of the culture and politics of the Names Project, and considered themselves too radical for what had become simply another exercise in AIDS kitsch. I found myself wondering about my own impetus for attending. Here I was flying cross-country for no other reason than this event, but pals in Boston or New York or Philadelphia couldn't be bothered. Why was this a command performance for me, yet they viewed it as an onerous task?

One friend infuriated me. About a dozen years earlier, Frank introduced me to Vince ("my best friend from the 'New York years,'" he'd told me) while he was visiting from the East Coast. Vince and I became fast friends and, as Frank's health declined, I leaned on him as close friends became accustomed to doing during the plague years. When Frank died, I longed for Vince's companionship in mourning, so it was difficult for me to hide my reaction when he informed me he was not flying to Los Angeles for the memorial service. At that time, I extracted a promise from Vince—I suppose now I forced it on him—that he would join me at the Quilt in October and we'd engage together in a ritual of farewell for Frank.

Two days before I headed East I found Vince's voice on my answering machine, bailing out from the Washington weekend. He and his lover had been traveling a great deal, were exhausted, and simply needed a weekend at home. It all made sense to me, but that didn't prevent a rage from erupting within, as I felt Frank was disrespected by Vince's action, and realized I would be at the Quilt without another close friend of Frank's.

My feelings of anger were unexpected and irrational. Early in the epidemic I had learned I had to cut friends some slack when dealing with AIDS deaths. After judging one man harshly for refusing to be a day-to-day caregiver for a close mutual friend suffering from dementia, I learned he'd been caring for sick friends constantly for two years and was about to go crazy from giving injections and changing diapers. All of us who were heavily impacted by AIDS reached our limits in attending funerals and memorials, and I learned people grieve in many ways. None of us was prepared for the morbidity we confronted, and judging others would only isolate me, leaving me alone with my losses.

I therefore flew east for Quilt Weekend in a conflicted state of both understanding and anger, knowing I'd be putting in much time at the Quilt and that much of it would be by myself. Ordinarily, this would be fine, but I knew that, because I used the Quilt as a ritual of unabashed grief, I'd need companions nearby. I wanted to visit dead friends' panels and sob undisturbed. Having a buddy close at hand protected me from spectators who might be alarmed at a big guy on his knees wailing, and from "grief monitors" who had kept trying to hug me at the last Quilt display.

STUFFING THE RED RIBBON RHETORIC

Fortunately, while in Washington I was staying with my old friend Tom, who'd befriended me in Boston in the 1970s, when we were young gay guys, dancing at the Sunday tea dance at Chaps and organizing gay and lesbian schoolworkers. Despite the significant cultural differences between us—Tom's Irish Catholic background left him less demonstrative than my own Eastern European Jewish background—I knew Tom and I brought similar feelings to the Quilt. As we stood on the sidelines during the opening ceremonies, we were watching our generation of gay men unfurled before us, and we were there to honor their lives. These were the men with whom we created identity and community in the 1970s and early 1980s; we'd danced, dated, tricked, and organized together. We were there to feel their presence surround us again, celebrate those never-severed connections, and again tell them good-bye.

Tom is a high-level appointee in the Clinton administration. A graduate student from out of town could spend the entire morning at the Quilt, but Tom had to go to work and could grab only a few hours to walk the pathways of the Quilt with me. While he was there, we scanned the index of the Quilt directory together, then rushed to specific locations to find old boyfriends, colleagues, and friends. I'd kneel down in front of an especially meaningful Quilt panel and immerse myself in conversation with a deceased pal. Inevitably this would attract observers. When the tears started and my babbling escalated, Tom would watch from a distance and warn off well-intentioned people who were drawn to comfort this blubbering boy. I was there to mourn publicly and I did not need to be held or comforted. The decimation of the epidemic in my life felt beyond being comforted or quelled.

When Tom took off for work, I was on my own, examining random swatches of fabric, marveling at the care that went into their handiwork, laughing at the humor threaded into this huge, colorful blanket spread over a space the size of many football fields stretching between the Washington Monument and the Capitol. Mostly I enjoyed the many references on the panels, some subtle, some not-so-subtle, to gay male sex cultures before the plague: a red handkerchief stitched into one panel, memorializing forever the deceased's passion for fist-fucking; photos of a man in leather chaps and vest, standing astride his prized Harley; quotations scrawled into Quilt panels from disco divas of our young years: Diana Ross, Donna Summer, and Gloria Gaynor.

I made daily visits to the Quilt throughout the weekend, stretching in time from an hour to half a day. Much of the sorrow stored inside my brain poured out that weekend. Yet during my visits to the Quilt, at the Candlelight AIDS March, and at the countless receptions, meetings, and conferences surrounding the weekend, something began to feel uncomfortable to me. Something felt different about visiting the Quilt this time from just a few years ago. I couldn't pin it down at first, and, as usual, I needed Tom to help me see the obvious.[2]

We attended the Candlelight AIDS March on Saturday night with Dennis, another friend from our dancing and organizing years, and his lover Donald. As we stood on the steps of the Capitol in the early evening sunlight, listening to the speeches and songs exhorting us to be strong and keep fighting the good fight, we began to make comments, dishing the rhetoric with which we'd become so familiar over the past fifteen years. "Our friends are not dead; they are with us tonight. Their spirits live on; they will never die," a speaker would plaintively tell the crowd.

"Sorry," I'd say loud enough for our small crowd to hear. "Our friends really are dead. They are no longer alive. They're gone, dead, kaput. AIDS kills. I swear, it really does. The worms crawl in and the worms crawl out. They are dead. Bye bye." Tom would chuckle but hush me up and go back to cruising the crowd.

"We must fight on; the cure is possible. It is right around the corner. We must be vigilant until we have the cure!" another speaker would exhort us.

Now it was Tom's turn. "Sorry, pal, we're not going to see a cure in our lifetime. Yeah, work for it all you want, but don't hold your breath. You've been saying the same line about the cure for a decade and a half!" We'd break into embarrassed laughter, try to muzzle our giggling, and join in the spirit of the event.

It was during this informal banter, while we were behaving like mischievous schoolboys, that I realized what was going on for me.

Something *was* different. An entire sea change had washed over AIDS work and gay communities throughout the nation over the past six months, yet the transformation of our communal life was only referred to here as a distraction, a trap lulling us into complacency. We'd all seen the headlines: fewer people were dying of AIDS, new drugs were bringing people back from the brink of death, the avalanche of corpses had subsided. Yet we were hearing the same pitches, singing the same songs, and being asked to share in the same war metaphors we'd embraced through the peak years.

I became aware of a conflict that emerged for me that evening, between old-school exhortations about the epidemic and the worlds we currently occupy. Only when I turned my brain off and let myself get intoxicated by the powerful culture of Quilt Weekend did all the talk of "crisis" and "cure" and "war" and "victory" seem meaningful. Most of the time, unable to shut off my thoughts, the red ribbon rhetoric grated on me like fingernails on a blackboard. The world of AIDS had changed dramatically over the past year, but few here acknowledged it, struggled to understand the changes, or found a way to welcome the transformation as something positive. From that moment on, it became impossible for me to sit comfortably through the familiar narratives of heroism and battles, crucifixion and resurrection.

For these rituals to remain meaningful to me, they will need to take a giant step into the post-AIDS era. For the Quilt to avoid becoming a vestige of the moment in which it was conceived, it has to be reconceptualized in a dramatically changed context. The work of rethinking, reinventing, and restructuring our work against HIV/AIDS must be taken on by the entire system we formed to respond to the epidemic. Organizations, rituals, publications, and entire systems will either swiftly be reconceived and reborn, or they surely will be abandoned as fossils of a painful past.

RESTRUCTURING HIV WORK FOR A POST-AIDS ERA

It is time for everyone involved in any part of what has come to be known as the "AIDS system" or "AIDS Inc." to take a collective deep breath and engage in serious review, analysis, and redesign of our efforts. While voices have been calling for AIDS service organizations (ASOs) to rapidly review and restructure their priorities, the kind of systemic change demanded necessitates deep self-reflection by governmental AIDS bureaus, grassroots AIDS activist groups, publications targeting people with HIV/AIDS, medical professionals in hospitals and health clinics, fund-raisers for AIDS groups, and self-help organizations of people with HIV/AIDS.

There are no quick and easy answers. The changes triggered in epicenter cities in the mid-1990s, initiated by the predicted dramatic fall-off of deaths and expanded by new treatments and large numbers of people with HIV living healthy lives, are rocking the foundation of the AIDS system. Nothing has gone unaffected and nothing is invulnerable to the fallout. This is because what it means to be a person living with HIV, or anyone involved in the AIDS system as volunteer, staff member, provider, or participant, is changing dramatically from what it was just five years ago. One journalist astutely observed:

> Change is scary, and we are entering a period of change that involves not just the facts of this particular virus, or of one particular sex act, but the identities gay men have constructed around AIDS in order to survive: HIV-negative, HIV-positive, PWA, AIDS activist, AIDS educator, service provider, fund-raiser. What do these roles mean anymore? Are they still relevant? What does it mean to be a "Person with AIDS" who isn't sick, or to be HIV-positive when no trace of virus can be found in your blood? What does it mean to have "unsafe" sex if you're not risking death? How are these new realities going to affect not just our sex lives, but every other aspect of our lives?[3]

Just as it is vitally important for prevention leaders to confront these powerful changes carefully in reconsidering their work, so must leaders in other areas—services, housing, fund-raising, information, treatment, activism, and rituals—closely analyze shifts occurring at this time and thoughtfully strategize about new directions for the future.

Gay men must play a leadership role in these conversations, as we have done through much of the past two decades on matters regarding HIV and AIDS. We must remember, however, that gay male communities do not share a singular experience of AIDS and that the diverse AIDS epidemics that have affected gay men throughout the nation may be distinct from the AIDS epidemics targeting other populations. Our own experiences in the epidemic must inform our thinking, but we must be humble enough to place our experiences in proper perspective. This is particularly true for gay men who inhabit gay neighborhoods in epicenter cities. Shifts are certainly occurring right now in the Castro, West Hollywood, and Chelsea, and they have both similarities and differences with the ways AIDS is changing in San Francisco's Mission District, South Central Los Angeles, and the South Bronx in New York. Learning to share power with other affected communities seems vital.

Planned change in the AIDS system is preferable to unplanned change, but not much easier. Epidemiological shifts and biomedical developments initiate major, complex sociocultural changes in the communities affected by HIV/AIDS. These changes may be recognized and responded to or they may go unrecognized and response may be avoided. The failure of organizations and systems to respond to sociocultural changes in their environments causes individual incidents of conflict to emerge that are often dramatically played out and understood only partially, stripped of the broader context. The failure to respond creates confusion among and between various constituencies and also results in dysfunctional interactions including undermining of leadership, scapegoating of organizations, the production of dualistic and polarized thinking, and the circulation of a great deal of free-floating finger-pointing and blaming.

This is precisely what has started to occur in the wake of dramatic changes that affect the entire AIDS system, nationally and locally, which have not been responded to in any serious way. A growing criticism of large AIDS organizations has emerged in epicenter cities, and groups such as AIDS Project Los Angeles, Gay Men's Health Crisis, and the San Francisco AIDS Foundation have been targeted as mega-bureaucracies out of touch with the people whom they were created to serve.[4] Key leaders in the fight against AIDS—particularly heterosexual women such as federal AIDS czar Patsy Fleming and San Francisco AIDS Foundation Executive Director Pat Christen—have been attacked, demonized, and targeted for harassment.[5] The AIDS Ride, an ambitious fund-raising effort conceived and directed by Dan Palotta, has been criticized, maligned, and taken to court.[6] Organizations, leaders, and campaigns that were exalted as saintlike in the mid-1980s, by the mid-1990s had been recast as vampires, draining the lifeblood of the community for personal gain.

This kind of internal critique and infighting is not new in either AIDS organizing or gay communities throughout the nation, nor is it limited to our communities. This has been an internally contentious epidemic since the day it began and it will continue to be so. Issues that circulate around the epidemic in gay communities—death, illness, and disability, as well as sex, drug use, race, and class—are likely to inspire heated debate and test the bonds of any romanticized version of "AIDS community" or "gay family." What is new this time around is that the terrain on which our civil wars are being waged is trembling underneath our feet as we debate, bicker, and take swipes at one another.

For example, the attacks on Pat Christen's leadership of the San Francisco AIDS Foundation have become among the most vitriolic and extreme, even in San Francisco, a community that traditionally has eaten its leaders alive. Critics have targeted her salary as their key concern and posted demeaning and sexist stickers with her likeness on them throughout the Castro.[7] They also have vocally castigated her at public events, and one small activist group dumped used kitty litter on her at a community forum. Perhaps because her loudest critics have a long history of choosing enemies within the AIDS system and engaging in protracted hate campaigns, the AIDS Foundation board and management have easily dismissed the criticisms and stood strongly in defense of her salary and organizational leadership.[8]

Yet the offensive launched against Christen is rooted, in part, in post-AIDS era changes that the AIDS Foundation would do well to acknowledge. Issues that may merit review constitute the underpinnings of the haphazard and often unethical attacks. One of these issues involves whether the changes occurring in the epidemic at this point necessitate the continued existence of a centralized, bureaucratized mega-organization or whether a new form of service delivery might increase efficiency and cut costs.

Critics have offered contradictory interpretations of what's wrong with AIDS services in San Francisco for years; they view any large AIDS organization that emerges as a worthy target for attack, yet they decry the multitude of small organizations that force clients to travel from one to another to receive services. Activists chide the AIDS service delivery system constantly for extensive duplication of services, yet when services are combined and situated in a single organization, that organization is attacked for being monocultural or becoming too large a bureaucracy. AIDS organizations, it seems, cannot win.

Does the assault on Christen's salary reflect increasing divisions based on economic class that are tearing at the once-unified constituency of people with AIDS? The newspaper spearheading media attacks on Christen, San Francisco's *Bay Area Reporter (B.A.R.)*, has long engaged in relentless campaigns critical of local AIDS groups that are large and bureaucratically organized and frequently fingers organizational leadership for attack, including me when I served as executive director of a local AIDS organization in the early 1990s. Yet the *B.A.R.* clearly shares the view of many people who question whether formal, large organizational structures are needed to support people with HIV. From this perspective, grassroots efforts such as the AIDS Emergency Fund, which provides cash grants to people with HIV in emergency situations, and small, underresourced groups such as AIDS Benefits Counselors, become seen as the models for service delivery. Despite the differences in scale and diversity of the services provided by these small groups and mega-organizations such as the AIDS Foundation, critics demand that corporate hierarchies be replaced by flatter organizational structures at these AIDS groups.

One can hear in the debates about Christen's salary petty disagreements or an emerging conflict between classes within gay communities. Few of the affluent donors of the AIDS Foundation may have a problem with the CEO of a $21 million organization taking home $131,000 plus benefits (in fact, some believe the executives of similar-sized corporations and nonprofits outside AIDS would be making much larger salaries), although less-affluent donors, as well as clients and community members who were raised working class or lower-middle class, might find such a salary obscene. While these differences have long existed within gay communities and occasionally flared in AIDS organizations, current trends, which make the experience of living with HIV increasingly different for poor people with HIV than for their affluent counterparts, may serve as an engine driving these concerns.

The trends that make for greater divisions between rich and poor in American culture, and certainly among people with HIV, are linked to post-AIDS changes that merit attention. As public benefits such as welfare and Medicaid are eroded and more people go without medical insurance, the spirit of optimism linked rhetorically in the media to protease inhibitors is, in many of parts of the nation, a class-bound spirit. In some states, public funding is not available to guarantee access to these medications for all.[9] And particular features of the treatments (their demand for regular compliance to schedules, predictable eating patterns, and refrigeration) make it more difficult for the homeless, substance abusers, and poor people to benefit (though not impossible, as some have claimed).[10] A redesigned AIDS system must seriously take into account the increasing ways class differences are implicated in AIDS care and treatment.

We have arrived at a moment when leaders of all parts of the AIDS system and those who hold as a priority the health and functionality of the system itself might initiate planning processes aimed at recognizing the biomedical, epidemiological, social, and cultural changes that have been occurring over the past few years. Perhaps because of their key position in the system and their long-standing identification as leaders in the fight against AIDS, ASOs, however large, unwieldy, and bureaucratic, might find themselves taking the lead in initiating a planned process of transformation.

AIDS SERVICE ORGANIZATIONS: RECONCEIVED, RESTRUCTURED, OR RETIRED?

An early shot in the battles emerging during the Protease Moment was boldly fired in Seattle in January 1997. While national publications had spent the previous three months discussing "The End of AIDS," it was left to local journalists and activists to bring the issue home to local AIDS systems. Who better than local bad-boy journalist Dan Savage to raise the hackles of the Seattle AIDS system?

In a cover story with the inflammatory title "Life After AIDS: How will the AIDS culture of death deal with protease inhibitors that make it a 'chronic manageable disease?'" published first in Seattle's *The Stranger*, then in other alternative weeklies around the nation, Savage takes on key structures of the local AIDS system for their failure to respond rapidly to changes he believes were triggered by protease inhibitors.[11] Savage aggressively targets local Seattle AIDS organizations and isn't shy about naming names. His thinking is broad and far-reaching and his searing analysis spares no sacred cows.

Perhaps most visionary is Savage's thinking about how AIDS organizations might change in a world in which HIV is no longer experienced as a crisis. In a city such as Seattle, where gay men continue to constitute the great majority of people with HIV, Savage argues that this population soon will have diminished need for support and services from ASOs, and the client base of such organizations will become primarily the poor, the addicted, and people with mental health diagnoses. This analysis may not be limited to Seattle, as it reflects what has happened first on the East Coast, where gay men no longer constitute the majority of new AIDS cases in many urban centers. Savage argues that AIDS becoming a chronic, manageable disease for middle-class gay men will greatly expedite a dramatic change in the gay population's relationship to AIDS organizations as clients, volunteers, and donors.

Savage holds up two options that AIDS organizations might consider in charting future directions. Using as an example Seattle's Chicken Soup Brigade (CSB), a group that has provided food, transportation, and volunteer support for people with AIDS, Savage reveals that, as requests for services from people with AIDS have declined, the group has changed its targeted client base to include poor people with HIV who are not diagnosed with AIDS. He argues that, given the effectiveness of the new treatments among many gay men, the direction CSB has taken "is a critical step away from the gay community," and toward "the needs of HIV-positive mothers, homeless people, and men and women with children."[12]

As an alternative to ASOs becoming service providers targeting poverty-based clients, Savage suggests they be transformed into multipurpose centers addressing a range of concerns facing lesbians and gay men:

> As AIDS gradually becomes someone else's problem, gays and lesbians will have not only the opportunity, but the responsibility to turn to other pressing problems facing "our own." For instance, breast cancer disproportionately affects lesbians. What about home-care services for ill lesbians not lucky enough to be HIV-positive and poor? And surely some of the gay community's time and money will have to be directed toward services for a soon-to-emerge class of gay and lesbian elderly.[13]

Savage could be criticized appropriately for glossing over ways in which class intersects with his analysis of these shifts, and the ways "taking care of our own," a theme he highlights as underpinning gay community AIDS efforts, is not about gays taking care of gays, but about middle-class gay men caring for their peers. Many of the homeless people with HIV whom he sees as potential continuing clients of CSB, in fact, may be poor gay men often on the fringes of gay ghetto life. Others might argue that Savage's preferred option (transforming AIDS organizations into gay service projects) could only be used in a city that currently lacks a gay and lesbian community services center. In other urban centers, many of the functions he suggests for the refitted AIDS organizations are already championed by existing queer-focused agencies.

But these were not the criticisms directed at Savage in the lengthy, furious letters to the editor that appeared over the next few weeks. Instead, local AIDS leaders sent letters that unabashedly reflect the conservative nature of the system and their reluctance to accept and respond to the transformations occurring during the current epidemic moment. Terry Stone, executive director of the Northwest AIDS Foundation, began his letter by refuting Savage's foundational argument that gay men have stepped beyond the crisis stage of the epidemic. He went on to insist that the role combination therapies will play in the long run is uncertain and that staff members of his organization have worked diligently to educate clients about protease inhibitors and ensure continued funding for the AIDS Prescription Drug Program. Marshaling dramatic facts about continuing infection and death rates, Stone presents a case for the continued need for ASOs during the Protease Moment:

> Some people are enjoying improved health because of pro- tease inhibitors. These individuals will encounter new prob- lems and challenges. They will need assistance grappling with return to work, housing problems, insurance/disability issues, continued drug access guarantees, and other issues in planning to live longer. New challenges will be present as we work with people whose AIDS diagnosis is compounded by mental ill- ness, poverty, and chemical dependency.[14]

Stone's letter typifies the response of many leaders of ASOs as they are confronted by post-AIDS shifts. He correctly cites a range of emerging needs that accompany the new treatments. Yet he fails to balance these new needs with acknowledgment that some preexist- ing services may no longer be heavily in demand. His entire letter resists acknowledging the need for a fundamental reconsideration of the mission, scope, and structure of his organization.

Likewise, John Leonard, director of Gay City Health Project, suggests that Savage's article might cause a "huge new wave of the epidemic," as post-crisis gay men "throw away their condoms." He goes on to paint a bleak scenario for gay men living through the Protease Moment:

> Take thousands of newly infected gay men and all the HIV- positive people now living longer, put most of them on pro- tease inhibitors, and what do you get? A large proportion of the gay community taking handfuls of pills that cause nausea, diarrhea, severe pain in the abdomen and limbs, and whose long-term side-effects are unknown. Add the fact that these drugs must be taken on a very strict regimen, and if patients miss even a few doses, the HIV in their system can develop resistance to the drugs. This means more and more people will be getting infected with drug-resistant strains of HIV that won't respond to the new treatments.[15]

While Leonard may be correct in mentioning side effects experi- enced by some men on protease inhibitors, and arguing that the long-term effects cannot yet be known, by creating a limited vision of community life for men on the treatments, he engages in a practice increasingly popular among leaders of AIDS organizations: dramatizing and exaggerating the circumstances of a minority of people on combination therapies in order to argue for the continued funding of ASOs. Rather than acknowledge the new treatments offer both opportunities and challenges, elucidate services that might be eliminated or reduced, and welcome a time when people with HIV do not need to turn to organizations for any kind of services, Leonard appears part of the collective circling of the wagons that many read as ASOs protecting their turf and maintaining their funding levels.

Leaders of AIDS organizations might reflect on these questions carefully before publicly responding to challenges such as Savage's. An alternative response came from Chuck Kuehn, executive director of Chicken Soup Brigade, the organization Savage targeted in his suggested redesign of AIDS services. Kuehn corrected three "errors and omissions" he found in Savage's writing about his organization but then moved on to articulate an openness to possibilities that may emerge from open community discussion over the coming months:

> Chicken Soup Brigade is excited about the promise of protease inhibitors and the accompanying dialogue. Will AIDS become a "manageable" disease? Can the immune system rebuild? If the viral load goes down, but the immune system can't rebound, will people living with AIDS remain in a semidisabled condition? How can we continue to pressure for a cure? And the question all the service organizations have been waiting to ask: Can we now safely think about shrinking our budgets and staff?[16]

When medical treatments result in a resumption of "normal life" for most people with HIV, maybe the mission of AIDS service groups should shift. Perhaps, as Savage suggests, they should become multipurpose queer agencies providing similar services—volunteer home care, medical information, support groups, bereavement services, food and shelter—to sick or poor gay people struggling with cancer, AIDS, multiple sclerosis, mental illness. Perhaps they should be transformed into organizations that assist all people in need, regardless of sexual identity or type of life-threatening illness. Or perhaps they should continue to focus on HIV/AIDS and gay men should simply relinquish ownership of the groups we founded in the 1980s. While leaders of AIDS organizations correctly assert that the success of new treatments and diminution of deaths have resulted in a greater number of living with people with HIV/AIDS who might need services, they are less eager to offer analyses of how the level, cost, frequency, and kind of care might be changing.[17]

Three things need to happen as stakeholders in the AIDS system initiate organized, planned processes to rethink their entire effort: (1) the leaders of local AIDS systems must open a dialogue with each other about ways in which the system must shift, including the merger or closure of organizations, to respond to contemporary changes in the epidemic; (2) local AIDS organizations must open a dialogue within their organizations, including their clients, volunteers, staff and donors, about ways to reconceive, redesign, restructure, or retire their organizations; and (3) gay men of all colors must participate in a conversation with other affected communities focused on shifts in ownership, power sharing or diminution, and ways to increase solidarity during the current changes.

A key element of these discussions must be whether ASOs need to remain providers of social services, switch over to focus on access to the new treatments, or balance the two. This is a conflict that has flared for ASOs since the Vancouver AIDS Conference began to change many people's thinking about the meaning of HIV and AIDS. Some have suggested that ASOs be shut down, defunded, or dismantled. Jerry Joshua De Jong, a long-time leader in gay health care and AIDS in the San Francisco Bay Area, wrote about protease inhibitors:

> It is time to make these drugs available, and the only way to do that nationwide is to dismantle the AIDS service industry and re-focus its priority of service. . . . It is time for a radical restructuring of what AIDS services mean. It is time to deliver medical services and not social services. It is time.[18]

In many people's minds, there is an emerging dichotomy between social services and treatment with the new drugs. Part of the fuel that drives the rage at ASOs, including the San Francisco AIDS Foundation, comes from treatment advocates who believe the ASOs could be doing a lot more to assist their clients with obtaining new treatments. A cover story in *San Francisco Weekly* titled "The AIDS Civil War: Behind the Pandemic's New Hope Lies a Bitter Rift," captured these emerging tensions in San Francisco.[19] While ACT UP/Golden Gate issued a letter to the editor insisting "It is disingenuous . . . to assert that there is 'An AIDS Civil War',"[20] quotations in the article from members of the group and others indicate otherwise. The story cites Jeff Getty, a visible leader of ACT UP/Golden Gate, acknowledging the need for both services and treatments, but adding:

> We are just warehousing people. It's time for the warehouses to start dispensing medicine. . . . If there isn't enough money, we will have to scale back on services to make sure that the drugs are paid for. . . . This is a disease first and foremost.[21]

Some service providers dealing with significant caseloads of clients who continue to be disabled or unable to get onto treatment regimens hear such comments as utopian fantasies coming from gay white middle-class men's limited worldview. Laura Strauss, a physician's assistant on the AIDS ward at San Francisco General Hospital, commenting on those advocating treatment instead of services in the same article, asked, "You know what I think about that point of view? It's elitist, selfish, and narrow-minded."[22]

This is one place where gay community organizing around AIDS ought to proceed very cautiously. While those who argue that the underclass will not benefit from the new treatments because of their inability to comply with strict regimens are rightfully accused of patronizing the poor, those who argue that the epidemic in gay ghettos is identical to AIDS in the indigent sections of the city are out of touch with reality.[23] More balanced approaches are necessary while both services and treatments are needed, sometimes by different populations of clients, and sometimes not.

This conflict was further exacerbated when ASOs and treatment activists wrangled over $100 million in emergency federal funding for the AIDS Drug Assistance Program.[24] ASOs successfully lobbied to have half of the allocation focus on expanding social services, though the original impetus for the new funding was to address many states' empty pockets for the new treatments. Jason Schneider, a former board member of Boston's AIDS Action Committee, alarmed at this move by ASOs and enraged because, in his eyes, "little has been offered by the large ASOs to these individuals [on the new treatments] facing huge life questions about relationships, work, and long-term health" proposed some changes:

> I propose that Massachusetts, long a leader in HIV care and treatment, create a model for re-structuring AIDS services as we enter the next century. The Department of Public Health's AIDS Bureau should convene a short-term community group. The group should consist of people with HIV and a limited number of representatives from organizations providing services to people with HIV. The group's goal should be: to determine what services are presently needed, which of these services are duplicated and which are not, to provide enhanced funding, if needed, to clinical and social organizations already doing an effective job of serving people with HIV and their loved ones, and to help ASOs return to their original missions of filling gaps in services.[25]

Schneider's blueprint for community planning is a good one and should be widely considered. One possible alteration worth examining might be to convene two separate committees, one entirely of people with HIV and the other with provider representatives, and have both come up with plans for a redesigned system meeting the contemporary needs of people with HIV. Once the plans are drafted, the two groups might sit down, discuss commonalities and differences, and together craft a plan for rapid implementation.

I make this suggestion because for years tensions have flared between people with HIV and providers about core issues related to service and treatment delivery systems. The late Victor D'Lugin, a pioneering activist and critic of the rigidity of AIDS organizations and systems, criticized the paternalism of professionals within the

AIDS system and argued that people with AIDS need to determine the priorities and processes of HIV-service delivery well before the new treatments arrived.[26] A model that allowed for the creation of autonomous plans might reveal whether there are truly different perspectives on major issues or if these are primarily politically-based rhetorical arguments. In any case, at this critical juncture, by allowing infected people to craft their own blueprint, we would reaffirm the movement's commitment to the empowerment of people with HIV begun at the Denver Summit in 1983.[27]

A disturbing tone appears in this discussion that accepts and expands the neoconservative representation of welfare that flared during recent debates on welfare reform in this nation. De Jong insists "It is time for AIDS service agencies to stop being the AIDS welfare network." Jeff Getty states "We shouldn't be creating a welfare system in the name of HIV. I wonder what's next? HIV-positive food stamps?" What's troubling about these remarks appearing during a time when the Right has successfully scapegoated welfare recipients "as a primary cause of economic and social problems in the U.S.," is that AIDS activists appear to buy into the argument that welfare is the root cause of our problems.[28] The AIDS welfare system that De Jong and Getty attack here was developed by gay men during the 1980s, often against the objections of the Right, who argued that people with HIV were being given services that people fighting other diseases were not given, usually including free food and home-delivered meals, the precise "HIV-positive food stamps" that seem to make Getty incredulous.

This conflict raises a series of uncomfortable but important questions. Should people with HIV who are doing moderately well in 1997—on the new treatments or without them—be offered a range of free or low-cost social services such as emotional support, practical assistance, disability benefits, and support groups? Or are resources better directed toward people with other infirmities or to people with HIV who are seriously ill or toward treatments rather than services? Should AIDS service groups gear up to assist previously sick people in finding jobs, maintaining their eligibility for Medicare, and confronting the psychological roller coaster that often accompanies improved health? Or is this simply an updated version of the "welfare system" some activists decry? Should people with HIV who are in government-supported, AIDS-related housing be forced to move out when their health conditions improve, get back to work and pay market rates for the housing, or continue to receive a free ride or subsidy?

An alternative way for AIDS leaders to respond to post-AIDS debates was suggested by Larry Kessler, the executive director of Boston's AIDS Action Committee. In an apparent response to Jason Schneider's challenge to call for ASOs to "return to their original mission of filling the gaps in AIDS services," Kessler published an opinion essay titled "Keeping hope alive" in a local gay newspaper.[29] Kessler began by articulating what he understood as the original and continuing mission of ASOs:

> Over the years, AIDS service organizations (ASOs) of all descriptions have remained remarkably true to a common mission: to prevent the spread of HIV while helping infected individuals to live longer, in better health and on their own terms.[30]

After providing examples of the progress made during the first two decades of AIDS, and highlighting the "unprecedented degree of hope" that has accompanied combination therapies, Kessler, drawing on lessons learned during his lengthy tenure in the trenches of the AIDS fight, explained:

> After years of skirmishes with this disease, you'll understand if we keep our guns drawn. The battle, at this point, hasn't let up. Services are still needed in our communities . . .

Kessler cataloged the continuing need for services of people with HIV and then confronted the economic barriers facing many people with HIV as they attempt to access the new treatments. He then cited an example of the ways in which his organization is changing in response to changing client needs:

> We have redesigned a support group that formerly focused on the issues faced by people leaving work. Now that group will also help people who are considering a return to the workplace.

The remainder of the letter slipped into familiar rhetoric ("Until HIV is eradicated, we cannot shut our door . . . ") and included a catalog of the new support services needed by an expanding case-load of protease babies. At the end of the letter, Kessler suggested the letter's defensive tone was in response to Schneider's criticisms of his organization. He wrote, "It would be a mistake, at this point, for us to use our talents to fight each other when the virus is out there mutating . . . "

Kessler's essay raises a number of issues ASOs might consider during a time when many of their clients are no longer experiencing AIDS as lethal, debilitating, or a crisis. Few thoughtful people are demanding ASOs close their doors at this time; they are aware that dramatic changes in the epidemic landscape result in all kinds of fallout for people with HIV. What they are asking is for ASO leadership to fundamentally rethink their groups' mission, objectives, structure, and services.[31] With few exceptions, they have become ossified as AIDS Inc. bureaucracies and they need to regain the responsiveness that characterized them during the early years. While Kessler should be praised for being one of the rare AIDS organization leaders responding to the current transformation by citing real changes his organization has made, he should be challenged to lead his organization into a bold revisiting of its mission, objectives, and structure. It's not simply whether AIDS groups need to initiate back-to-work programs, support groups for men who are not succeeding on combination therapies, and separate counseling projects for people newly infected with HIV. Beyond changing programs, organizations and systems need to explore core questions about purpose, mission, and objectives for the new era.

These changes have started to occur throughout the nation. In Arizona, the Tucson AIDS Project, Shanti, and People with AIDS Coalition, organizations with a long history of interorganizational competition, have merged into the Southern Arizona AIDS Foundation. In Wisconsin, the AIDS Resource Center of Wisconsin and Green Bay's Center Project, Inc. merged in April 1997.[32] In California, the San Diego AIDS Foundation closed its doors suddenly, facing a debt of almost $1 million.[33] Under the watchful eye of the media,[34] AIDS Inc. is beginning a period of self-reflection and reinvention. If we're lucky, the system will retain some of the stability needed to continue to serve large numbers of needy clients, but gain increased flexibility in terms of services delivered, populations served, and paradigms and models utilized.

Can AIDS organizations and the entire AIDS system adapt itself to the changes in both the epidemic and the event known as AIDS? Is it possible for groups created to help people leave employment and move onto public benefits to transform themselves and help people find employment and get off some of their benefits? What role will gay men play in the upcoming changes, as we become a shrinking part of the population of people with AIDS throughout the United States?

A multiyear process of deliberation should tackle these tough questions under the watchful eyes of the media, affected communities, and people with HIV/AIDS.

WHAT ELSE HAS TO CHANGE?

ASOs are not the only part of the AIDS system that needs to change. The functioning of governmental AIDS bureaus needs to be fundamentally reconsidered, as do the forms of organizations that serve people with HIV, and these groups' relationships to broader community-based health services and the emerging managed care system. For example, we might want to encourage the integration of AIDS care services into the broader health care system, and let go of the separate system of autonomous organizations and services we've organized. Yet even institutions that have enjoyed tremendous community support cannot see themselves as exempt from this moment of self-reflection, untouchable by the shifts occurring now. A number of additional organizations should seriously consider transforming themselves for the post-AIDS era.

ACT UP

The tenth anniversary of the AIDS Coalition to Unleash Power (ACT UP) in March 1997 was marked with celebrations, street actions, and dozens of news articles in the gay and mainstream press. *The Washington Blade* headlined its front-page story, "After

10 years, ACT UP now fights dwindling membership."[35] San Francisco's *Bay Area Reporter*'s cover story was titled "ACT UP: Ten years on the front lines of an epidemic."[36]

The articles highlight ACT UP's considerable achievements of the past decade and offer various explanations for the waning of its membership and influence over the past few years. Yet few discussed how grassroots political activism, organized through ACT UP or otherwise, should be adapted to the post-AIDS era. How can we recharge our activism as we approach the third decade of AIDS?

Indeed, ACT UP chapters have been in the forefront of the continued use of the crisis construct of AIDS. ACT UP Golden Gate's letter to the editor, referenced above, chides the *San Francisco Weekly* in what many have begun to see as their usual guilt-tripping fashion:

> We are surprised to see that *SF Weekly* is interested in our struggles for AIDS services. Perhaps this concern will lead to stories about AIDS, an area in which *SF Weekly*'s reporting has been abysmal. Your Phoenix-based, corporate bosses may not know it, but this epidemic is still a crisis in San Francisco. Shame on you and your corporate parent for attempting to divide a fragile community of sick people.[37]

How much longer will it be possible to recycle representations of the epidemic that are a dozen years old and that no longer fit the contemporary context? Can people with HIV/AIDS in San Francisco be collectively described as "a fragile community of sick people" with any authenticity or honesty? What makes AIDS "still a crisis in San Francisco," besides the convenient rhetorical flourish and activists' failure to reinvent their efforts in a changing world?

Explanations offered for the dwindling number of ACT UP chapters and low participation in the surviving ones—deaths of many of the original ACT UP members, burnout facing others, transfer of former street activists into full-time workers in the AIDS system (some would call this co-optation), infighting and splits that tore at specific chapters—never seem to include the obvious: the group's failure to shift out of the 1987 epidemic moment in which it was conceived and adopt strategies, tactics, and representations appropriate to the 1990s.

We need a revitalized ACT UP, perhaps under a new name and augmenting its original organizing and political protest tactics with new ones that can grapple with the continuing biomedical condition of AIDS and the host of social issues that it exposes (racism, sexism, and homophobia in heath care, the demonizing of queers, addicts, and youth of color, the sex panic sweeping the nation in the guise of AIDS prevention). We certainly need ACT UP to continue to focus on ensuring augmented funding of the AIDS Drug Assistance Program and, if nothing else, forcing states to change policies that restrict client access and reduce the number of HIV-related drugs included in the program.[38] Moreover, we need a group that will understand the need to place our work against AIDS in a more general context of health care concerns. We need an activist group concerned with gay men's health issues.

ACT UP can be more than a simple grassroots critic of public officials, holding them publicly accountable as lobbyists negotiate tough issues at the bargaining table. At some point, ACT UP's simplistic chants and repeated demands for more AIDS funding will be challenged by internal forces who have made their own transitions into a post-AIDS era. Local funders might seriously explore whether fighting for additional funding for services or prevention continues to be the proper priority or whether it is time to initiate an ACT UP agenda for the new millennium.[39] Such an agenda could attract mass participation and might include disparate demands such as FDA approval of condoms (including the "female condom") for gay men, the funding of drug treatment on demand, and the expansion of efforts to develop a vaccine against HIV.[40]

Project Inform and AIDS Treatment News

At least two remarkable projects emerged from San Francisco in the 1980s that have been widely praised for their unique role in the international effort against AIDS. Project Inform, a community-based organization led by Martin Delaney, and *AIDS Treatment News*, a publication founded and led by John James, both translate complex biomedical and treatment information into language many nonscientists (including most people with HIV) can understand. Project Inform's town meetings have toured the nation and provided thousands of people with HIV with the latest information about treatments. If ASOs can be faulted for not responding to the new treatments swiftly after the Vancouver conference, Project Inform should be praised for immediately taking its show on the road and holding public meetings disseminating key findings from the International AIDS Conference from coast to coast.

We need the work of these two organizations now as much as ever. We have moved into a post-AIDS stage, in part, because of the considerable efforts of Project Inform, *AIDS Treatment News*, and smiliar grassroots efforts. As new treatments go through the drug approval process pipeline, these organizations, and other similar efforts, must remain vigilant, calling the shots as they see them, and, as much as possible, ducking the nasty internecine warfare that plagues community-based AIDS efforts. There is much we do not know about protease inhibitors and the long-term effects of triple combination therapies. These groups will continue to ensure that research is appropriately targeted and prioritized, and that findings are put to the service of people with HIV. Buyer's clubs may also have an important, though changing, function amid the changes of the Protease Moment.[41]

In my earlier book, I called for the establishment of a prevention-focused effort modeled on Project Inform. No one to my knowledge has taken up this idea and yet I continue to believe it should be at the top of any priority list for post-AIDS efforts in the area of prevention and education. If we are truly going to create a framework for safer promiscuity for gay men, we need to ensure that the proper research is being done, findings are disseminated in an accessible manner, and gay men are supported as they grapple with new data. As Project Inform tours the nation meeting with people who are interested in learning about treatments to combat HIV, we need to develop a prevention-focused effort that tours the nation and convenes town hall meetings that give gay men and others the latest information about transmission and sexual risk.

Project Inform and *AIDS Treatment News* should be supported to keep doing good work during the post-AIDS period. Their continued funding must be near the top of our priority list. Energetic activists seeking to initiate an important project would be wise to adapt the publications of these organizations and their methods of popular education to an era in which prevention of HIV and the improvement of the overall health of gay men is a true priority.

World AIDS Day and Other Rituals of Loss

During the late 1980s and early 1990s, as AIDS deaths in epicenter cities crested, a variety of rituals emerged that offered hard-hit communities opportunities to come together in grief. In San Francisco, we have the opportunity to participate in the annual AIDS Candlelight Vigil at the end of May and World AIDS Day activities on December first. We can visit the AIDS Memorial Grove in Golden Gate Park or attend any of the AIDS memorial services hosted at many churches and synagogues in the city. Latino communities may observe AIDS through annual Posadas, walks that honor the dead and support those living with HIV.[42]

Several years ago, I had to stop attending these activities because I felt uncomfortable. It became painful to hear the same speeches and repeat the same exhortations we've shouted for many years. With rare exception, unscripted expressions of grief were replaced by what felt like broken-record texts about loss, sorrow, and the need to continue the good fight. Politicians began to seize center stage and leave people with HIV/AIDS and grassroots community leaders on the side. It felt too predictable and too unreal.

There have been times when I've argued that rituals of grief should be scrapped: the AIDS vigils should end, the mass memorial services in churches should cease, the World AIDS Day observations should be boycotted out of existence. While some have insisted that grief is a poor substitute for rage and action, I have long recognized the need for communal grief rituals, particularly when specific communities were undergoing enormous suffering under a cataclysm of corpses. My reasons for ending these rituals were more humble: I simply felt they'd become trite and had grown to substitute hollow rhetoric for sincere expressions of loss. While I'm not opposed to cruising or laughter, I saw more of them than I saw tears during the last AIDS Candlelight Vigil I attended.

I no longer campaign for these rituals to end. The current epidemic moment's offer of a space to breathe allows backlogged grief to come surging forward in surprising ways. We may need these rituals now more than ever. I believe, however, that the organizers of these rituals face a simple choice: either keep the rituals up-to-date with the contemporary experiences of hard-hit communities in their areas, or accept that they will diminish in meaning for many people. World AIDS Day should be a crucial vehicle reminding Americans that the epidemic is not the same in every place and that, while many gay men might be experiencing post-AIDS shifts, this is not the case for much of the Third World, nor for much of the poor population (including poor gay men) in the United States. Organizers must develop innovative and creative ways to keep these observances fresh and relevant under changing contexts.

As the number of participants in annual rituals declines, many within what is referred to as "the AIDS community" complain that people have lost interest in the epidemic and moved on to other concerns and interests. This simplifies and demeans what is truly happening. Certainly many people now experience and understand AIDS in new ways that make rituals conceived in the 1980s less meaningful to them. Others have recreated their lives and awarded AIDS a less prominent position. Organizers concerned about attracting larger crowds might take the time to reconceptualize and redesign their rituals to more effectively meet people where they are in the present epidemic moment.

The Names Project AIDS Memorial Quilt

Shortly before Gay Pride Week in June 1997, San Francisco newspapers announced that the Names Project/AIDS Memorial Quilt was cutting its staff by 20 percent due to a dramatic drop in fund-raising revenues.[43] The organization eliminated or reduced to half-time sixteen staff and six contract positions. The organization's budget went from $5.2 to $4.7 million. Perhaps most surprising was the fact that the number of AIDS panels arriving each week had declined from sixty-eight in earlier years to thirty-eight. Attendance at displays of the Quilt had fallen by 50 percent and sales from T-shirts and other Quilt memorabilia were down 59 percent. A spokesperson for the Names Project told the press:

> We are delighted that the quilt is not growing as quickly as it was. This is what we've all been longing to hear. AIDS is no longer a death sentence. The layoffs are difficult news, coming

out of extraordinary good news. . . . AIDS organizations have always said that they exist to put themselves out of business. Increasingly, this is not just a figure of speech.[44]

While AIDS organizations must be prepared to shut their doors when and if they are no longer needed—because people with HIV no longer need services, or a cure and vaccine have been developed, or because other entities now more readily meet the needs of HIV-infected people—the Names Project/AIDS Memorial Quilt is different in important ways from an ASO. I believe the post-AIDS period must protect the work of the past decade that has created the Quilt, but that such efforts will face severe challenges in the coming years.

This is a critical time for the Quilt's leadership to rethink their mission. Flagging public support does not mean people have been duped into putting their money and energies elsewhere; it means the mission of the Quilt is no longer as meaningful to many people as it was a decade ago.

I do not think I am unusual among gay men when I acknowledge that the Quilt remains meaningful to me at the close of the 1990s, but in new ways. When close friends die, as Frank and Dick died last summer, or Greg just a few weeks ago, I do not even think about who's going to design what Dan Savage refers to as their "little piece of glory." Seven years ago, this very issue might have been contentiously debated during memorial services and often several quilt panels were produced for a single individual by several different factions of friends. During visits to the Quilt, friends and I have joked about the differences between panels produced by gay friends and those stitched by the family back in Kansas and those crafted by colleagues at work. Over recent years, quilting seems to have become a less pressing matter for the survivors. In fact, during my recent visit to the Quilt, I was stunned to note that many gay men who had died since 1993 weren't represented by a single panel—no one had sewn a panel for them! This included not only my personal friends, but also several prominent gay writers and politicos.

I am not sure whether large numbers of gay men still find the Quilt meaningful as a day-to-day ritual for collecting and memorializing our dead. Perhaps other communities do. If so, the ongoing function of expanding the Quilt seems like an important project for those communities to assume, direct, and fund. For me, the Quilt remains meaningful as a piece of history, as material evidence of what happened to my gay generation, as a memorial to our identities and cultures of the 1970s and 1980s. I want to make sure nothing ever happens to those panels. I certainly do not want to see them burned, as some have suggested, although I understand how the Quilt has come to symbolize a "death sentence" conceptualization of AIDS which many abhor.[45] I want them preserved forever and displayed on occasion.

It might be wise for the Quilt's overseers to choose a date two decades after the first cases were documented, perhaps the year 2000, and declare the original Quilt completed, sew on the final panels, and preserve it for posterity. A separate, spin-off project could begin a second quilt, almost like a movie: *AIDS Quilt II: The Sequel.* In this way, the original event of AIDS as understood, developed, and produced in hard-hit gay male communities might be captured and preserved, and a new event of AIDS, currently under construction by several communities, might be reflected in the new quilt.

I do not make this suggestion lightly or without understanding it will disturb some people, infuriate others. Still, there should be no piece of the AIDS system left unexamined in our efforts to reconceive AIDS work in this current epidemic moment. We must understand the final days of AIDS Inc. as the end of the rigid system set up to respond to the biomedical realities of AIDS of the 1980s and the sociocultural experience of crisis, and the return to a more flexible, responsive system. If the Quilt is to avoid being seen as out of touch with the times, and if all AIDS organizations and rituals are to avoid closure due to failure to move with the times, now is the time to talk seriously about organizational redesign and systemic restructuring.

Epilogue:
Alive in My Own Life Story

The post-AIDS period in gay cultures has brought many changes to my life, but one of them is not an absence of illness and death due to HIV disease. Open Hand, the local meals-on-wheels program for people with AIDS, still rings my doorbell and drops off a dinner dish when my next-door neighbor is unable to respond to their knocking. Some of the friends who join me for tea at Pasqua continue to cycle through various illnesses and cope with the gap between the public perception that AIDS has been cured and the reality of their bodies and blood work. I continue to assist with HIV-prevention campaigns, contribute financially to my favorite community organizations, and comfort friends who discover that they are now HIV positive.

So what's changed? HIV is no longer central to my daily life. It's there, but in a diminished capacity—present but not overwhelmingly so. Other issues now claim a larger portion of my energy and attention. I remain a political activist and a health advocate, and feel a lifelong commitment to social justice movements. HIV is one of my causes, but one among many. It is something I want to continue to work against, but it has joined a long list of scourges, such as child abuse, misogyny, racism, and poverty.

I'm happy to be a part of the lesbian, gay, bisexual, and transgender health movement, aiming to tackle a wide range of threats to the well-being of our communities. When I see advertisements for the new Gay, Lesbian, Bisexual, and Transgender Health Access Project, sponsored by the Massachusetts Department of Public Health, I am inspired with a vision for the future.[1] Reading about the Brothers for Sisters Campaign, a program aimed at generating support from gay men for lesbian services at Lyon-Martin Women's Health Clinic in San Francisco, I feel a small sense of hope that men will consider women's health needs as worthy of their active support.[2] Picking up the Sunday *New York Times* to read that New York's Community Health Project is converting an old warehouse into a 27,000-square-foot clinic, leaves me filled with excitement about the future health of our communities.[3] In my early activist years in the 1970s, I never dreamed gay clinics would own entire buildings, lesbian characters would star in television sitcoms, and openly gay men would be elected to Congress. Seeing change in my lifetime makes it difficult for me to be a pessimist about social change movements. My opportunities and position in the world are different today because of the movements we've created and stuck with through good times and bad.

HIV has been a primary influence on how my midlife years are structured. Having spent a decade working full-time in AIDS and gay organizations, I've returned to my original career as an educator and hope to complete my doctorate in the field in the next few months. I spend my time working in schools, researching new reform initiatives, and investigating the intersection of race/gender/ sexual identity in classrooms. If AIDS had never happened, I think I would have gone to graduate school in my thirties rather than my forties, but in the post-AIDS era I've returned to a life interrupted and gotten back on track. At other times, I feel that the years of intensive work on AIDS weren't an interruption at all and instead were an integral, necessary part of my development as an educator and activist. It was a key part of my own maturation process.

Another way HIV continues to influence my everyday life involves the social circles I inhabit. Although much of my time is spent in gay male environments, I increasingly maintain close and important friendships with people who are not gay men. Part of this is related to the deaths of several peers which created large voids in my life that have gone unfilled. I find it difficult to make new friends in midlife and increasingly my gay male friends are in their twenties and early thirties. My women friends—lesbians, bisexuals, and heterosexuals—continue as central to my life, and several straight men I've met through graduate school have become important to me.

Increasingly my life focuses around my lover. This is something I have resisted for a long time. I've always structured my primary relationship in a manner that ensured a great deal of independence and allowed for autonomous friendship networks. Because he is positive and I am negative, I felt it was wise to preserve my autonomy and ensure that, should something happen to him, I could count on a foundation of friendship to carry me forward.

Our struggles about sex, geography, and communication, have brought us closer together. After almost a year of couples counseling focused on where we would live, we made the decision to remain in San Francisco. I began to let go of my dreams of returning to New England and finally allow myself to consider San Francisco home. This has not been easy, but steady progress has been made. I became open to buying a home together and putting down roots. Again we ran into conflict as I wanted to live in a small, rustic cottage and my lover wanted to live in the heart of the Castro. Without a great deal of effort, we discovered a sweet cottage, perfect for the two of us. To my lover's delight, it's located about 100 feet from the corner of Castro and 18th streets, the crossroads of this gay neighborhood. To my delight, it is on the same block as the Cove Cafe, and just a two-minute walk to Pasqua.

LEAVING BEHIND THE FUNEREAL FEELINGS

Crispin and I were immersed in the month-long process of moving into the cottage when the tragic death of Princess Diana occurred. As we drove down Market Street to the Castro that Sunday morning, we passed a lone drag queen, dolled up to resemble Diana, who appeared to be heading off to church. It was only after we'd parked and ambled down Castro Street that we came upon a makeshift shrine to Diana rapidly being assembled on the corner of 18th and Castro. Similar shrines had sprouted up there when gay heroes such as Leonard Matlovitch or icons such as Lucille Ball had died. I was only surprised to see that the large shrine to Diana featuring cards, letters, photographs, and drawings had been erected so quickly. A large banner festooned the shrine proclaiming "Princess Diana: You Will Always Be Our Queen of Hearts."

I love that I live in a neighborhood that acknowledges deaths through the informal, grassroots process of creating these shrines. Over the following few days, the shrine expanded enormously and stretched down the length of the building. People chalked epitaphs into the sidewalk and left bowls of fruit, flowers, and votive candles. The cards attached to the wall touted Diana's achievements and thanked her for her open embrace of gay people. "You touched the hand of a man with AIDS while others were afraid," read one card, signed with a large heart. Another simply promised, "We love you always—The Boys," while another stated, "Princess Diana— You are unforgettable. Love always, John and Jay." One sign drawn up with magic markers offered a cautionary note: "Seatbelts Save Lives: Rest in Peace Diana—The Best Queen England Never Had."

An e-mail address was posted for the London Gay Community Center, "to send condolences and expressions of your grief." The Sisters of Perpetual Indulgence announced a memorial candlelight march from the Castro down to the British Consulate. The event attracted 15,000 people, who marched under the banner "Diana: Queen of Our Hearts." A local gay pride festival occurring a few weeks after Diana's death was renamed in her honor. Gay newspapers throughout the nation featured tributes, editorials, and pages of recollections of the princess.[4]

A week after her death, the shrine to Diana continued to expand. Television crews from all over the world filmed people drawn to the shrine: reading the tributes, writing their own, kneeling in prayer, wiping away tears. I told Crispin that I feared the shrine would become a permanent fixture. Queens thrive on such tragedies, I reasoned, and Diana's untimely death gave us a new reason to wear black and take out the handkerchiefs. When the shrine remained the day following Diana's funeral and gay men continued to pack the sidewalk, dropping off bouquets and cards, I became edgy. Was this going to be another funeral without end?

I strolled out of the new cottage a day later and headed for Pasqua, passing the corner of 18th and Castro. I failed to notice that the shrine had been disassembled and carted off. It was only after I seated myself on the bench in front of the coffeehouse and began to sip my tea that I noticed something was different. A man in the seat in front of me let out a sigh of relief and gestured across the street. "Thank god they took down that hideous shrine to Diana!" he insisted. " Now the girl can finally rest in peace."

The intense period of mourning following Diana's death in which some gay men immersed themselves is a tribute to our communal consciousness about celebrities who care for our kind. By engaging in a concentrated communal experience of grief and then returning to the land of the living, gay men did something with Diana which many of us cannot do with AIDS: we gave ourselves permission to leave behind our funereal feelings and return to life. We let go of the comfortable familiarity of tragedy and the drama of crisis.

LEARNING TO FUCK AGAIN

My sex life has changed enormously in the post-AIDS era, as the fear and guilt that suffused my erotic encounters during the 1980s and early 1990s diminished. Turning forty moved me to question the position sex held in my life and reexamine some of my desires. I hoped sex would remain in a prominent position in my life, and that possibilities for fulfilling encounters would continue. I found myself considering moving in some new sexual directions and exploring activities that had not previously been central to my erotic life.

My sexual tastes have been surprisingly stable through most of my life. I developed strong fetishes and interests in specific activities even before I first had sex with a man. Some of the things that attract me powerfully today—physical characteristics such as body hair, thick forearms, big hands; specific acts of surrender and control—were key parts of my adolescent masturbatory fantasies. I would sit in synagogue as a twelve-year-old boy and focus my attention intensely on men with beards, my eyes darting to their throats and hands, curiously drawn to body hair. When I messed around with other boys, I was excited by rope games, rubbing against each other's bellies, and talking dirty and in detail about precisely what we were doing.

Fucking never seemed to interest me, even after coming out in the 1970s. I tried to get fucked a few times and the experience was painful and exhausting. The idea of being overpowered and taken by a masculine brute excited me, but technical difficulties down below neutralized the appeal. I might have penetrated a dozen men before the epidemic's arrival, but an aversion to being inside someone else's anus reduced my interest in fucking other guys. My pre-AIDS sexual activities usually ranged from rough sex to S/M, with a heavy emphasis on kissing and getting blown.

My sexual practices changed little during the early years of the epidemic. I marveled at my good fortune: AIDS increased the popularity of the acts I enjoyed and diminished the appeal of those I didn't. Fewer men I approached in bars were looking to get fucked and more were seeking to blow me. Lists of safer sex activities actually promoted the kinky practices in which I'd become skilled—bondage, dirty talk, fantasy role-playing, discipline, and uniforms. Many men, encouraged to abandon specific penetrative practices, moved gingerly toward the fantasy world of kink, and I found myself sought after despite my relative youth and inexperience. In the mid-1980s, as AIDS exerted a powerful influence, fear of infection and mass death and the stigma of disease permeated my sex life. I was determined to find ways to remain sexually active, yet it often felt as if I were tiptoeing between land mines.

Anal sex crept into my fantasy life slowly during the late 1980s. Repeated cultural messages telling me to "Wear a Rubber Every Time," and "Use Condoms—100 Percent" may have heightened my interest in fucking and created powerful new meanings of anal sex for me. As fucking and getting fucked asserted themselves increasingly in my daydreams, I wondered whether my own desires emerged from transgression. Was the now-forbidden nature of anal sex sparking new desires within me? Did I want to fuck guys now because it was dangerous? Was there something about illness, death, and prohibition that got me hard?

Fucking continued to occupy larger and larger portions of my sexual fantasies and eventually made cameo appearances in my sex life. I didn't actually fuck or get fucked by men; instead I talked about it a lot in my encounters. I'd confess to partners that I don't like to fuck guys, so if anal sex was what they were looking for, they might try another man. Sometimes I'd let them know that I enjoyed talking about fucking guys, but I was clear that my cock was not going to enter their butts. AIDS-related prohibitions lent credence to my boundaries and I met men who enjoyed a verbal narrative of getting fucked, and could be quite happy with nothing more than one of my fingers poking up their holes. I liked it when a man would talk about fucking me, perhaps even pushing his dick up against my ass, encouraging me to imagine it inside me; those who tried to enter me, however, found the doors tightly locked.

By 1993, I noticed myself cruising men who'd never before interested me and moving into new sexual activities. Was it the changing trajectory of the epidemic? Was it the approach of my fortieth birthday? Was it the influence of a lover with great versatility and wide-ranging tastes? I no longer restricted my erotic gaze to one or two narrow types—the Castro clones or macho bears—and now also pursued younger men, smooth bodies, even blondes! I had a new and powerful attraction to Asian men, quite different from the big, hairy Jewish or Italian studs who had previously dominated my erotic imagination. Whereas once the men with whom I'd slept were often a decade or two older than I (I recall insisting men younger than I didn't know how to have sex), I now found myself sleeping with men of all ages. I still enjoyed older men, now the group of men in their forties, fifties, and sixties, but I also found myself sexing with younger men, including several in their early twenties.

Somehow I also lost some of my rigidity around sex roles. Previously I'd found the top/bottom dynamic to be very exciting and almost all of my encounters followed a choreography of domination/submission. I never switched roles in a sexual encounter; I also found it difficult to move from one role to another in separate encounters with the same man. Now I found a flexibility creeping into my sexual repertoire that was entirely new. I could be the man in control one day and then be the one who was controlled at my next interlude with the same man. I also began switching roles during a single encounter. I started blowing guys myself, something I'd rarely done and never fully enjoyed, then moved into mutual simultaneous cocksucking. I even began enjoying myself when guys whom I'd been topping turned the tables and I suddenly found myself bound and gagged.

I explained these changes to myself in a number of ways. I had often wondered about my penchant for constantly reenacting a narrow sexual script and finding it satisfying. Had I finally exhausted the power of that scenario? Having been in gay men's sex cultures for twenty years, had I used up all my Tom of Finland-oriented fantasies? I considered whether the aging process may have influenced these shifts, and whether the broad range of men that now attracted me wasn't simply a by-product of waning sexual appeal as a middle-aged gay man living in the gay ghetto. Yet I still felt attractive, had little trouble attracting partners, and found that my broadened interests delivered wider opportunities to me.

I slowly became aware that I had been profoundly influenced by a dozen years of unceasing manipulation of my desires through the vast discourse of AIDS prevention. I, along with most other urban gay men, had been bombarded with messages on billboards, radio stations, T-shirts, and posters. Messages we received from our peers during sexual encounters may have been even more influential. Some of these interpersonal and often unspoken messages adhered to the dictates of prevention and some of them violated them. In either case, I began to realize that erotic desires and practices are not inbred genetic qualities, but are constantly reinvented and turned on their heads through complex social and cultural processes.

In 1996, I started fucking guys, something I had not done in about a dozen years. This shift in my sexual practices came upon me quickly; it was not a decision I consciously pondered for a long time. The desire to fuck had developed over a number of years, but I relegated it to the realm of fantasy, telling myself it was not wise to develop a new and active interest in anal sex during the HIV epidemic. I only began to consider buttfucking a serious option during the summer of 1996.

I attribute this shift to two important changes. First and foremost was the cultural shift in our thinking about HIV that emerged from the Vancouver conference. The dramatic shift from despair to hope, and the powerful discourse about HIV infection moving toward becoming chronic and manageable, seemed to make it less frightening to consider fucking again. I can't say that I consciously thought to myself, "Eric, it's okay to fuck now because (a) fucking with a condom does not present a huge risk for the man doing the fucking; and (b) HIV is becoming chronic and manageable, so if I get infected it's not such a big deal." Instead, the news from Vancouver quietly moved me to a place where fulfilling my desire to fuck guys seemed reasonable. I have not yet altered my prohibition about getting fucked myself; lingering fears of pain and HIV lead me to relegate that activity to the world of virtual sex (via telephone or cyberspace).

The second influence on my interest in fucking was my immersion in a range of new scholarship focused on the meanings men make of anal sex. I had engaged in a number of international meetings with scholars, prevention workers, and researchers and had become transfixed by work exploring the meanings derived from particular sexual acts. A paper from the Netherlands titled "Viewed from Behind: Anal Sex in the AIDS Era," by Marty PN van Kerkhof, Onno de Zwart, and Theo Sandfort[5] initiated powerful discussions about the meanings fucking and getting fucked have for gay men and the complex negotiations—verbal, body, spiritual, and emotional—that occur during sex. Looking back, I believe I was drawn to this work because of my dawning interest in fucking, but something about having public conversations about anal sex drew me closer to the act of fucking men.

During the fall and winter of 1996, I began fucking guys. Two of my regular partners were willing to assist, but both were small men, who experienced much discomfort as I attempted to gently thrust into them. As much as I enjoyed fantasies of forced fucking, I did not want to hurt men in ways they didn't find pleasurable, and I was concerned that my inexperience and the difference in size between us might do some damage.

I began obsessing on fucking guys. Soon this became the sole act dominating my fantasies. I began looking at men's butts with great intensity and, when I'd meet a new partner, focus all my energies on getting my dick into his hole. I often felt like a young puppy, humping against anything in my path.

Eventually I took out a personal advertisement in a local gay paper seeking a "teacher" who would assist me in developing my fucking skills. I received twenty-seven replies in one week and, after a protracted process of screening, met with Michael, a lawyer who worked in the financial district, who was willing to help me out. For a period of three months, Michael came over once a week during lunchtime and eased me into fucking. He taught me how to properly use condoms, how to open up a guy's butt gently, and how to position myself in a way that allowed me easier access. Because I found him attractive—and because he was willing to indulge some of my dirty sex talk—this became a successful partnership. He enjoyed showing me how to fuck, and I enjoyed gaining a small measure of confidence with the act.

I now understand the appearance of fucking as an increasingly central act in my erotic imagination in new ways. Perhaps some psychologists would argue I'd successfully repressed my interests in the act for a number of years as a defense mechanism during the plague years. I think something else has happened: fucking has taken on new meanings for me derived specifically from AIDS prevention discourse. Thus I find that I channel a range of power issues into my fucking activities. My interest in fucking is often about pretending I'm forcing a man to do something he either does not want to do, or feels he shouldn't be doing. This verges on rape fantasies and sometimes explicitly enters that arena.

I am well aware I step into "edge" territory here, but I do not believe my interests, fantasies, or practices are uncommon. I have found that the idea of anal sex without a condom is a great turn-on for me, and have brought this fantasy into my sex life while refusing to engage in unprotected anal sex. To make the matter a bit more heretical, I have had sex with men who are uninfected and who are aware I am uninfected, yet who enjoy the fantasy that I am HIV-positive and about to fuck them without a condom. I have played out these narratives, first through phone sex, then through actual sexual encounters. For me, such playacting is preferable to actual unsafe practices.

What does this look like? I regularly have sex with a butcher named Jack. I met him one evening at the Eagle, a leather bar in the South of Market district, and was pleased when he asked for my phone number. We began having sex together every few weeks. He has great legs, a great, hairy butt, and a very sexy, Southern drawl. He is also HIV positive and has struggled with several serious infections over the past three years. I have not actually fucked Jack yet and am not sure if I want to penetrate him with my cock. Despite his strong, sinewy body, he strikes me as vulnerable, even fragile, and I wonder whether buttfucking—not a central part of his own sexual repertoire—is in the best interest of his health right now.

During one of our first encounters, I found myself laying on top of his prone and naked body, with my hard cock wedged flat against the cheeks of his butt, and my lips chewing on the nape of his neck. As he growled like a puppy, his ass began to rock against me, jarring me into a fucking motion against him. He had already told me that getting fucked was not going to happen, so I felt comfortable, without additional conversation, moving into a specific scenario. I began to push my dick against him as I wrapped my arms tightly around his muscular frame. I bent my lips to his ear and whispered, "I am gonna fuck you now, kid. Yep, I'm gonna put my big hard dick up your tight butt and I'm gonna do it whether you want it or not. No condom, no lube, no nothing. I'm just gonna fuck you hard and hold you down while I do it."

Jack's eyes opened wide and he turned a bit to look at me, seeking reassurance. I immediately demonstrated such reassurance, by sliding my cock along the upper ridge of his ass and his lower back, and grunting as if I were actually inside him. "I'm fuckin' you now, boy, fuckin' you hard and dirty," I said gruffly. "And nothing's gonna make me stop till I shoot my sperm deep into you, right up your tight little butt."

At this point, Jack began groaning with pleasure and whispered deeply in his hoarse voice, "Yeah, daddy, fuck your boy. Fuck me hard. I want to feel that sperm in me, Sir. Fuck me hard!" I rode him, hard and rough, yet, at the same time, gentle and loving. As I shouted and groaned and went crazy with abandon, energy rushed to my groin and I felt my cock begin to ejaculate and cover his back and butt with semen.

THE KIND WHO CAN'T FORGET

There is a song by Mary Chapin Carpenter, one of my favorite country/folk singers, with the lyrics, "This world is kinder to the kind that won't look back."[6] I find myself agreeing with the lyrics a lot these days. I am the kind that can't forget. I am the kind that looks back too much.

My lover and I attended the San Francisco Gay Men's Chorus spring concert focused entirely on songs by Abba. As a major fan of Abba, I eagerly anticipated the event and planned my schedule to ensure I'd be in town. The concert hall was packed, the spirit was high, and the performance was terrific. Yet every few minutes, one

Abba song or another would spin me back in time, flipping me back and forth between memory and regret. "Dancing Queen" would bring me back to tea-dance in Provincetown with Don, and Paul, and Steven, all long gone now due to AIDS. "Lay All Your Love on Me" shot me back to dancing at Probe in West Hollywood with Frank and Daniel. How embarrassing to find myself teary-eyed at "Fernando," a song we'd all mocked when it was popular among teenage girls!

The post-AIDS years have brought a bit of relief from my tendency to revel in a romanticized version of the past and use nostalgia as a trigger for memories, yet I still find myself wrestling a great deal with the cultures we created before AIDS changed everything. Do I miss them? Am I glad they are over? Were they good times or did they destroy us, or both? I fear I may spend the rest of my life cycling through those memories and trying to sort out what happened and why my friends aren't here any more. I'm glad whenever I feel myself moving on, becoming engaged with current issues and participating in contemporary movements. Much of my life is ahead of me, and an obsessive focus on the past can only keep me disengaged from the present moment.

I find relief in dance. For much of my life, gay dance clubs have served as arenas of celebration for me, taking me out of my own head, putting my body in motion, and freeing my spirit. During the peak years of the epidemic, dancing became painful; tunes rang in my head but couldn't drown out the rising terror. The music died as I crashed amid the horrors of those years and channeled my manic energies into efforts to fight AIDS.

I started dancing again as the post-AIDS era dawned. My reconnection to music and movement has been key to my personal revival and, to my mind, the regeneration of our communities. An astounding novel by Jack Fritscher focused on pre-AIDS San Francisco, takes its title from the Eagles' refrain:

> Some dance to remember.
> Some dance to forget.[7]

For a while, I danced to remember the good times. Then I danced to forget the past. And some nights I moved back and forth between one and the other in a jumble of confusion. Now I dance to revel in the present and be alive in my own life story.

About two years ago, Pleasuredome, a Sunday night dance club, began featuring 1970s disco music from 9 to 11, before the young crowds arrived and the music became high-energy, house, or some other type of contemporary dance music. I dropped in to see who was dancing, expecting a few dinosaurs like myself, working out our painful memories. I didn't think it would be a pretty sight.

But the dance floor was packed with a diverse range of people, dancing to Donna Summer and Candi Staton and Vicki Sue Robinson. There were twenty-one-year-old dykes who knew all the words to "Born to be Alive," and fifty-five-year-old fan dancers taking to the stage. When Sylvester started wailing the room came alive and everyone broke out in smiles. I knew this was a place I could dance.

So I dance now, a few times a month, at Pleasuredome. I have new friends I meet on the dance floor and my feet come alive to the music of the past. Sometimes I'll stay at the club after the music changes and the boys with shaved bodies and ripped abs take over. It's their music, not mine, but I'm learning to dance to it. I have even learned some of the lyrics.

Notes

Chapter 1

1. Lois Pearlman, "Activist Says AIDS Is No Longer a Killer," *The Slant* (San Rafael, CA), November, 1996, 1.

2. Richard Shumate, "It's Good Bad News," *Bay Windows* (Boston), n.d., 1; Patricia Field, "Hospice Closing Is Bittersweet," Letter to the editor, *Bay Windows*, January 23, 1997, 7; Dennis Conkin, "SF HIV Care Residence to Expand," *Bay Area Reporter* (San Francisco), December 5, 1996, 17; Tom McGeveran, "Agape to Open Second Home for Latino PWAs," *focusPOINT* (Minneapolis), December 11, 1996, 1; Debbie Carvalko, "AIDS Housing Shortage Critical in CT," *Bay Windows*, November 7, 1996, 22; Mona Shah, "Sierra Project Celebrates 10 Years With Visions of Hope," *The Lesbian News*, September 1997, 20.

3. Associated Press, "Debate Over Gay Sex Clubs Heats Up in NYC," *Bay Windows*, April 13-19, 1995, 1, 22.

4. Rene Beauchamp, "Bring Back the Bathhouses—or Relight the Restaurants!," *Bay Area Reporter*, November 28, 1996.

5. Sean Strub, "S.O.S.," *POZ*, August 1997, 18; David May, "I Bought the Plot—Now What?," *San Francisco Frontiers*, May 22, 1977, 17-18; David Dunlap, "Surviving with AIDS: Now What?", *The New York Times*, August 1, 1996.

6. David Dunlap, "Surviving with AIDS: Now What?", *The New York Times*, August 1, 1996.

7. See Bob Nelson, "AIDS Is Now an Epidemic for the Poor," *San Francisco Examiner*, April 21, 1997, A17.

8. Centers for Disease Control and Prevention, *HIV Surveillance Report: U.S. HIV and AIDS Cases Reported Through December 1996*, 8 (2). See also "Morbidity and Mortality Weekly Report Chart" published in *The Washington Blade*, June 5, 1995, 31; Lisa Keen, "Gay and Bi Men Account for 40% of Cases," *The Washington Blade*, July 18, 1997, 26.

9. Lawrence K. Altman, "U.N. Reports 3 Million New H.I.V. Cases Worldwide for '96," *The New York Times*, June 28, 1996, A6.

10. Deaths of people with AIDS from strange cancers continue to occur. See Lawrence K. Altman, "Surviving with AIDS Is One Problem: Cancer Is Yet Another," *The New York Times*, May 6, 1997, B10.

11. Mitchell H. Katz, "AIDS Epidemic in San Francisco Among Men Who Report Sex with Men: Successes and Challenges of HIV Prevention," *Journal of Acquired Immune Deficiency Syndrome and Human Retrovirology*, 14(Supple-

ment 2): S38-S46, 1997; New York City Department of Health, Office of AIDS Surveillance, "AIDS Surveillance Update," First Quarter 1997; San Francisco Department of Public Health, "AIDS Surveillance Report," June 1997, 7.

12. Lawrence K. Altman, "AIDS Deaths Drop 19% in U.S., Continuing a Heartening Trend," *The New York Times*, July 15, 1997, 1; Bob Roehr, "AIDS Deaths Down, Problems Up," *Bay Area Reporter*, July 17, 1997, 1; "AIDS Toll Drops Overall—Minorities Still Hit Hard," *San Francisco Chronicle*, July 15, 1997.

13. See Susan Sontag, *AIDS and Its Metaphors* (New York: Farrar, Strauss, and Giroux, 1988).

14. Cindy Patton's work best elucidates this process. See Cindy Patton, *Sex and Germs: The Politics of AIDS* (Boston: South End Press, 1985); Also *Inventing AIDS* (New York: Routledge, 1990), and *Fatal Advice: How Safe-Sex Education Went Wrong* (Durham, NC: Duke University Press, 1996).

15. Frank Browning was among the first to document the rebirth of gay male sexual subcultures in the early 1990s. See Frank Browning, *The Culture of Desire* (New York: Crown, 1993).

16. I am speaking here of Hunter Madsen, Marshall Kirk, Andrew Sullivan, and others. This is best documented in Urvashi Vaid, *Virtual Equality: The Mainstreaming of Gay and Lesbian Liberation* (New York: Doubleday, 1995).

17. Wayne Hoffman, "Skipping the Life Fantastic: Coming of Age in the Sexual Devolution," in Dangerous Bedfellows (Eds.), *Policing Public Sex* (Boston: South End Press, 1996), 337-354.

18. Ron Stall, Don Barrett, Larry Bye, Joe Catania, Chuck Frutchey, Jeff Henne, George Lemp, and Jay Paul, "A Comparison of Younger and Older Gay Men's HIV Risk-Taking Behaviors: The Communications Technologies 1992 Cross Sectional Survey," *Journal of Acquired Immune Deficiency Syndrome*, 5:682-687.

19. Michael T. Wright, "The Self-Interest of AIDS Workers and the Future of the AIDS Service Movement," paper presented at the National Lesbian and Gay Health Conference/National HIV-AIDS Forum, July 1997, Atlanta, 3. Reprinted by permission.

20. For one striking example by a twenty-two-year-old gay man see Wayne Hoffman, "AIDS Generation Gap Is Closing," *The Washington Blade*, January 29, 1993.

21. I am indebted here to the work of Cindy Patton, who first identified the ways in which the constant sense of emergency which circulates around AIDS "becomes a system of control in itself." See Cindy Patton, *Inventing AIDS* (New York: Routledge, 1990), 107-109.

22. David Halperin, personal communication of his lecture notes, October 29, 1997. The class is Sociology 1161, "Sexuality, Culture, and Communication". The University of New South Wales, Sydney, Australia.

23. Mitchell H. Katz, "AIDS Epidemic in San Francisco Among Men Who Report Sex with Men: Successes and Challenges of HIV Prevention," *Journal of Acquired Immune Deficiency Syndrome and Human Retrovirology*, 1997, 14(Supple-

ment 2): S39-S40; National Centre in HIV Social Research: *Sydney Men and Sexual Health,* Report C1 (Darlinghurst, Australia: Macquarie University, 1995), 33.

24. There are notable exceptions among prevention organizations, which are discussed in Chapter 7. While a few groups have worked in earnest to shift paradigms, I find most prevention for gay men in 1998 continues to operate covertly out of oppressive models of colonization marked by rigid professionalism, narrow understandings of how sexual desires and activities are constituted, and social marketing campaigns that depend upon a foundation of guilt extant in gay cultures.

25. See Scott Holmberg, "The Estimated Prevalence and Incidence of HIV in 96 Large U.S. Metropolitan Areas," *American Journal of Public Health,* 86(5), May 1996, 642-654; also, Thomas Mills, Ron Stall, Joseph Catania, and Thomas Coates, "Interpreting HIV Prevalence and Incidence Among Americans: Bridging Data and Public Policy," *American Journal of Public Health,* 87(5), May 1997, 864-865.

26. Mitchell H. Katz, "AIDS Epidemic in San Francisco Among Men Who Report Sex with Men: Successes and Challenges of HIV Prevention," *Journal of Acquired Immune Deficiency Syndrome and Human Retrovirology,* 14(Supplement 2): S38-S46.

27. Interview with G.B., August 28, 1996, Provincetown, MA.

28. R.W. Connell, J. Crawford, G.W. Dowsett, S. Kippax, V. Sinnott, P. Rodden, and R. Berg, "Danger and Context: Unsafe Anal Sexual Practice Among Homosexual and Bisexual Men in the AIDS Crisis," *The Australian and New Zealand Journal of Sociology,* 26(2):187-208 (1990); R.W. Connell, M.D. Davis, and Gary W. Dowsett, "A Bastard of a Life: Homosexual Desire and Practice Among Men in Working-Class Milieux," *The Australian and New Zealand Journal of Sociology,* 29(1):112-35 (1993); R.W. Connell, G.W. Dowsett, P. Rodden, M.D. David, L. Watson, and D. Baxter, "Social Class, Gay Men and AIDS Prevention," *Australian Journal of Public Health* 15(3): 178-189 (1991).

29. Gary Dowsett and David McInnes, "'Post AIDS': Assessing the Long-Term Social Impact of HIV/AIDS in Gay Communities," paper presented at the XI International Conference on AIDS, Vancouver, July 8, 1996. Reprinted by permission.

30. XI International Conference on AIDS, *Abstracts* I., (Vancouver: International AIDS Society, 1996), 51.

31. Dowsett and McInnes, "'Post AIDS': Assessing the Long-Term Social Impact of HIV/AIDS in Gay Communities," 3-4; see also Gary Dowsett, *Practicing Desire: Homosexual Sex in the Era of AIDS,* (Stanford, CA: Stanford University Press, 1996).

32. Ibid.

33. Ibid.

34. National Centre in HIV Social Research, *Sydney Men and Sexual Health,* Report C1 (Darlinghurst, Australia: Macquarie University, 1995), 33; Mitchell H. Katz, "AIDS Epidemic in San Francisco Among Men Who Report Sex with Men:

Successes and Challenges of HIV Prevention," *Journal of Acquired Immune Deficiency Syndrome and Human Retrovirology,* 14(Supplement 2).

35. *Holy Bible, Contemporary English Version* (New York: American Bible Society, 1995), Ezekiel 37, 877-878. For thoughtful commentary on this passage, see Elie Wiesel, *Sages and Dreamers* (New York: Simon & Schuster, 1991), 80-98; also, Louis Ginzberg, *Legends of the Bible* (Philadelphia: Jewish Publication Society, 1978). I thank Reverend Jim Mitulski for leading me to this passage.

Chapter 2

1. Andrew Sullivan, "When AIDS Ends," *The New York Times Magazine,* November 10, 1996; Dan Savage, "Dan Savage on the End of the AIDS Crisis," *The Stranger* (Seattle), January 16, 1997; Bernard Garver, "I Have a Reason to Be Here," *Parade Magazine,* April 6, 1997; John Leland, "The End of AIDS," *Newsweek,* December 2, 1996; John Gallagher, "Back in the Running," *The Advocate,* December 24, 1996.

2. Gay City in Seattle, for example, held a forum titled "The End of AIDS: Hope or Hype," on May 29, 1997, which focused on "What every gay man, positive and negative, needs to know about the impact of the new AIDS drugs on the gay community." See *Volunteer Voice: A Newsletter for Volunteers and Friends of Gay City,* May 1997, 1.

3. For a more complete discussion of this period, see Eric Rofes, *Reviving the Tribe: Regenerating Gay Men's Sexuality and Culture in the Ongoing Epidemic,* (Binghamton, NY: Haworth Press, 1996), 97-224.

4. Ibid., 294-295.

5. Ibid.

6. See William J. Mann, "Perfect Bound," *Frontiers,* January 13, 1994, 82-86. See also Lynette A. Lewis and Michael W. Ross, *A Select Body: The Gay Dance Party Subculture and the HIV/AIDS Pandemic* (London: Cassell, 1995), 166-191.

7. Charles Winick, "AIDS Obituaries in *The New York Times,*" *AIDS & Public Policy Journal* (Fall 1996):148-152 offers an interesting perspective on tracking AIDS deaths in one mainstream newspaper.

8. Jane Rosett, "Dressed for Arrest: The Day the Suits Seized the Street," *POZ,* (May 1997): 48.

9. Mitchell H. Katz, "AIDS Epidemic in San Francisco Among Men Who Report Sex with Men: Successes and Challenges of HIV Prevention," *Journal of Acquired Immune Deficiency Syndromes and Human Retrovirology,* 1997, 14 (Supplement 2):539-540.

10. Dan Savage has discussed this dynamic, wondering why he and I maintain similar analyses, yet he is attacked and I am applauded. See Dan Savage, "Shooting the Messenger," *The Stranger,* June 19, 1997, 26.

11. Letter from S.T., March 4, 1997.

12. Dan Savage, "Life After AIDS," *The Stranger,* January 17, 1997, 8-13.

13. Ibid., 8. Reprinted by permission of Dan Savage.

14. John Leonard, letter to the editor, *The Stranger,* February 6, 1997, 4.

15. Robert Wood, letter to the editor, *The Stranger,* February 6, 1997, 6.

16. Terry M. Stone, letter to the editor, *The Stranger,* February 13, 1997, 9.

17. Irving Sambolin, letter to the editor, *The Stranger,* February 13, 1997, 9.

18. Interview with E.T., November 17, 1997, Los Angeles, CA.

19. See David May, "I Bought the Plot—Now What?," *San Francisco Frontiers,* May 22, 1997, 17-18; Also Sean Strub, "S.O.S.," *POZ,* August 1997, 18; see also Paul Reed's powerful chapbook, *Back from the Brink: Reflections on Illness, Renewal and Hope* (San Francisco: House of Lillian, 1996).

20. This flyer appeared in a doorway adjacent to Daddy's Bar on Castro Street on December 23, 1996.

21. Nightsweats & T-cells advertisement, *Bay Area Reporter,* November 21, 1996.

22. This flyer appeared in Dr. Lisa Capaldini's Castro Street office.

23. Peter Freiberg, "Viatical industry in 'utter chaos'," *The Washington Blade,* February 14, 1997, 1, 17. See also Wilbanks & Associates, Inc. advertisement, "Viatical Settlements: The Game Has Changed," *Bay Area Reporter,* November 14, 1996.

24. Herbert G. McCann, "Insurance available for some with HIV," *San Francisco Examiner,* April 15, 1997 discusses Guarantee Trust Life Insurance in Glenview, IL, which "specializes in insuring high-risk individuals."

25. Dennis Conklin, "SF HIV Care Residence to Expand," *Bay Area Reporter,* December 5, 1996, 17; Tom McGeveran, "Agape to Open Second Home for Latino PWAs," *focusPOINT* (Minneapolis), December 11, 1996, 1; Debbie Carvalho, "AIDS Housing Shortage Critical in CT," *Bay Windows,* November 7, 1996, 22; Richard Shumate, "It's Good Bad News," *Bay Windows,* n.d., 1; Patricia Field, "Hospice Closing Is Bittersweet," letter to the editor, *Bay Windows,* January 23, 1997, 7; Edwin McReady, letter to the editor, "The Abrupt Closing of Chris Brownlie House," *Edge,* October 30, 1996, 23; Christopher Jones, "Combination Therapies Reduce Hospital Stays," *Washington Blade,* January 31, 1997, 29.

26. Kim Painter, "AIDS Deaths Drop 13% in First Decline," *USA Today,* February 28, 1997, 1.

27. Ibid., 1.

28. Ibid., 1.

29. David Perlman, "AIDS Deaths Drop Across Nation," *San Francisco Chronicle,* February 28, 1997, 1. Copyright *San Francisco Chronicle.* Reprinted by permission.

30. Ibid., 1.

31. David Brown, "AIDS Toll Falls by Half in New York," *The Washington Post,* January 25, 1997, A1.

32. Ibid., A10.

33. "The Declining AIDS Toll," editorial, *San Francisco Examiner,* March 5, 1997. Copyright 1997 by the *San Francisco Examiner.* Reprinted by permission.

34. I credit activist with Gregg Consalves for suggesting this metaphor for the current epidemic moment. See Pacific Resources for Education and Learning,

"Multiculturalism in the Gay Community: Consciousness-Raising for Managed Care" (Honolulu: Pacific Resources for Education and Learning, July 28, 1997), 18.

35. Andrew Sullivan, "When Plagues End: Notes on the Twilight of an Epidemic," *The New York Times Magazine,* November 10, 1996, 52-62, 76-77, 84. Copyright 1996 by *The New York Times.* Reprinted by permission.

36. Ibid., 10.

37. Sullivan, "When Plagues End"; Robert Nesti, "Settling into a New Life, with New Hope," *Bay Windows,* November 29, 1996, 1, 20.

38. Tony Valenzuela, "Me and HIV," *Gay and Lesbian Times,* November 16, 1995, 2-5; Tony Valenzuela, "HIV Positive and Twentysomething," *Gay and Lesbian Times,* December 14, 1995, 39, 41; Sue Fox, "I Just Didn't Think That I Would Get It So Young," *The Washington Blade,* March 3, 1995, 10; Wayne Hoffman, "Skipping the Life Fantastic: Coming of Age in the Sexual Devolution," in Dangerous Bedfellows (Eds.), *Policing Public Sex* (Boston: South End Press, 1996), 337-354.

39. Sullivan, "When Plagues End," 57-58.

40. G. Galland, letter to the editor, *The New York Times Magazine,* December 1, 1996, 20.

41. John Leland, "The End of AIDS?" *Newsweek,* December 2, 1996, 64-75.

42. Ibid., 64-66. See also Bernard Garzer, "I Saw I Had a Future," *Parade Magazine,* April 6, 1997, 4-7; Jim Howley, "Empower Yourself," *The Advocate,* May 27, 1997, 13; John Gallagher, "Back in the Running," *The Advocate,* December 24, 1996, 22-30.

43. John D'Emilio, "The End of AIDS? Not Exactly," *Direct Report: A Publication of the National Gay and Lesbian Task Force,* March 1997, 3.

44. Urvashi Vaid, "Hope versus Hype," *The Advocate,* December 24, 1996, 80.

45. Bruce Mirken, "Hope, Hype and Survival," *Bay Windows,* December 26, 1996, 5.

46. "The Media Is the Message," *POZ,* August 1997.

47. *The Advocate*, March 18, 1997, 30-36.

48. See *Bay Windows,* November 7, 1996, 11. For full information see press packet, "Be Smart About HIV," October 1996 (Glaxo Wellcome, Blue Bell, PA).

49. Advertisement in the *Bay Area Reporter,* January 8, 1998, 23.

50. Advertisement in *The Advocate,* March 18, 1997, 24.

51. Advertisement in *The Advocate*, July 22, 1997, 26.

52. John Lauritsen and Ian Young (Eds.), *The AIDS Cult: Essays on the Gay Health Crisis* (Provincetown, MA: Asklepios, 1997); Ian Young, *The Stonewall Experiment: A Gay Psychohistory* (London: Cassell, 1995).

53. See Centers for Disease Control and Prevention, *HIV Surveillance Report: U.S. HIV and AIDS Cases Reported Through December 1996,* 8(2). For popular media coverage, see Bernard Garzer, "I Saw I Had a Future," *Parade Magazine,* April 6, 1997, 4-7.

54. Jeff Levi, "Rethinking HIV Counseling and Testing," *AIDS & Public Policy Journal,* Winter, 1996, 164-168.

55. See Chandler Burr, "The AIDS Exception: Privacy vs. Public Health," *Atlantic Monthly,* June 1997; Also Wayne Hoffman, "Contact Tracing for the HIV Infected?," *Bay Windows,* June 12, 1997, 6-7; Lynda Richardson, "Progress on AIDS Brings Movement for Less Secrecy," *The New York Times,* August 21, 1997, 1.

56. Catherine Hanssens, "Skin Deep," *POZ,* August 1997; for additional evidence of the continuing precarious legal status of HIV positives, see Lisa Keen, "Decision on HIV Bias Called 'Very Disturbing'," *The Washington Blade,* August 29, 1997, 1.

57. *The American Heritage Dictionary of the English Language,* Third Edition (Boston: Houghton Mifflin, 1992).

58. See Daniel Harris, *The Rise and Fall of Gay Culture* (New York: Hyperion, 1997), 219-238.

59. See Michael Wright, "The Self-Interest of AIDS Workers and the Future of the AIDS Service Movement," paper presented at the National Lesbian and Gay Health Conference/National HIV/AIDS Forum, July 1997, Atlanta, 3. Reprinted by permission.

60. The research for this book occurred over two years and consists of in-depth one-on-one interviews with over seventy gay and bisexual men of varying races, generations, and locations; interviews with an additional thirty-seven men in three small group settings; reviews of medical and other scientific publications focused on HIV and gay men; examination of key texts including mainstream magazines, gay newspapers, and organizational records; a small survey completed during the winter of 1996-97 by twenty-four men on protease inhibitors; participant observer research at several HIV-related conferences and public meetings; and analyses of advertisements and other representations of gay men's contemporary experience of HIV/AIDS. Some of the men interviewed are quoted in this book, but only their initials are provided and details of their lives have been altered to assure anonymity. Other men interviewed are not quoted in the final text, but they contributed significantly to my thinking on the topics covered in this book and I appreciate their willingness to speak with me about a range of personal issues. In relating information from my interviews with community leaders, I have used their real names whenever granted permission.

61. Interview with R.G., April 24, 1996, San Francisco, CA.

62. Interview with A.W., April 15, 1996, San Francisco, CA.

63. "New Survey Shows One in Three Gay Men Do Not See HIV as a Crisis," *Wisconsin Light,* October 23, 1997, 3.

64. Interview with S.M., May 2, 1996, Berkeley, CA.

65. Interview with M.M., June 23, 1996, San Francisco, CA.

66. Interview with E.T., November 17, 1997, Los Angeles, CA.

67. Metropolitan Community Church/San Francisco has constructed such a ritual, by organizing an evening to recount the oral history of this deeply affected congregation's involvement with AIDS.

Chapter 3

1. See M. Jane Taylor, "National Gay, AIDS Groups See CFC Donations Dip 10 Percent," *The Washington Blade,* August 15, 1997, 14; See also Peter Freiberg, "Early Signs of Funding Fatigue?" *The Washington Blade,* August 8, 1997, 12; "The Coming Sunset on AIDS Funding Programs," *Project Inform Perspective,* July 1997, 1; Laurie Fitzpatrick, "Bingo," *Art and Understanding,* July 1997, 36-41.

2. John James, "AIDS Treatment Activism: Turning to Service," *San Francisco Bay Times,* April 3, 1997, 16; Peter Freiberg, "After 10 Years, ACT UP Now Fights Dwindling Membership," *The Washington Blade,* March 14, 1997, 1.

3. Advertisement, *San Francisco Frontiers,* July 3, 1997, inside cover.

4. Advertisement, *San Francisco Chronicle,* July 19, 1997, A18.

5. Sighted at several Castro district establishments, including the Cove Cafe and Market Street Gym.

6. Cynthia Laird, "Over 25,000 Walk for AIDS; Largest Event Ever Raises $3.5 Million," *Bay Area Reporter,* July 24, 1997, 14; Monique Fields, "New Hope, Same Resolve," *San Francisco Chronicle,* July 21, 1997, A13.

7. Advertisement, *San Jose Gay Pride Magazine,* 1997, 13.

8. Advertisement, *The Advocate,* June 10, 1997, 38.

9. Advertisement, *Bay Area Reporter,* June 26, 1997, 90.

10. Advertisement, *Bay Area Reporter,* July 17, 1997, 36.

11. Gary Dowsett, "Living Post-AIDS," *National AIDS Bulletin* (Australia), March-April 1996, 22. Reprinted by permission.

12. Interview with K.S. in Milwaukee on May 21, 1997.

13. Gone are Sheldon Andelson, Rand Schrader, Steve West, Bob LeMieux, Alan Goodman, Randy Klose and Duke Comegys. Gone are Gabe Kruks, Gustavo Vega-Correa, Ron Shigaki, Hugh Rice, Jeff Campbell, and Bob Lien.

14. Walt Odets, *In the Shadow of the Epidemic: Being HIV-Negative in the Age of AIDS,* (Durham, NC: Duke University Press, 1995; Will I. Johnston, *HIV-Negative: How the Uninfected Are Affected by AIDS* (New York: Insight Books, 1995).

15. Steven Schwartzberg, *A Crisis of Meaning: How Gay Men Are Making Sense of AIDS* (New York: Oxford, 1996).

16. Michael Wright, *Und Wir Uberleben* (Berlin: Deutsche AIDS-Hilfe, 1996).

17. See *National Directory of Resources for HIV-Negative Gay Men* (New York: RJM Charitable Trust, 1997).

18. Andy Humm, opening remarks, The First National Forum on and for HIV-Negative Gay Men, Atlanta, July 1997.

19. Alex Carballo-Dieguez, "Where We've Come Since the 1994 Dallas Conference on HIV-Negative Gay Men," the First National Forum on and for HIV-Negative Gay Men, Atlanta, July 1997.

20. Conversation with B.C. in Atlanta, Georgia, July 26, 1997. The video was Ioannis Mookas and David Deitcher's *Only Human: HIV-Negative Gay Men in the AIDS Epidemic* (New York: Nitty Gritty Productions, 1997), which is a moving portrait of this population.

21. Tony Valenzuela, personal communication, August 25, 1997.

22. John Peterson, interview, Atlanta, Georgia, July 29, 1997.

23. Fred Kuhr, "Reaching Out: MOCAA Plans Service Project for Playground in Mattapan," *Bay Windows,* June 12, 1997, 3; Cynthia Laird, "NTFAP AIDS Campaign Targets Men of Color," *Bay Area Reporter,* January 16, 1997, 25; Viet Dinh, "One-Year Grant Will Help Develop and Distribute AIDS Information to Gay Asians," *The Washington Blade,* August 1, 1997, 5; Ta'Shia Asanti, "Black Lesbian Pride on Malibu Beach," *Lesbian News* (Los Angeles), August 1997, 17.

24. Interview with G.G., Chicago, May 24, 1997.

25. Interview with J.G., Atlanta, Georgia, July 26, 1997.

26. Interview with D.S., Boston, August 26, 1996.

27. Interview with M.R.D., San Francisco, January 7, 1997.

28. Ibid.

29. Ibid.

30. Wayne Hoffman, "Skipping the Life Fantastic: Coming of Age in the Sexual Devolution," in Dangerous Bedfellows (Eds.), *Policing Public Sex* (Boston: South End Press, 1996), 351-352.

Chapter 4

1. See Jeff McMillan, "Preventing AIDS in Rural America," *Chronicle of Higher Education,* November 15, 1996, A10; Pamela DeCarlo, *What Are Rural HIV Prevention Needs?* (San Francisco: Center for AIDS Prevention Studies, UCSF, May 1997); Rural Center for the Study and Promotion of HIV/STD Prevention, "Fact Sheet: HIV/AIDS in Rural America," a joint project of Indiana University and Purdue University, 1996.

2. See Tom Aloisi and Jim Dickinson, National Lesbian and Gay Health Conference Preconference Institute on Rural MSM, July 1997, Atlanta, 1.

3. Ibid.

4. Interview with D.K. in Milwaukee, Wisconsin, on May 21, 1997.

5. Interview with N.N. in Warm Springs, Oregon, on January 18, 1997.

6. Interview with R.D. in Austin, Texas, on August 7, 1996.

7. Interview with N.N. in Warm Springs, Oregon, on January 18, 1997.

8. Interview with R.E. in Madison, Wisconsin, on May 22, 1996.

9. Kimberley Murphy, "Utah Bill Would Ban Gay Clubs in Schools," *San Francisco Examiner,* April 19, 1996, A2; Associated Press, "Utah High School Students Protest Club Ban," *Bay Windows,* March 7, 1996, 1; Don Terry, "Suit Says Schools Failed to Protect a Gay Student," *The New York Times,* March 29, 1996; Austin Lewis, "The School for Scandal," *San Francisco Frontiers,* December 19, 1996, 12.

10. Interview with H.D. in Warm Springs, Oregon, on January 19, 1997.

11. Interview with A.C. in Warm Springs, Oregon, on January 18, 1997.

12. Interview with H.C. in Warm Springs, Oregon, on January 18, 1997.

13. Interview with K.F. in San Diego, California, on August 12, 1996.

14. Rural Caucus Report, AAPHR Summit on HIV Prevention for Gay Men, Bisexuals and Lesbians at Risk, Dallas, TX, July 17, 1994.

15. Interview with H.C. in Warm Springs, Oregon, on January 18, 1997.

16. Interview with J.E. in Warm Springs, Oregon, on January 19, 1997.

17. Interview with J.J. in Madison, Wisconsin, on May 23, 1996.

18. Interview with N.D. in Seattle, Washington, on July 16, 1996.

19. Interview with M.N. in Dallas, Texas, on August 9, 1996.

20. Interview with H.D. in Warm Springs, Oregon, on January 19, 1997.

21. Interview with N.N. in Warm Springs, Oregon, on January 18, 1997.

22. Interview with R.N. in Dallas, Texas, on August 9, 1996.

23. Interview with R.J. in Montague, Massachusetts, on March 22, 1997.

24. Interview with D.K. in Milwaukee, Wisconsin, on May 21, 1997.

25. Interview with J.E. in Warm Springs, Oregon, on January 19, 1997.

26. Interview with C.H. in Austin, Texas, on August 7, 1996.

27. See Dennis Conkin, "SF Gays Put the Camp into Camping at Rainbow Gathering," *Bay Area Reporter,* July 31, 1997, 14-15.

28. Austin Lewis, "O Where Have You Been Billy Club?," *San Francisco Frontiers,* November 21, 1996, 25. Copyright 1996, *San Francisco Frontiers.* Reprinted by permission.

29. Ibid., 27.

30. *The Billy Times,* 3(2), August 1997, 1-3.

31. See Tim Kingston, "The Year of the AIDS Cocktail," *San Francisco Frontiers,* December 19, 1996, 10; John Gallagher, "HIV Hiding in Plain Sight," *The Advocate,* March 18, 1997, 44; Lisa Keen, " 'Real World' Wrestles with AIDS Treatments," *The Washington Blade,* December 13, 1996, 1; Steven Scheibel, Bradford Saget, and Terry Rowley, "Protease Inhibitors—Hype, Hyperbole, Reality," *Bay Area Reporter,* February 6, 1997, 6; Mark Baker, "Don't Let 'Friendly Fire' Be the Cause for Losing the War on AIDS," *Provincetown Positive,* May 1997, 1; Tim Kingston, "New Era or False Dawn?" *San Francisco Frontiers,* September 26, 1996, 10.

32. At a recent workshop examining the impact of new treatments on people with HIV, Dr. Marshall Forstein, medical director of mental health and addiction services at Boston's Fenway Community Health Center, and Dr. John Weekly, a psychiatrist at the Howard Brown Memorial Health center in Chicago, offered early and tentative findings. These doctors found that a wide range of complex issues have emerged in the wake of the new treatments and that, in some ways, contemporary HIV mental health work is reminiscent of "the early days of HIV care, when we were starting the first groups for people with AIDS."

33. Sheryl Gay Stolberg, "Despite New AIDS Drugs, Many Still Lose the Battle," *The New York Times,* August 22, 1997, 1.

34. Dan Savage, "Shooting the Messenger," *The Stranger,* June 19, 1997, 26-27.

35. Interview with S.B. in San Francisco on November 16, 1996.

36. Lynda Richardson, "A Gap in the Resumé," *The New York Times,* May 21, 1997, A15.

37. Cynthia Laird, "New Leaf Expands Substance Abuse Program," *Bay Area Reporter,* July 24, 1997, 5; see also Joseph Amico and Joseph Neisen, "Sharing

the Secret: The Need for Gay-Specific Treatment," *The Counselor,* May/June 1997, 27-31.

Chapter 5

1. The first quotation is from Anita Bryant and Bob Green, *At Any Cost* (Old Tappan, NJ: Fleming H. Revell Company, 1978), 110; the second is from Larry Kramer, "Sex and Sensibility," *The Advocate,* May 27, 1997, 59.

2. The first quotation comes from Tim LaHaye, *The Unhappy Gays* (Wheaton, IL: Tyndale House, 1978), 35; the second is from Michelangelo Signorile, *Life Outside: The Signorile Report on Gay Men: Sex, Drugs, Muscles, and the Passages of Life* (New York, HarperCollins, 1997), xxxiii. Copyright © 1997 by HarperCollins Publishers. Reprinted by permission.

3. The first quotation is from Anita Bryant and Bob Green, *At Any Cost,* 114. The second is from Barbara Adler, Rev. Michael A. Backlund, Michael Bala, Kristen Balmann, Richard Bargans, Patrick Barresi, Al Baum, Michael Baum, Michael Bettinger, Joe Brewer, et al., "Making the Best of It," *San Francisco Frontiers,* June 5, 1997, 2. Reprinted by permission.

4. Larry Kramer, "Sex and Sensibility," *The Advocate,* May 27, 1997, 59.

5. George A. Rekers, *Growing Up Straight* (Chicago, Moody Press, 1982), 53.

6. Larry Kramer, "Sex and Sensibility," 65.

7. Rekers, *Growing Up Straight,* 29.

8. Signorile, *Life Outside,* xviii. Reprinted by permission.

9. LaHaye, *The Unhappy Gays,* 54.

10. Gabriel Rotello, *Sexual Ecology: AIDS and the Destiny of Gay Men* (New York: Dutton, 1997), 286.

11. Rekers, *Growing Up Straight,* 29.

12. Rotello, *Sexual Ecology,* 10.

13. The gay press gave significant coverage to the twentieth anniversary of the campaign, although few other sources acknowledged the occasion. See Wendy Johnson, "Anita Bryant's Legacy Haunts Dade County," *The Washington Blade,* June 27, 1997, 14; David Bianco, "When We Had to Bear Anita Bryant," *Bay Area Reporter,* June 12, 1997, 12; "Anita's Legacy," *The Advocate,* June 24, 1997, 16; Peter Freiberg, "The Turning Point in the War," *The Washington Blade,* May 23, 1997, 18.

14. Signorile, *Life Outside*; Rotello, *Sexual Ecology*; Larry Kramer, "How Can We Be Gay Now?" *LGNY,* July 6, 1997, 1, 28-29; Kramer, "Sex and Sensibility," 59-70.

15. Michael Bronski (Ed.), *Taking Liberties: Gay Men's Essays on Politics, Culture, and Sex* (New York: Masquerade Books, 1996), 1.

16. Kramer, "How Can We Be Gay Now?", 28.

17. I discuss this more fully in a section called "Displacing the Utopian Vision of Prevention," in *Reviving the Tribe,* 208-211.

18. Scott D. Holmberg, "The Estimated Prevalence and Incidence of HIV in 96 Large US Metropolitan Areas," *American Journal of Public Health,* 86(5), May

1996, 642-654. A year later, several prominent AIDS researchers critiqued Holmberg's report regarding statistics on the number of men who have sex with men in particular cities, and argued "Holmberg's point estimates are consistently 10% to 20% below the point estimates obtained" from their methodology. See Thomas C. Mills, Ron Stall, Joseph Catania, and Thomas Coates, "Interpreting HIV Prevalence and Incidence Among Americans: Bridging Data and Public Policy," *American Journal of Public Health,* May 1997, 87(5), 864-865.

19. Kramer, "Sex and Sensibility," 17; Karen Arneson, "The Normal Heart vs. Cooler Heads," *The New York Times,* July 9, 1997, A17.

20. Kramer, "Sex and Sensibility," 59.

21. Ibid., 64.

22. Ibid., 65.

23. Ibid., 65.

24. Jeffrey Meyers, *D.H. Lawrence: A Biography* (New York: Knopf, 1990); Keith Sagar, *The Life of D.H. Lawrence* (New York: Pantheon, 1980).

25. Stephen McCauley, *The Object of My Affection* (New York: Simon and Schuster, 1987); Stephen McCauley, *The Man of the House* (New York: Simon and Schuster, 1996); E. Lynn Harris, *Just as I Am* (New York: Doubleday, 1994); E. Lynn Harris, *Invisible Life* (New York: Anchor, 1994); Michael Cunningham, *Flesh and Blood* (New York: Farrar, Strauss, & Giroux, 1995); Michael Cunningham, *A Home at the End of the World* (New York: Farrar, Strauss & Giroux, 1990); Melvin Dixon, *Vanishing Rooms* (New York: Dutton, 1994); Carter Wilson, *Treasures on Earth* (New York: Alfred A. Knopf, 1980); David Leavitt, *The Lost Language of Cranes* (New York: Alfred A. Knopf, 1986); Douglas Sadownick, *Sacred Lips of the Bronx* (New York: St. Martin's, 1994); Lev Raphael, *Dancing on Tisha B'av* (New York: St. Martin's 1990); William Mann, *The Men from the Boys* (New York: Dutton, 1997).

26. John Preston, *Winter's Light: Reflections of a Yankee Queer*, Michael Lowenthal (Ed.), (Hanover, NH: University Press of New England, 1995). See also *Franny, the Queen of Provincetown* (Boston: Alyson, 1983); *My Life as a Pornographer and Other Indecent Acts* (New York: Masquerade Books, 1993); *A Member of the Family: Gay Men Write About Their Families* (New York: Dutton, 1992); *Hometowns: Gay Men Write About Where They Belong* (New York: Dutton, 1991).

27. Andrew Holleran, *The Beauty of Men* (New York: William Morrow, 1996).

28. Michael Bronski (Ed.), *Flashpoint: Gay Male Sexual Writing* (New York: Maqsquerade Books, 1996), 11-12.

29. Kramer, "Sex and Sensibility," 65.

30. Rotello, *Sexual Ecology;* Signorile, *Life Outside;* Andrew Sullivan, *Virtually Normal* (New York: Knopf, 1995); John Rechy, "Gay Sex: Dangerous Climax," *The Advocate,* October 14, 1997, 67; Jonathan Capeheart, "Getting Undressed, Going Undercover," *New York Daily News,* February 6, 1995; Duncan Osborne, "Time for Gays to Say No to Unsafe Sex," *New York Daily News,* November 20, 1994; Dan Perreten, "Keep It Zipped, Boys," *Windy City Times,* September 16, 1997; see an interview with Perreten in Terry Wilson, "On the

Record," *Chicago Tribune,* August 24, 1997; Duncan Osborne, "Time for Gays to Say No to Unsafe Sex," *Daily News,* November 19, 1994, 39; Ian Young, *The Stonewall Experiment* (London: Cassell, 1995).

31. *The Advocate,* July 8, 1997.

32. David Heitz, "Men Behaving Badly," *The Advocate,* July 8, 1997, 26.

33. I am grateful to Michael Scarce for pointing this out.

34. "Kramer strikes a nerve," *The Advocate,* June 24, 1997, 6.

35. Robert Tannenbaum, "Wake-Up Call," *The Advocate,* June 24, 1997, 4.

36. John Eller, letter to the editor, *The Advocate,* June 24, 1997, 6.

37. Ron Akanowicz, letter to the editor, *The Advocate,* June 24, 1997, 8.

38. Jo Schwartz, letter to the editor, *The Advocate,* June 24, 1997, 6.

39. Vivian Sanchez, letter to the editor, *The Advocate,* June 24, 1997, 6.

40. Mary McKenna, letter to the editor, *The Advocate,* June 24, 1997, 6.

41. Larry Kramer, "How Can We Be Gay Now?" *LGNY,* July 6, 1997, 29. Copyright 1997 by *LGNY.* Reprinted by permission.

42. Lisa Duggan and Nan D. Hunter, *Sex Wars: Sexual Dissent and Political Culture* (New York: Routledge, 1995); see also Carole Vance (Ed.), *Pleasure and Danger: Exploring Female Sexuality* (Boston: Routledge and Kegan Paul, 1984).

43. Starla C. Muir, "Time to Grow Up, Boys, & Spare Your Brother's Life," *2002* (Seattle), July 1996, 8. Reprinted by permission of Starla Muir.

44. Lisa Duggan, "Lesbians, Feminism, and Sex Panics," *LGNY,* August 17, 1997, 10. Copyright 1997 by *LGNY.* Reprinted by permission.

45. Ibid., 10. For other thoughtful responses to Larry Kramer's suggestion that lesbians get angry at gay men see Kate Kendell, "A Faustian Choice," *San Francisco Frontiers,* August 28, 1997, 35; Ann Pellegrini, "Lesbianism Lite," *New York Blade News,* October 24, 1997, 27; Paula Martinac, "Lesbians Getting Hit from Other Side of the Rainbow," *Between the Lines* (Detroit), September 1997, 9. Jeanne Bergman circulated a powerful response to Kramer on an e-mail list, which criticized him for haranguing lesbians while simultaneously targeting his proposed gift to Yale only for academic projects focused on gay men. She ended with the terse suggestion, "Kramer can suck my dick."

46. Michael Antisdale, letter to the editor, *The Advocate,* June 24, 1997, 8.

47. Les Daniels, letter to the editor, *The Advocate,* June 24, 1997, 6.

48. Alan Cantwell, Jr., letter to the editor, *The Advocate,* June 24, 1997, 6.

49. John Lauritsen, letter to the editor, *The Advocate,* June 24, 1997, 8.

50. Michael Wakefield, letter to the editor, *The Advocate,* June 24, 1997, 6.

51. Lawrence Mass (Ed.), *We Must Love One Another or Die: The Life and Legacies of Larry Kramer* (New York: St. Martin's, 1997). It has often seemed to me that Kramer puts forth a message by using this particular quote which suggests that all of those who have died of AIDS did so because they failed to love others—eerily familiar to much of the Louise Hay analysis of disease early in the epidemic which was experience by many people with AIDS as blaming the victim.

52. See Michael Bronski, *Culture Clash: The Making of Gay Sensibility* (Boston: South End Press, 1984); Daniel Harris, *The Rise and Fall of Gay Culture* (New York: Hyperion, 1997).

53. Kramer, "How Can We Be Gay Now?," 28. Kramer attempted to deliver this speech at the San Francisco Lesbian and Gay Freedom Day Rally on Saturday, June 28, 1997, after publishing it a week earlier in a New York gay paper. An eyewitness report from Bob Schoenberg (personal communication, July 10, 1997) explains that Kramer was met by chanting protesters who held up signs, including one that simply read "Passé." Kramer initially grew silent, then chastised the protesters by saying, "You're the problem. They have destroyed New York and I am sad to see you're also destroying San Francisco." He then switched to a less controversial portion of his speech and left the stage after one more salvo to the protesters. Another report from Todd Wohlfarth (personal communication, July 8, 1997), a protester, explained that "It wasn't a planned protest at all. We were sitting on 'tranny hill,' a hill overlooking the main stage, . . . He was awful! . . . I just went up to the stage and screamed 'Randy Shilts said the same things and look where he is!' Other people (mostly in my party) were booing him and heckling him." Because the protest caused Kramer not to present his full speech, he was given time on the stage late in the day on Sunday.

54. Wayne Hoffman, speech presented at Creating Change Conference, November 15, 1997, San Diego, California.

55. *The Advocate*, August 19, 1997; see Steve Howard, p. 15; Rudy Galindo, p. 21; Dan Hawes, p. 60; Dwight McBride, p. 29; Darren Carter, p. 76; Jamie Nabozny, 67.

56. Signorile, *Life Outside*.

57. Michelangelo Signorile, "Beyond the Good Gay, Bad Gay Syndrome," *Newsday,* August 18, 1997.

58. Signorile, *Life Outside,* xxi.

59. Denise L. Eger, "A Celebration of Gay Culture," *EDGE Magazine*, July 23, 1997, 18. Denise L. Eger. Copyright 1997, *EDGE Magazine,* published by EDGE Publishing, Inc. Reprinted by permission.

60. Ibid., 18.

61. Michael Kimmel and Michael Messner (Eds.), *Men's Lives* (New York: Macmillan, 1992); R.W. Connell, *Masculinities* (Berkeley, CA: University of California Press, 1995); Mairtin Mac an Ghaill, *The Making of Men: Masculinities, Sexualities, and Schools* (Buckingham, UK: Open University Press, 1994); Mairtin Mac an Ghaill (Ed.), *Understanding Masculinities* (Buckingham, UK: Open University Press, 1996).

62. For useful qualitative research into circuit culture, see Lynette A. Lewis and Michael W. Ross, *A Select Body: The Gay Dance Party Subculture and the HIV/AIDS Pandemic* (London: Cassell, 1995).

63. Jim Eigo, "Recognition of Sexual Rights Is Fundamental AIDS Prevention," letter to the editor, *LGNY,* August 4, 1997, 14.

64. Ibid., 1. Jim Eigo. Reprinted by permission.

65. Greg Rider, "The Outsider: An Interview with Michelangelo Signorile," *Art and Understanding*, August 1997, 35.

66. Cynthia Laird, "No More Coffee in the Castro?" *Bay Area Reporter*, April 10, 1997, 1; See also Cynthia Laird, "Supes Freeze Juice and Coffee in the 'Hood," *Bay Area Reporter*, April 17, 1997, 22.

67. "Best Place to Listen to Tales of Leather and Lace," *SF Weekly*, June 25, 1997, 57. For a take on New York City's "lounge scene," another new sector of gay social sites, see Brendan Lemon, "New Lease on Leisure," *The Advocate*, February 18, 1997, 72.

68. Barbara Adler, Rev. Michael A. Backlund, Michael Bala, Kristen Balmann, Richard Bargans, Patrick Barresi, Al Baum, Michael Baum, Michael Bettinger, Joe Brewer et al., "Making the Best of It," *SF Frontiers*, June 5, 1997. Reprinted by permission.

69. Ibid., 1.

70. In his weekly sex advice column, Dan Savage addressed a letter from a similar gay man who wrote under "Lonely Horny Hurt Stud-Boy," and complained, "All I got out of the gay world was heartache, burnt by gold diggers and a lot of shitty lovers." Savage's lengthy and wise analysis argues, "After making a series of bad choices, whether out of gay naiveté or plain old stupidity, disillusioned young gay men will, like Stud-Boy here, blame the 'gay family' rather than take responsibility for their own fucked-up lives." See Dan Savage, "Savage Love," *SF Weekly*, July 23, 1997, 95.

71. Adler et al., "Making the Best of It," *SF Frontiers*, June 5, 1997. Reprinted by permission.

72. Kevin Phillips, *The Politics of Rich and Poor* (New York: Random House, 1990); Joe R. Feagin and Hernan Vera, *White Racism* (New York: Routledge, 1995); Michael Omi and Howard Winant, *Racial Formation in the United States* (New York: Routledge, 1994).

73. Adler et al., "Making the Best of It," *SF Frontiers*, June 5, 1997, 3. Reprinted by permission.

74. John Peterson, "Black Men and Their Same-Sex Desires and Behaviors," in Gilbert Herdt (Ed.), *Gay Culture in America: Essays from the Field* (Boston: Beacon Press: 1992), 147-164; Joseph Carrier, "Miguel: Sexual Life History of a Gay Mexican American," in Gilbert Herdt (Ed.), *Gay Culture in America: Essays from the Field*, 202-224; Allen Drexel, "Before Paris Burned: Race, Class, and Male Homosexuality on the Chicago South Side, 1935-1960," in Brett Beemyn (Ed.), *Creating a Place for Ourselves: Lesbian, Gay, and Bisexual Community Histories* (New York: Routledge, 1997), 119-144; Brett Beemyn, "A Queer Capital: Race, Class, Gender, and the Changing Social Landscape of Washington's Gay Communities, 1940-1955," in Brett Beemyn (Ed.), *Creating a Place for Ourselves*, 183-210; John D'Emilio, *Making Trouble: Essays on Gay History, Politics, and the University* (New York: Routledge, 1992); John Sears, *Growing Up Gay in the South* (New York: Harrington Park Press, 1991); Cathy Cohen, "Contested Membership: Black Gay Identities and the Politics of AIDS," in Steven Seidman (Ed.), *Queer Theory/Sociology* (Cambridge, MA: Blackwell, 1996),

362-394; Josh Gamson, "Must Identity Movements Self-Destruct? A Queer Dilemma," in Steven Seidman (Ed.), *Queer Theory/Sociology* (Cambridge, MA: Blackwell, 1996), 395-420; Essex Hemphill (Ed.), *Brother to Brother: New Writings by Black Gay Men* (Boston: Alyson, 1991).

75. Adler et al., "Making the Best of It," *SF Frontiers*, June 5, 1997, 2. Reprinted by permission.

76. Judith Herman, *Trauma and Recovery* (New York: Basic Books, 1992); see also Susan Brownmiller, *Against Our Will: Men, Women, and Rape* (New York: Simon & Schuster, 1975); K. Sarachild, "Consciousness-Raising: A Radical Weapon," in *Feminist Revolution,* ed. K. Sarachild (New York: Random House, 1978), 145; Ellen Bass and Laura Davis, *The Courage to Heal: A Guide for Women Survivors of Child Sexual Abuse* (New York: Harper & Row, 1988).

77. Ignacio Martin-Baro, *Writings for a Liberation Psychology* (Cambridge: Harvard University Press, 1994), 189. Copyright 1994 by the President and Fellows of Harvard College. Reprinted by permission of Harvard University Press.

78. Ibid., 120-121.

79. Kevin Phillips, *The Politics of Rich and Poor* (New York: Random House, 1990).

80. Jay A. Levy, "The Transmission of HIV and Factors Influencing Progression to AIDS," *American Journal of Medicine,* 95:95 (July 1993).

81. For further discussion of this, see chapter 6.

82. Suzanne Pharr, *In the Time of the Right* (Berkeley, CA: Chardon, 1996), 67.

83. Gabriel Rotello, "An Open Letter to Sex Panic," *LGNY*, August 4, 1997, 16; Michelangelo Signorile, "Anatomy of a Smear Campaign," *LGNY,* August 4, 1997, 15.

84. Jim Eigo, "Recognition of Sexual Rights Is Fundamental AIDS Prevention," letter to the editor, *LGNY,* August 4, 1997, 1. Reprinted by permission. See Michael Warner, "Media Gays: A New Stonewall," *The Nation,* July 14, 1997, 15-19.

85. Eric Rofes, *Reviving the Tribe* (Binghamton, NY: The Haworth Press, 1996), 253.

86. Margot Hornblower, "Great Xpectations," *Time,* June 9, 1997, 58.

87. Larry Kramer, "How Can We Be Gay Now?," *LGNY,* July 6, 1997, 1. Copyright 1997 by *LGNY.* Reprinted by permission.

88. Ibid., 28. Reprinted by permission.

89. My analysis here is focused on the men who signed the statement. A significant number of female health care workers also signed the statement. Confidential sources have suggested to me that the work of writing and editing the piece was primarily done by gay men.

90. Personal correspondence, May 12, 1997. Reprinted by permission of Dan Savage.

91. Rofes, *Reviving the Tribe.*

92. One social worker who has written insightfully about his own experiences with aging is Paul Zak in "Gay Male Midlife: Aging Well? or Aging . . . Well!?" unpublished manuscript. Novelist Robert Glück has started a monthly column in

San Francisco's *Bay Area Reporter* on being gay and middle-aged. See "New to Age," *Bay Area Reporter,* October 23, 1997, 42.

93. Adler et al., "Making the Best of It," *SF Frontiers,* June 5, 1997, 2. Reprinted by permission.

94. Personal correspondence, May 12, 1997. Reprinted by permission of Dan Savage.

95. I am indebted to Todd Wohlfarth for helpful descriptions of Trannyshack and Litterbox.

96. Rofes, *Reviving the Tribe,* 262.

97. Fran Lebowitz, "The Impact of AIDS on the Artistic Community," *The New York Times,* September 13, 1987, section 2, 22. Copyright ©1987 by Fran Lebowitz. Reprinted by permission of William Morris Agency, Inc. on behalf of the author.

98. Richard Rodriguez, *Days of Obligation: An Argument with My Mexican Father* (New York: Viking, 1992), 26-47.

99. Deborah Peifer, "M Is for M.D.—Lisa Capaldini Knows What Ails Us," *Bay Area Reporter,* June 26, 1997, 46. Reprinted by permission.

Chapter 6

1. Gabriel Rotello and Michelangelo Signorile, while holding somewhat distinct perspectives, are representative of one side of the current debates. For Rotello's support for state regulation and action, and use of public shaming and demonization of specific subcultures, see *Sexual Ecology: AIDS and the Destiny of Gay Men* (New York: Dutton, 1997), 86-89, 195-202, 259-260; also Gabriel Rotello, "For Sale: State of the Art Unsafe Sex," *Newsday,* January 26, 1995, A38; Gabriel Rotello, "Sex Clubs Are the Killing Fields of AIDS," *Newsday,* April 28, 1995, A42; Gabriel Rotello, "Unsafe Sex Clubs: Safe from Crackdowns," *Newsday,* January 12, 1995, A33; Gabriel Rotello on *All Things Considered,* National Public Radio, with host Joe Neel, June 1, 1995; Gabriel Rotello, "Last Word," *The Advocate,* October 15, 1997, 70; Gabriel Rotello, "An Open Letter to Sex Panic," *LGNY,* August 4, 1997, 16-19, 27. For Signorile's support for state regulation and action, and use of public shaming and demonization of specific subcultures, see Michelangelo Signorile, *Life Outside: The Signorile Report on Gay Men: Sex, Drugs, Muscles, and the Passages of Life* (New York: HarperCollins, 1997), xvii-xxx, 19-30, 74, 94-102, 127-130; also Michelangelo Signorile, "Monitoring the Bathhouses," *The Washington Blade,* Readers' Forum, September 8, 1995, 37; Michelangelo Signorile, "Anatomy of a Smear Campaign," *LGNY,* August 4, 1997, 15; Greg Rider, "The Outsider: An Interview with Michelangelo Signorile, author of *Life Outside,*" *Art and Understanding,* August 1997; Michelangelo Signorile, "Bareback and Reckless," *Out,* July 1997, 36; Michelangelo Signorile, "A Troubling Double Standard," *The New York Times,* August 16, 1997, 21.

The other side might be represented by Sex Panic!. See Douglas Crimp, Ann Pellegrini, Eva Pendleton, and Michael Warner, "Sex Panic! Highlights Threats Facing Queer New York," *LGNY,* August 4, 1997, 14, 19; also Jim Eigo, "Get Used to Sex Panic!," letter to the editor, August 4, 1997, 10; Jim Eigo, "Recognition of Sexual Rights Is Fundamental to AIDS Prevention," *LGNY,* August 4, 1997, 14.

2. Lou Chibbaro, Jr., "Nude Dancing Ban Closes Wet," *The Washington Blade*, October 25, 1996, 6; Lou Chibbaro, Jr., "Gay Bar's Liquor License Pulled for Three Months," *The Washington Blade*, September 27, 1996, 8; Lou Chibbaro, Jr., "Mayor Allows Green Lantern to Remain Open," *The Washington Blade*, October 4, 1996, 10; Lou Chibbaro, Jr., "Video Store Removes Gay Sex Paraphernalia," *The Washington Blade*, October 25, 1996, 12; Dawn Leach, "Park Rangers Said to Be Entrapping Gays," *Gay People's Chronicle*, August 29, 1997; Jeff Epperly, "Bathroom Sex: A Relic of the '70s," *Bay Windows*, September 21, 1995, 6; Daniel Robbins, "Back Bay Arrests," *Bay Windows*, August 17, 1995; Susan Ryan-Vollman, "Restroom Arrests at Back Bay Station Trigger Concern," *Bay Windows*, August 3, 1995, 1; Fred Kuhr, "He's Here, He's Queer; and He Doesn't Understand What the Fuss Was About," September 12, 1996, 1, 22; Dan Quinn, "Back to the Baths," *The Advocate*, April 1, 1997, 51; Tony Valenzuela, "Sex Panic: The Assault on Consensual Gay Sex," *Gay & Lesbian Times* (San Diego), May 22, 1997, 43-48; Tony Valenzuela, "Sex Panic: Public Sex In Closed Quarters: The Bathhouse/Sex Club Debate," *Gay & Lesbian Times*, May 29, 1997, 46-51; Tony Valenzuela, "The Policing of Go-Go Dancers and Adult Businesses," *Gay & Lesbian Times*, June 5, 1997, 46-49; Tony Valenzuela, "Boys for Rent," *Gay & Lesbian Times*, June 12, 1997, 51-55; Tony Valenzuela, "The Acts and Consequences of Public Sex," *Gay & Lesbian Times*, June 19, 1997, 46-53; Tony Valenzuela, "Liberty and Responsibility: Forging a Pro-Sex Revival in the Ongoing Epidemic," *Gay & Lesbian Times*, June 26, 1997; Ed Jahn, "Mission Hills Residents Seek to Retake Presidio Park," *San Diego Union-Tribune*, March 31, 1997; Ann Rostow, "SF Health Department Begins Sex Club Crackdown," *Bay Times*, March 6, 1997, 3, 10; Community United for Sexual Privacy, "Statement of Purpose and Principles" (San Francisco, CA, 1997); "Sex and the City," Editorial, *San Francisco Examiner*, June 17, 1997, A16; Community United for Sexual Privacy, "Why We Want Bathhouses," *Bay Area Reporter*, January 16, 1997, 6; Phil Julian, "You Cannot Be Trusted," *San Francisco Frontiers*, March 13, 1997, 4; "Fight for Your Fucking Rights," Editorial, *Bay Area Reporter*, April 17, 1997, 6; Arthur Bruzzone, "The 'Risks' of Sex Club Regulations," *San Francisco Chronicle*, October 30, 1996.

3. Estelle Freedman, "'Uncontrolled Desires': The Response to the Sexual Psychopath, 1920-1960," in Kathy Peiss and Christina Simmons (Eds.), *Passion and Power: Sexuality in History* (Philadelphia: Temple University Press, 1989), 199-240; Gayle Rubin, "Thinking Sex: Notes for a Radical Theory of the Politics of Sexuality," in Henry Abelove, Michele Aina Barale, and David Halperin, *The Lesbian and Gay Studies Reader* (New York: Routledge, 1993).

4. George Chauncey, Jr., "The Postwar Sex Crime Panic," in William Graebner (Ed.), *True Stories from the American Past* (New York: McGraw-Hill, 1992, 160-178.

5. Ibid., 163.

6. Gayle Rubin, "Thinking Sex: Notes for a Radical Theory of the Politics of Sexuality," in Henry Abelove, Michele Aina Barale, and David Halperin, *The Lesbian and Gay Studies Reader* (New York: Routledge, 1993), 25; See also Lisa

Duggan, "Sex Panic," in Lisa Duggan and Nan Hunter (Eds.), *Sex Wars: Sexual Dissent and Political Culture* (New York: Routledge, 1995) 74-79.

7. Ibid., 25.

8. Allan Bérubé, "A Century of Sex Panics," in *SEX PANIC!* (New York: Sex Panic!, 1997), 4-8.

9. See for example, "Sex, Morality and the Protestant Minister," *Newsweek,* July 28, 1997, 62. Also, "Louisiana Couples Can Sign Up for Stricter Marriage Vows," *San Francisco Chronicle,* August 15, 1997, A6; Northwest AIDS Foundation, "'Parental Rights' Bills Hit Olympia," *Seattle Gay News,* February 14, 1997, 16; "The Trouble with Premarital Sex," cover story, *U.S. News and World Report,* May 19, 1997; Tamar Lewin, "Study Criticizes Textbooks on Marriage as Pessimistic," *The New York Times,* September 17, 1997, A21.

10. Mubarak S. Dahir, "Sudden Visibility," *The Advocate,* April 15, 1997, 35; Todd S. Purdum, "Registry Laws Tar Sex-Crime Convicts with Broad Brush," *The New York Times,* July 1, 1997, A1, A11; Ron Lazar, "Megan's Law Provides Dangerous Data for Better or for Worse," *Bay Area Reporter,* August 21, 1997, 24; Daniel Tsang, "A Sex-Crime Law for the Dark Ages," *Los Angeles Times,* September 18, 1996, B9; Bill Andriette, "America's Sex Gulags," *The Guide,* August 1997, 2-5. Thanks to the work of the ACLU and gay legal groups, this may be changing. See Peter Freiberg, "States Ease Registration Laws That Swept Up Gays," *The Washington Blade,* November 21, 1997, 19.

11. I am aware this book argues that the crisis period of AIDS for gay men has ended, while positing that a crisis focused on gay men's sex is beginning. Although I believe some who share my belief that a moral panic is emerging are simply transferring the crisis construct of AIDS onto sex in order to continue to hold onto an emergency mind-set, for others the linkage is not occurring.

12. David Waggoner, editor of *Art and Understanding,* has used the term "New Puritans." See David Waggoner, "Summer Complaint," *Art and Understanding,* July 1997, 6. Edmund White has chosen to call his critics "prudes." See Edmund White, "The Joy of Gay Lit," *Out,* September 1997, 112.

13. Sara Miles, "And the Bathhouse Plays On," *Out,* July/August 1995, 128.

14. Michelangelo Signorile, *Life Outside: The Signorile Report on Gay Men: Sex, Drugs, Muscles, and the Passages of Life* (New York: HarperCollins, 1997), xxii, xxiii; Larry Kramer, "How Can We Be Gay Now?," *LGNY,* July 6, 1997, 28; Johnny Ray Huston, "Clubbed to Death," *San Francisco Bay Guardian,* May 7, 1997, 55; Andrew Sullivan, "When Plagues End," *The New York Times Magazine,* November 10, 1996, 55; David Spivey, "Holocaust Offers Lessons for Those Who Won't Speak Out About Unsafe Sex, Drug Abuse," *Southern Voice,* December 4, 1997, 11. See also Mary Curtius and Michael Ybarra, "Gay Party Tour: More Harm Than Good?" *Los Angeles Times,* October 13, 1997.

15. Doors, cubicles, lighting, and patterns of traffic have all taken on tremendous symbolism. See John Lindell, "Public Space for Public Sex," in Dangerous Bedfellows (Eds.) *Policing Public Sex* (Boston: South End Press, 1997); "Sex and the City," Editorial, *San Francisco Examiner,* June 17, 1997, A16; San Francisco Department of Public Health, "Addendum to the Commercial Sex Club Ordi-

nance, Health Department Regulations" draft document, October 10, 1996; Cynthia Laird, "A Candid Conversation with Dr. Sandra Hernandez," *Bay Area Reporter*, July 24, 1997, 16; Sandra Hernandez, "On Conflicting Expectations and Demands," *Bay Area Reporter*, May 15, 1997, 6; Sara Miles, "And the Bathhouse Plays On," *Out*, July/August, 1995.

16. Scott Holmberg, "The Estimated Prevalence and Incidence of HIV in 96 Large U.S. Metropolitan Areas," *American Journal of Public Health*, 86(5), May 1996, 642-654. John Whyte, Ernie Green, Marcia Polansky, and Chris Bartlett, *Men's Survey Report: Assessing the Knowledge, Attitudes, Beliefs, and Behaviors Regarding HIV* (Philadelphia: AIDS Information Network, 1997), 19-34.

17. Signorile, *Life Outside*, xxi-xxiii, 94.

18. Mitchell Katz, "AIDS Epidemic in San Francisco Among Men Who Report Sex with Men: Successes and Challenges of HIV Prevention," *Journal of Acquired Immune Deficiency Syndromes and Human Retrovirology*, 14(Supplement 2): S38-S46; Jose Zuniga, "For Black Gays, the Numbers Get Worse," *The Washington Blade*, June 9, 1995, 1; Cynthia Laird, "San Francisco AIDS Cases, Deaths Continue to Drop," *Bay Area Reporter*, October 23, 1997, 1, 26.

19. Signorile, *Life Outside*, xviii.

20. Rubin, "Thinking Sex," 25.

21. Miles, "And the Bathhouse Plays On," 87; Amy Pagnozzi, "Gay Group Measures Prevention in Lives," *Daily News*, February 15, 1995; Jonathan Capehart, "Getting Undressed, Going Undercover, *Daily News*, February 13, 1995; Gay and Lesbian HIV Prevention Activists, "Gay Group to City Hall: 'Make Sex Clubs Safe!'," Press release, March 9, 1995; Duncan Osborne, "Time for Gays to Say No to Unsafe Sex," *Daily News*, November 19, 1994; Mark Schoofs, "Beds, Baths, and Beyond," *The Village Voice*, March 28, 1995, 13; Jorge Morales, "Curtains for New York Sex Clubs?," *The Advocate*, March 21, 1995, 20; Peter Freiberg, "Gay Community, City Officials Face Off Over Sex Businesses," *The Washington Blade*, October 20, 1995, 14; "Limiting Sex Shops, Responsibly," Editorial, *The New York Times*, October 27, 1995, A14; Peter Freiberg, "In New York, a Battle Erupts Over Gay Sex Establishments," *The Washington Blade*, May 26, 1995; Andy Humm, "Closing Unsafe Sex Clubs," *LGNY*, June 4, 1995; Alan Klein, "The Right to Fuck Ourselves?," *LGNY*, June 4, 1995, 12; David Dunlap, "Crackdown on Gay Theaters and Clubs," *The New York Times*, April 16, 1995; Mireya Navarro, "The Indelicate Art of Telling Adults How to Have Sex," *The New York Times*, May 16, 1993; Andrew Jacobs, "Of Vice and Men," *New York*, March 27, 1995, 24; "Debate over gay sex clubs heats up in NYC," *Bay Windows*, April 13, 1995, 1.

22. Signorile, *Life Outside*; Gabriel Rotello, *Sexual Ecology: AIDS and the Destiny of Gay Men* (New York: Dutton, 1997).

23. Jim Eigo, "Get Used to Sex Panic!," letter to the editor, *LGNY*, August 4, 1997, 10; Douglas Crimp, Ann Pellegrini, Eva Pendleton, and Michael Warner, "Sex Panic! Highlights Threats Facing Queer New York," *LGNY*, August 4,1997, 14, 19; Richard Goldstein, "Attack of the Pier Sluts," *Village Voice*, September 16, 1997, 62.

24. Michelangelo Signorile, "Anatomy of a Smear Campaign," *LGNY*, August 4, 1997, 15; Gabriel Rotello, "An Open Letter To Sex Panic," *LGNY*, August 4, 1997, 16-19; Michelangelo Signorile, as recorded in Greg Rider, "The Outsider—An Interview with Michelangelo Signorile," *Art and Understanding*, August 1997, 35.

25. Sex Panic!, "Queer New York Is Being Shut Down!!!," flyer, June 1997.

26. Paul Schindler, "From the Editor," *LGNY*, August 4, 1997, 3; Paul Schindler, "From the Editor: Pride, But Not in Lockstep," *LGNY*, July 6, 1997, 3.

27. Duncan Osborne, "Dramatic Drop in City Drive Against Adult Businesses in 1997," *LGNY*, August 4, 1997, 1; Gabriel Rotello, "An Open Letter To Sex Panic," *LGNY*, August 4, 1997, 16-19.

28. Sheryl Gay Stolberg, "Gay Culture Weighs Sense and Sexuality," *The New York Times*, November 23, 1997, section 4, p. 1.

29. Richard Nolan, "Self-Defeating Choices," letter to the editor, *The New York Times*, November 30, 1997, WK8.

30. David Smith, "Fighting for Rights," letter to the editor, *The New York Times*, November 30, 1997, WK8.

31. Larry Kramer, "Gay Culture, Redefined," *The New York Times*, December 12, 1997.

32. Ibid.

33. Jimmy van Bramer, "Guiliani's Dubious, Panicked Thrust at Messinger Over Sex Shops," *LGNY*, October 12, 1997, 1.

34. Jake Stevens and Christine Quinn, "Anti-Violence Project Clarifies Arrest Tally," letter to the editor, *LGNY*, August 4, 1997, 10.

35. Liz Highleyman, "Women's Sexuality Conference Under Fire in New York State," *Bay Area Reporter*, November 13, 1997, 18; Editorial, "Free Speech at New Paltz," *The New York Times*, November 11, 1997.

36. Ann Rostow, "SF Health Department Begins Sex Club Crackdown," *Bay Times*, March 6, 1997, 3, 10; Community United for Sexual Privacy, "Statement of Purpose and Principles," San Francisco, 1997; "Sex and the City," Editorial, *San Francisco Examiner*, June 17, 1997, A16; Community United for Sexual Privacy, "Why We Want Bathhouses," *Bay Area Reporter*, January 16, 1997, 6; Phil Julian, "You Cannot Be Trusted," *San Francisco Frontiers*, March 13, 1997, 4; "Fight for Your Fucking Rights," Editorial, *Bay Area Reporter*, April 17, 1997, 6; Arthur Bruzzone, "The 'Risks' of Sex Club Regulations," *San Francisco Chronicle*, October 30, 1996; "Amending Part II, Chapter V of the San Francisco Municipal Code (Health Code) By Adding Article 27, Encompassing Sections 27.1 through 27.24, to Require a Permit for the Operation of a Commercial Sex Club," draft, Board of Supervisors, San Francisco, October 10, 1996; Ann Rostow, "Mayor Brown Will Not Back Sex Club Ordinance," *Bay Times*, November 14, 1997, 10; Jim Zamora, "Sex Club Owners Welcome License Program," *San Francisco Examiner*, November 13, 1996, 1; Liz Highleyman, "Sex Club Operation Restricted," *Bay Area Reporter*, November 21, 1996; "Your Sex, Your Responsibility," Editorial, *OutNOW!* (San Jose), October 29, 1996, 15; Rachel Gordon, "Mayor Pushes for Debate on Licensing Sex Clubs," *San Francisco*

Examiner, October 23, 1996, A9; Rene Beauchamp, "Bring Back the Bathhouses—or Relight the Restaurants," *Bay Area Reporter*, November 28, 1996.

37. Sandra R. Hernandez, "On Conflicting Expectations and Demands," *Bay Area Reporter*, May 15, 1997, 6; Cynthia Laird, "A Candid Conversation with Dr. Sandra Hernandez," *Bay Area Reporter*, July 24, 1997, 16-17; Mike Pierce, "Monitoring Katz," letter to the editor, *San Francisco Frontiers*, February 27, 1997, 10; Steve Johnson, "Enough Is Enough!," letter to the editor, *San Francisco Frontiers*, February 27, 1997, 10; Stephen O. Murray, "Department of Public Health Mendacity," *Bay Area Reporter*, May 29, 1997, 7; Luke Adams, "Time for Them to Go," *Bay Area Reporter*, May 29, 1997, 7; Will Roscoe, "Vertical Sex in the Mosh Pits," *Bay Area Reporter*, October 31, 1996, 11.

38. Reid Condit, "NY: Saunatized for Your Protection," letter to the editor, *Bay Area Reporter*, July 31, 1997, 8.

39. Lauren Hauptman, "Penis in the Morning: Speak Softly, and Don't Expose Your Big Stick," *San Francisco Frontiers,* October 9, 1997, 4; Laura Federico, "People Are Talking: The Great Penis Debate," *San Francisco Frontiers,* November 6, 1997, 12; Mark Mardon, "Penis Flap Grows Larger," *Bay Area Reporter,* October 23, 1997, 1.

40. Allan Bérubé, "The History of Gay Bathhouses," *Coming Up!*, December, 1984; Allan Bérubé, "Don't Save Us from Our Sexuality," *Coming Up!*, April 1984.

41. Telephone conversation with Gayle Rubin, June 23, 1997.

42. Bérubé, "The History of Gay Bathhouses"; Bérubé, "Don't Save Us from Our Sexuality."

43. Joseph Hanania, "Crackdown in Clubland," *Out*, July 1997, 31-34. Reprinted with permission.

44. Ibid., 31-34; also, Jamie Wolters, "Party Crashers II: Have Efforts to Stop Silverlake Cruising Gone Too Far?," *Frontiers/Los Angeles*, November 29, 1996, 22-23; Jeff Still, "Panting After Sex," Interview with Brian Miller, *Frontiers/Los Angeles*, November 29, 1996, 47.

45. Goldberg's activist history extends back to the Free Speech Movement at Berkeley in the 1960s. See W.J. Rorabaugh, *Berkeley at War* (New York: Oxford University Press, 1989), 24.

46. Beth Shuster, "Gay Men's Sex Club Closes, Citing Exhausting Fight with City Council," *Los Angeles Times,* November 22, 1997; Tracy Sypert, "Going Legit," *Frontiers,* November 14, 1997, 17; "Mayor, Citing Complaints, Vetoes 'Sex Club' Variance," *The Washington Blade,* November 28, 1997, 16; Beth Shuster and Jim Newton, "Riordan's Veto Blocks Sex Club," *Los Angeles Times,* November 15, 1997, B1, B3; Bettina Boxall, "Future of Sex Clubs May Hinge on Zoning," *Los Angeles Times,* October 27, 1997.

47. Lou Chibbaro, Jr., "Nude Dancing Ban Closes Wet," *The Washington Blade*, October 25, 1996, 6; Lou Chibbaro, Jr., "Gay Bar's Liquor License Pulled for Three Months," *The Washington Blade*, September 27, 1996, 8; Lou Chibarro, Jr., "Escort Service Searched by Police," *The Washington Blade*, August 15, 1997, 5; Lou Chibbaro, Jr., "Mayor Allows Green Lantern to Remain Open," *The*

Washington Blade, October 4, 1996, 10; Lou Chibbaro, Jr., "Video Store Removes Gay Sex Paraphernalia," *The Washington Blade*, October 25, 1996, 12; Lou Chibbaro, Jr., "Police, Building Inspectors 'Visit' Crew Club," *The Washington Blade*, April 18, 1997, 14; Hastings Wyman, Jr., "It's Time to Close Gay Bathhouses," *Bay Windows*, June 22, 1995, 6, 11; "Gay Club Vows to Officials That No Sex Will Take Place on Site," *Bay Windows*, May 11, 1995, 10; Mickey Wheatley, "In Defense of Gay Sex Clubs," *The Washington Blade*, April 21, 1995; "GLAA seeks investigation of 'raids'," *The Washington Blade*, January 10, 1997, 6; Lou Chibbaro, Jr., "Police Chief Puts Two Gay Bars on 'Hit' List," *The Washington Blade*, March 21, 1997, 8; Lou Chibbaro, Jr., "Gay Bars Form Guild to Fight 'Harassment'," *The Washington Blade*, April 25, 1997, 14; Lou Chibbaro, Jr., "Bar Closed During Crackdown," *The Washington Blade*, March 28, 1997, 6; Lou Chibbaro, Jr., "Fairfax County Man Charged with Violating Virginia's Sodomy Law," *The Washington Blade*, July 11, 1997, 5; M. Jane Taylor, "20 Arrested for 'Lewd Acts' in Annapolis Bookstore," *The Washington Blade*, July 11, 1997, 5; Lou Chibbaro, Jr., "Liquor Board Says Wet Must Go Dry," *The Washington Blade*, October 18, 1996, 5; even nudity at the gay pride parade is causing some gay people to express outrage, see Matthew Bachteler, "Modesty Please," letter to the editor, *The Washington Blade*, June 27, 1997, 31.

48. Jeff Epperly, "Bathroom Sex: A Relic of the '70s," *Bay Windows*, September 21, 1995, 6; Daniel Robbins, "Back Bay Arrests," *Bay Windows*, August 17, 1995; Susan Ryan-Vollman, "Restroom Arrests at Back Bay Station Trigger Concern," *Bay Windows*, August 3, 1995, 1; Jeff Epperly, "Gross Stupidity at a Great Parade," *Bay Windows*, June 13, 1996, 6; Rachel Keegan, "Controversy Over Pride: Whose Community Is It?" *Sojourner*, 19; Fred Kuhr, "He's Here, He's Queer; and He Doesn't Understand What the Fuss Was About," September 12, 1996, 1, 22.

49. Dan Quinn, "Back to the Baths," *The Advocate*, April 1, 1997, 51.

50. "Nightclub Raided by Vice Officers," *Miami Herald*, August 15, 1997; Also "Undercover Detectives Arrested 21 Men for Lewd and Lascivious Behavior," Reuters, August 15, 1997; Police Release the Names of 20 Arrested in Gay Nightclub Raid, *The Washington Blade*, August 22, 1997, 14.

51. Richard Mohr, "Parks, Privacy, and the Police," *The Guide* (Boston), January 1996.

52. Judith Dobrzynski, "San Antonio Cuts Subsidies for the Arts by 15 Percent," *The New York Times,* September 13, 1997, 17.

53. "Police Raid San Diego Private Club in Sensational Action," *IN Newsweekly* (Boston), December 15, 1996, 20; Neal Putnam, " 'Slave Number One' Speaks Out," *Update* (San Diego), December 25, 1996, A11; Neal Putnam, "Did the Punishment Fit the Crime?," *Update*, March 5, 1997, A11; Tony Valenzuela, "Sex Panic: The Assault on Consensual Gay Sex," *Gay & Lesbian Times* (San Diego), May 22, 1997, 43-48; Tony Valenzuela, "Sex Panic: Public Sex in Closed Quarters: The Bathhouse/Sex Club Debate," *Gay & Lesbian Times*, May 29, 1997, 46-51; Tony Valenzuela, "The Policing of Go-Go Dancers and Adult Businesses," *Gay & Lesbian Times*, June 5, 1997, 46-49; Tony Valenzuela, "Boys for

Rent," *Gay & Lesbian Times*, June 12, 1997, 51-55; Tony Valenzuela, "The Acts and Consequences of Public Sex," *Gay & Lesbian Times*, June 19, 1997, 46-53; Tony Valenzuela, "Liberty and Responsibility: Forging a Pro-Sex Revival in the Ongoing Epidemic," *Gay & Lesbian Times*, June 26, 1997; Ed Jahn, "Mission Hills Residents Seek to Retake Presidio Park," *San Diego Union-Tribune*, March 31, 1997.

54. David Dunlap, "AIDS Agency's Message Questioned Over Drug Use at Fire I. Fund-Raiser," *The New York Times*, August 17, 1996, 22. Copyright © 1996 by The New York Times Company. Reprinted by permission.

55. Ibid., 22. Quotation from Louis Bradbury, president of the board of Gay Men's Health Crisis. Copyright 1996 © by The New York Times Company. Reprinted by permission.

56. See T.J. Sullivan, letter to the editor, *The Advocate*, November 12, 1997, 6; also Mike Varady, letter to the editor, *The Advocate*, November 12, 1997, 6; also "Morning Sickness," *The Advocate*, September 3, 1996, 16. For a more nuanced view, see Michael Shernoff, "Use or Abuse? Deciding When Drugs or Alcohol Become a Problem," *LGNY*, May 25, 1997, 10.

57. Gabriel Rotello, "A Deal with the Devil," *The Advocate*, October 15, 1996, 96. Copyright 1996 by Liberation Publications, Incorporated. Reprinted by permission.

58. See for example, Paul Schindler, "Two Community Forums Tackle Drugs, Alcohol and Controversy," *LGNY*, November 17, 1997; Liz Highleyman, "Stop AIDS Hosts Crystal Forum," *Bay Area Reporter*, March 27, 1997, 1.

59. Alan Brown, "Crime of the Scene," in *Electric Dreams*, New Haven, July 1997. Copyright 1997 by EDreams. (EDreams@aol.com)

60. Joyce Peyre, "Say No to Drugs," *Bay Windows*, November 21, 1996, 7.

61. Gabriel Rotello, *Sexual Ecology: AIDS and the Destiny of Gay Men* (New York: Dutton, 1997).

62. Joshua Oppenheimer, "Unforgiving Errors," *Gay Community News*, Summer 1997, 40-45; Richard Goldstein, "Big Science," *Out*, May 1997, 62-65; Jim Eigo, "Sexual Ecology: An Activist Critique," unpublished review, 1-14; William Leap, "The Greening of AIDS," *Lambda Book Report*, May 1997, 14-16; Rodger McFarlane, "Painful Truths," *POZ*, June 1997, 60; Daniel Kevles, "A Culture of Risk," *The New York Times Book Review*, May 25, 1997, 8; Linnea Due, "Histrionics," *Bay Area Reporter*, May 15, 1997, 44; Louis Bayard, "Sexual Ecology," *The Washington Blade*, April 11, 1997, 40; Mark Schoofs, "The Law," *The Village Voice*, April 5, 1997.

63. Advertisement, *Bay Windows*, July 3, 1997, 14.

64. Peter Jay, in an op-ed piece in *The Baltimore Sun* (July 20, 1997) cites Rotello's book to argue, "Rotello shows how [the AIDS epidemic's] successful treatment was aborted by gay political pressure with the complicity of mainstream liberal institutions. The former resulted in useful public-health initiatives such as mandatory HIV testing being labeled 'homophobic.' The latter's role [pushed] ultimately groundless propaganda messages—that the use of condoms could achieve 'safe sex' . . . " Jay's piece blames the killing spree of Andrew Cunanan

on "gay culture." See also conservative writer David Horowitz, "Right On!," *Salon Magazine On-Line*, April 14, 1997; Leonard Larsen, "Gays Still Mostly Responsible for Ongoing AIDS Epidemic," *Desert News,* December 7, 1997, which, while not citing Rotello, is constructed upon his central arguments.

66. Rotello, *Sexual Ecology,* 48.

67. Ibid., 86-89.

68. Ibid., 48-49.

69. Signorile, *Life Outside*, xxiii.

70. Alan Brown, "Tales of the Circuit," *Circuit Noize,* Spring 1997, 22. Reprinted by permission.

71. Ibid., 75-132; also see Jim Leatherman, letter to the editor, *The Advocate*, November 12, 1996, 6; Larry Kramer, "How Can We Be Gay Now?" *LGNY,* July 6, 1997, 28; Johnny Ray Huston, "Clubbed to Death," *San Francisco Bay Guardian*, May 7, 1997, 55; David Heitz, "Men Behaving Badly," *The Advocate*, July 8, 1997, 26-29.

72. Signorile, *Life Outside,* 31-32.

73. This poster was sighted at the corner of Castro and 18th Streets on June 26, 1997.

74. Eric Rofes, "Making Our Schools Safe for Sissies," in Gerald Unks (Ed.), *The Gay Teen* (New York: Routledge, 1995), 79-84; Gary Alinder, "My Gay Soul," in Karla Jay and Allen Young (Eds.), *Out of the Closets: Voices of Gay Liberation* (New York: Douglas/Links, 1972); Paul Monette, *Becoming a Man* (San Francisco: Harper, 1992).

75. For a seminal analysis of this dynamic, see William Mann, "Perfect Bound," *Frontiers*, January 13, 1995, 82-86. For an interesting perspective on Signorile's discussion of masculinity, see Stephen H. Miller, "Is Masculinity the Culprit?," *Bay Windows*, June 19, 1997, 6-7; also see Michael Denneny, "Hymn to a Gym," *POZ*, May 1997, 52.

76. Peter McQuaid, "Circuit Queen for a Day," *Out*, August 1997, 30. Copyright 1997 by OUT Publishing Inc. Reprinted by permission.

77. For a discussion of class and the bear subculture, see Eric Rofes, "Academics as Bears: Notes on Middle-Class Eroticization of Workingmen's Bodies," in Les Wright (Ed.), *The Bear Book* (Binghamton, NY: The Haworth Press, 1997), 89-99.

78. David Dean, "The Bigger They Come . . . ," letter to the editor, *Out*, August 1997, 12.

79. Jon Catanese, "Back to Bad Habits," letter to the editor, *The Advocate*, April 1, 1997, 8.

80. William Stosine, "Ordinary Gay Lives," letter to the editor, *The New York Times,* July 31, 1997.

81. Lynette Lewis and Michael Ross, *A Select Body: The Gay Dance Party Subculture and the HIV/AIDS Pandemic* (London: Cassell, 1995). Copyright 1995 by Cassell Academic, London, England. Reprinted by permission.

82. Ibid., 133. Reprinted by permission.

83. Ibid., 160. Reprinted by permission.

84. Ibid., 210. Reprinted by permission.

85. I am grateful to Ray Crossman and Chris Dillehay (personal communication, August 20, 1997) for this report from the Saint-at-Large White Party, February 15, 1997, at Roseland in New York City; music by Warren Gluck, lights by Richard Sabella. Roseland is reputed to have the largest wooden dance floor in the country.

86. Christian Hart, "The Circuit: Drugged-Out Party Boys, or Neo-Tribal Spirituality?" *Circuit Noize*, Winter 1997, 31.

87. Michael Warner, "Why Gay Men Are Having Risky Sex," *The Village Voice*, January 31, 1995; Michelangelo Signorile, "HIV-Positive, and Careless," *The New York Times*, February 27, 1995; see also Michelangelo Signorile, "Negative Pride," *Out*, March 1995.

88. Stephen Gendin, "Riding Bareback," *POZ*, June 1997, 64-66. Copyright 1997 by POZ Publishing, LLC. Reprinted by permission.

89. Henry Wallengren, letter to the editor, *POZ*, August 1997, 24.

90. Ted Gancarz, letter to the editor, *POZ*, August 1997, 24; see also Paul Schindler, "Loose Logic from Bareback Stephen," *LGNY*, May 25, 1997, 3.

91. Paul Harris, "Riding Bareback," *San Francisco Bay Times,* August 21, 1997, 9.

92. Robert Marra, "Bareback Busted," letter to the editor, *POZ*, August 1997, 24; Bill Strubbe, "Positive and Unprotected," *SF Weekly*, July 9, 1997, 10; Michelangelo Signorile, "Bareback and Reckless," *Out*, July 1997, 36-40; Christian Matthews, "Fucking Without a Condom," *San Francisco Bay Times,* October 30, 1997, 18; Paul Schindler, "Loose Logic from Bareback Stephen," *LGNY,* May 25, 1997, 3.

93. Richard Tafel, "Dangerous Rhetoric Threatens Gays," *The San Francisco Chronicle,* January 7, 1998, 23.

94. Eric Rofes, *Reviving the Tribe* (Binghamton, NY: The Haworth Press, 1996), 173-179; Ilan Meyer discusses this as "the virtuous gay man" syndrome which he sees as utilizing "the kind of implicit reasoning typical of abused or maltreated children." See Ilan Meyer, "Self Oppression as Virtue," a statement circulated in New York City at Sex Panic! meetings, June 1997.

95. See Robert B. Hays, Susan M. Keegles, and Thomas J. Coates, "High HIV Risk-Taking Among Young Gay Men," *AIDS*, 4(9):901-907 (1990); Ron Stall, Don Barrett, Larry Bye, Joe Catania, Chuck Frutchey, Jeff Henne, George Lemp, Jay Paul, "A Comparison of Younger and Older Gay Men's HIV-Risk-Taking Behaviors: The Communications Technologies 1989 Cross-Sectional Survey," *Journal of the Acquired Immune Deficiency Syndrome* 5:682-687 (1992); Jane Gross, "Second Wave of AIDS Feared by Officials in San Francisco," *The New York Times*, December 11, 1993.

96. Richard Elovich, "Four Percent and Counting . . ." an open letter to the gay community, New York: Gay Men's Health Crisis, November 11, 1997, 1.

97. Rofes, *Reviving the Tribe*, 178.

98. Douglas Crimp, "The Attack on Sexual Liberation," flyer passed out at Sex Panic! meeting, June 1997, 1. Reprinted by permission.

99. I am grateful to Chris Bartlett from Philadelphia's AIDS Information Network, SafeGuard's Project for the discussion of AIDS as metaphor for gay men's health.

100. Mark Schoofs, "Who's Afraid of Reinfection," *POZ*, May 1997, 60-63, 78; David Menadue, "Reinfection: Is It a Myth?" *Positive Living* (Melbourne, Australia), June 1997, 3.

101. Ilan Meyer, "Self Oppression as Virtue," a statement circulated in New York City at Sex Panic! meetings, June, 1997.

102. Allan Brandt, *No Magic Bullet: A Social History of Venereal Disease in the United States Since 1880* (Oxford, UK: Oxford University Press, 1985).

103. Gayle Rubin, "Sexual Politics, the New Right, and the Sexual Fringe," *The Leaping Lesbian,* Spring 1978, 6-7; Andrew Hodges and David Hutter, *With Downcast Gays* (London: Pomegranate Press, 1974); Dennis Altman, "Sex: The New Front Line for Gay Politics," (1982), in Mark Blasius and Shane Phelan (Eds.), *We Are Everywhere: A Historical Sourcebook of Gay and Lesbian Politics* (New York: Routledge, 1996), 529-534.

104. See Audre Lorde, "Uses of the Erotic: The Erotic as Power," in *Sister Outsider* (Freedom, CA: Crossing Press, 1984); Albert Memmi, *The Colonizer and Colonized* (New York: Orion Press, 1965).

105. Lillian Hellman, *Scoundrel Time* (Boston: Little, Brown, 1976).

106. James Baldwin, "If Black English Isn't a Language, Then Tell Me, What Is?" in *Rethinking Schools: An Urban Education Journal,* Fall 1997, 16. Baldwin's discussion of black English, which is pertinent to current debates over Ebonics, offers much that is useful to gay men's current debates on sex cultures.

Chapter 7

1. National Institutes of Health, "Interventions to Prevent HIV Risk Behaviors" (February 11-13, 1997) Draft Consensus Development Statement. Bethesda, MD.

2. Ibid., 4.

3. Ibid., 10-11.

4. See Peter Keogh, "HIV Prevention Amongst Gay Men: Personal Strategies and Community Responses," oral presentation for DAH satellite panel, Vancouver, July 1996; also Darryl O'Donnell, paper presented at the Third AFAO Gay Men's Education Conference, Sydney, Australia, May 1996, 4-15; Ralph Bolton and Merrill Singer, "Rethinking HIV Prevention: Critical Assessments of the Content and Delivery of AIDS Risk-Reduction Messages," *Medical Anthropology,* 14:139-143, 1992; Dwayne Turner, *Risky Sex: Gay Men and HIV Prevention* (New York: Columbia University Press, 1997), 128-147.

5. Mark Schoofs, "Learning from Each Other or Monogamy: Pleasures and Pitfalls," speech presented at the National Lesbian and Gay Health Conference, Atlanta, July 26, 1997, 2. Reprinted by permission.

6. Gayle Rubin, "Thinking Sex: Notes for a Radical Theory of the Politics of Sexuality," in Henry Abelove, Michele Aina Barale, David M. Halperin (Eds.), *The Lesbian and Gay Studies Reader* (New York: Routledge, 1993), 13-14.

7. Michelangelo Signorile, *Life Outside* (New York: HarperCollins, 1997), 213.

8. Daniel Geer, *Gay Men and Monogamy,* a thesis submitted to the faculty of San Francisco State University (May 1996). See also Daniel Geer, "Gay Men and Monogamy," *Bay Area Reporter,* October 16, 1997, 14.

9. Ibid., 33.

10. Philip Blumstein and Pepper Schwartz, *American Couples* (New York: William Morrow, 1983); David McWhirter and Andrew Mattison, *The Male Couple* (Englewood Cliffs, NJ: Prentice Hall, 1984).

11. This is the stated purpose of the national gay couples' group. See Cynthia Laird, "Gay Couples Club Provides Social Outlet," *Bay Area Reporter,* June 26, 1997, 99; also, Claudia Figueroa, "Bay Area Therapist Makes Book on Gay Couples' Longevity," *Bay Area Reporter,* February 13, 1997, 15. I am grateful to Merle Yost for apprising me of the existence of several groups of gay couples throughout the nation. (Merle Yost, personal communication, August 22, 1997).

12. Bonds Limited, organizational brochure, San Francisco, 1997.

13. Jim Eigo, "The Attack on Safer Sex," flyer distributed June 1997, Sex Panic! forum, New York City.

14. AIDS Council of New South Wales, Inc., "Talk Test Test Talk" brochure, n.d.

15. Susan Kippax, J. Crawford, and M. Davis, "Sustaining Safe Sex: A Longitudinal Study of a Sample of Homosexual Men," *AIDS* 7:257-263 (1993). Also see Susan Kippax, "A Commentary on Negotiated Safety" 96-97; Ron Gold, "Dangerous Liaisons: Negotiated Safety, the Safe Sex Culture, and AIDS Education," 102-103; Rachel Sharp, Nick Crofts, Gary Sattler, Laurie Marcus, John Meade, Jack Wallace, and Ruth Wood, "Negotiated Safety? Sexual Practices Among Young Gay Injecting Drug Users," 106-113; all in *Venereology,* 9(2), April-June 1996. In a paper published in 1997, a leading U.S. AIDS prevention research center suggests negotiated safety might be a useful technique to consider. See Colleen C. Hoff, "Differences in Sexual Behavior Among HIV Discordant and Concordant Gay Men in Primary Relationships," *Journal of Acquired Immune Deficiency Syndromes and Human Retrovirology,* 14:72-78 (1997).

16. AIDS Council of New South Wales, Inc., "Talk Test Test Talk" brochure, n.d.

17. Michelangelo Signorile, "A Troubling Double Standard," *The New York Times,* August 16, 1997, 21; Matt Foreman, "Plainclothes Cops Have No Place at the Party," letter to the editor, *LGNY,* September 14, 1997, 32. See also letters to the editor responding to Signorile's piece, under the headline, "Morning Party Is a Place to Prevent AIDS," *The New York Times,* August 23, 1997, 20.

18. Ibid.

19. Mark Schoofs, "Learning from Each Other or Monogamy: Pleasures and Pitfalls," speech presented at the National Lesbian and Gay Health Conference, Atlanta, July 26, 1997, 2-3. Reprinted by permission.

20. Eric Rofes, "Gay Lib vs. AIDS: Averting Civil War in the 1990s" (1990), in Mark Blasius and Shane Phelan (Eds.), *We Are Everywhere: A Historical Sourcebook of Gay and Lesbian Politics* (New York: Routledge, 1997); Keith Clark, "The 'Re-Gaying' of AIDS," *OutNOW!* (Silicon Valley, CA), 1.

21. Lawrence Mass, "The Lost World in the Oral Sex Debates: The Other STD's," *LGNY,* June 22, 1997, 10. Copyright 1997 by *LGNY.* Reprinted by permission. See also John Gallagher, "Forgotten But Not Gone: Other Sexually Transmitted Diseases," *The Advocate,* July 8, 1997, 35.

22. Hank Wilson, "Poppers (Nitrite Inhalants) and HIV: Immunosuppression, Seroconversion, Unsafe Sex," ACT UP Golden Gate, San Francisco, September 1997.

23. Centers for Disease Control and Prevention, *HIV/AIDS Surveillance Report,* 8(2), Atlanta, December 1996.

24. National Lesbian and Gay Health Association, *1997 Conference Program Book,* Atlanta, July 1997.

25. In Australia, a national men's health movement and a national gay men's health movement exist. See *Male Out* 3 (June 1997). The publication includes articles on foreskin restoration, aging, bisexuality, and a list of "healthy websites."

26. Robin Hardy, "Accentuate the Positive," letter to the editor, *Village Voice,* March 21, 1995, 6.

27. See Wendy Johnson, "Two Northeastern States Allot Funds for Gays," *The Washington Blade,* September 19, 1997, 21.

28. Wendy Johnson, "Massachusetts Governor OKs Funding for Gay Youth Programs," *The Washington Blade,* September 19, 1997, 21.

29. Wendy Johnson, "Pride Day to Serve as Fundraiser for Clinic," *The Washington Blade,* August 15, 1997, 1.

30. See The Medical Foundation, *Health Concerns of the Gay, Lesbian, Bisexual, and Transgender Community,* Second Edition (Boston: Massachusetts Department of Public Health, June 1997).

31. Gay Men's Health Crisis, *Rethinking HIV Prevention—Beyond 2000,* New York, 1.

32. Ibid., 1.

33. Ibid., 1.

34. Stephen Soba, "Beyond 2000: Rethinking HIV Prevention for Gay Men," *The Volunteer,* Gay Men's Health Crisis, New York, May/June 1997, 10.

35. Duncan Osborne, " . . . But Forum Still Reflects Harm Reduction Philosophy," *LGNY,* August 4, 1997, 4, 16. Copyright 1997 by *LGNY.* Reprinted by permission. Gabriel Rotello offers a critique of harm reduction, see Gabriel Rotello, *AIDS and the Destiny of Gay Men* (New York: Dutton, 1997), 110-111, 184-185. So does Troy Masters in "For Gay Men, a Cultural Change?" *The New York Times,* letter to the editor, July 30, 1996, A14.

36. Daniel Castellanos, speech given at First National Forum on and for HIV-Negative Gay Men, July 1997, Atlanta, sponsored by National Lesbian and Gay Health Association. Reprinted by permission of Daniel Castellanos.

37. The SafeGuards Project, "Promoting Gay and Bisexual Men's Health into the New Millennium," organizational document, Philadelphia, PA, 1997, 1.

38. Ibid., 4.

39. Ibid., 4.; See also The SafeGuards Project, "Report on SafeGuards Programmatic Development Retreat," Philadelphia, PA, March 29, 1997.

40. The SafeGuards Project, "Promoting Gay and Bisexual Men's Health into the New Millennium," 4.

Chapter 8

1. Mitchell Katz, "AIDS Epidemic in San Francisco Among Men Who Report Sex with Men: Successes and Challenges of HIV Prevention," *Journal of Acquired Immune Deficiency Syndromes and Human Retrovirology*, 14(Suppl. 2): S38-S46, 1997; New York City Department of Public Health, *AIDS Surveillance Update*, first quarter 1997, 2.

2. Bruce Bawer, "The Morning After Is Too Late for Safe Sex," *The New York Times,* June 15, 1997.

3. B.R. Simon Rosser, "The Effects of Using Fear in Public AIDS Education on the Behaviour of Homosexually Active Men," *Journal of Psychology and Human Sexuality*, 4(3):123, 1991; also see Dwayne Turner, *Risky Sex: Gay Men and HIV Prevention* (New York: Columbia University Press, 1997), 130-133.

4. Gabriel Rotello, *Sexual Ecology* (New York: Dutton, 1997), 188-189.

5. Rotello, *Sexual Ecology,* 233-261.

6. Alex Carballo-Dieguez, "The Difficult Road of Safer Sex for Latin-American Gay Men," in Stephen Ball (Ed.), *Survival Strategies for HIV-Negative Men,* Special issue of *Journal of Gay and Lesbian Social Services* (in press).

7. Thomas J. Coates and Michael Shriver, "In the Race for a Cure, Prevention Must Persist," *The Washington Blade*, November 29, 1996, 31. Reprinted by permission of Thomas J. Coates and Michael Shriver.

8. Sara Miles, "And the Bathhouse Plays On," *Out*, July/August 1995.

9. Cynthia Laird, "Got Condoms? Supes Call for Wider Distribution," *Bay Area Reporter*, February 13, 1997, 1.

10. I am grateful to Michael Scarce for spurring my thinking on activism focused on anal pleasures and rights. See Michael Scarce, *Smearing the Queer: Gay Male Sexual Health and Medical Science* (Binghamton, NY: The Haworth Press, in press).

11. The *Bay Area Reporter* has editorialized about the FDA's lack of effort on developing anal microbicides. See "It's Still Prevention," editorial, November 14, 1996, 6. Clark Taylor has also called for research into microbicides. See Clark L. Taylor, "Bringing Safe Sex Up to Date," *Bay Area Reporter*, May 22, 1996, 6.

12. Dan Savage devoted an entire column to the female condom. See "Savage Love," *SF Weekly*, July 30, 1997, 87; also, Mike Salinas, "Reality Approach Cuts STD Rate in Thailand, UN Finds," *Bay Area Reporter*, August 28, 1997, 28; I am grateful to the work of Michael Scarce and Chris Bartlett for heightening my awareness of the politics of this condom. See Michael Scarce, *Smearing the Queer: Gay Male Sexual Health and Medical Science* (Binghamton: The Haworth Press, in press), particularly the chapter on "Gay Men and the Female Condom: Is Rectal Reality Getting a Bum Wrap?"

13. Paul Recer, "AIDS Expert Says Vaccine Unlikely," *San Francisco Examiner,* May 14, 1997, 9.

14. Fred Kuhr, "Repeal of Archaic Sex Laws Is Topic of Beacon Hill Hearing on June 11," *Bay Windows,* June 19, 1997, 1; Lisa Keen, "Court Strikes Down Montana's Sodomy Law," *The Washington Blade,* July 18, 1997, 23; Sean Cahill, "These are not just personal conversations," In *Newsweekly,* June 22, 1997.

15. Robert Fisher and Peter Romanofsky, *Community Organization for Urban Social Change: A Historical Perspective* (Westport, CT: Greenwood Press, 1981); Sarah Archer, Carole Kelly, and Sally Ann Bisch, *Implementing Change in Communities* (St. Louis: Mosby, 1984).

16. Gary Dowsett has written a critique of the concept of "community development," especially as applied to gay men. See Gary Dowsett, "Living Post-AIDS," *National AIDS Bulletin* (Australia), March-April 1996, 23.

17. Gay City Health Project, "Welcome to Gay City," brochure, Seattle, 1995.

18. John Peterson, speech at first National HIV-Negative Forum, Atlanta, July 1997.

19. Craig Washington, interview, July 29, 1997, Atlanta.

20. Craig Washington, "Second Sunday," *Venus,* October/November 1996, 9.

21. Craig Washington, interview, July 27, 1997, Atlanta.

22. John Peterson, interview, July 29, 1997, Atlanta.

23. Craig Washington, interview, July 27, 1997, Atlanta.

24. John Peterson, interview, July 29, 1997, Atlanta.

25. Amitai Etzioni, *The New Golden Rule: Community and Morality in a Democratic Society* (New York: Basic Books, 1996); Amitai Etzioni (Ed.), *New Communitarian Thinking* (Charlottesville, VA: University Press of Virginia, 1995).

26. Joe Conason, Alfred Ross, and Lee Cokorinos, "The Promise Keepers Are Coming: The Third Wave of the Religious Right," *The Nation,* October 7, 1996, 11-12. Reprinted with permission from October 7, 1996 issue of *The Nation* magazine.

27. See "Heavenly promises," *U.S. News & World Report,* October 2, 1995, 68-70; "A 'Men Only' Club That Women Love," *National Enquirer,* n.d.; Laurie Goodstein, "Men Pack RFK on Promise of Renewal," *The Washington Post,* May 28, 1995; Chris Bull, "Searching for the Promised Land," *The Advocate,* September 30, 1997, 31-32.

28. "NGLTF Exposes Divisive Policies of "Promise Keepers," press release, National Gay and Lesbian Task Force, Washington, DC, May 24, 1995, 2.

29. Gay City Health Project, "Welcome to Gay City," brochure, Seattle, 1995.

30. Rotello, *Sexual Ecology,* 260.

31. Ibid., 260.

Chapter 9

1. See Frontdesk, "Absentee Vote," *POZ,* November 1996.

2. For coverage of this weekend, see Wendy Johnson, "You Can't See the Quilt Without Being Changed," *The Washington Blade,* October 18, 1996, 1.

3. Dan Savage, "Life After AIDS" *The Stranger*, January 16, 1997, 11. Reprinted by permission of Dan Savage.

4. Tommi Avicolli Mecca, "Boycott, Anyone?" *San Francisco Frontlines*, July 1997, 16; Doug Sadownick, "Flesh & Blood & APLA: The Rise and Fall and Rise and Fall (and Rise?) of an AIDS Agency," *Frontiers* (Los Angeles), January 28, 1994; Sara Miles, "The Party Is Over," *Out*, July 1997, 76.

5. See Cynthia Laird, "Pat Gets Raise, After Raise, After Raise . . . " *Bay Area Reporter*, June 12, 1997, 1; "Christen Charity," Editorial, *Bay Area Reporter*, June 12, 1997, 6; Dennis Conkin, "ACT UP/SF vs. SFAF: A Real Shitfight," *Bay Area Reporter*, October 24, 1996, 1.

6. David France, "Wheels of Fortune—Will the Real AIDS Ride Founder Please Stand Up?," *Out*, October 1997, 104-107, 150.

7. "Dump Fat Cat Pat" stickers were put up all over the Castro on newspaper boxes, bus stations, kiosks, in December 1996.

8. Tommi Avicolli Mecca, "Boycott, Anyone?" *San Francisco Frontlines*, July 1997, 16; Dennis Conkin, "Interview with Paul Wisotzy, San Francisco AIDS Foundation Board President," *Bay Area Reporter*, January 2, 1997; Cynthia Laird, "Is It Time for the SF AIDS Foundation to Downsize?" *Bay Area Reporter*, January 2, 1997, 1.

9. Kai Wright, "ADAPs Are Struggling, According to New Study," *The Washington Blade*, July 25, 1997, 25.

10. Jerry Joshua De Jong, "Time to conquer AIDS, Inc." *Bay Area Reporter*, January 9, 1997. A recent study by the Gay Men's Health Crisis found almost 75 percent of the clients surveyed who were being treated with protease inhibitors missed taking a dose at least once in the previous three months. See Mark Sullivan, "Study Finds Many Miss Doses of HIV Medicine," *The Washington Blade,* December 18, 1997, 23.

11. Dan Savage, "Life After AIDS," *The Stranger*, January 16, 1997, 8-13.

12. Ibid., 12.

13. Ibid., 13. Reprinted by permission of Dan Savage.

14. Terry Stone, letter to the editor, *The Stranger*, February 13, 1997, 9.

15. John Leonard, letter to the editor, *The Stranger*, February 6, 1997, 4.

16. Chuck Kuehn, letter to the editor, *The Stranger*, February 6, 1997, 6.

17. Tom Nolan, director of Project Open Hand in San Francisco, is one of many executive directors pointing this out. See Michael Dougan, "AIDS Meal Program Jubilant at New Site," *San Francisco Examiner*, A1, A8.

18. Jerry Joshua De Jong, "Time to Conquer AIDS, Inc."

19. George Cothran, "The AIDS Civil War," *SF Weekly*, February 19, 1997, 12-18.

20. The General Membership of ACT Up [sic] Golden Gate, "Uncivil War," *SF Weekly*, March 5, 1997, 3.

21. Cothran, "The AIDS Civil War," 14.

22. Ibid., 18.

23. Jerry Joshua De Jong, "Time to Conquer AIDS, Inc."

24. Jason Schneider, "What's Happened to AIDS Organizations," *Bay Windows*, November 29, 1996, 6.

25. Ibid., 7.

26. Victor D'Lugin, "The Trouble with Angels," *Metroline* (Hartford, CT), March 2, 1995.

27. See Michael Callen (Ed.), *Surviving and Thriving with AIDS: Hints for the Newly Diagnosed* (New York: People with AIDS Coalition, Inc., 1987), 128.

28. Suzanne Pharr, *In the Time of the Right: Reflections on Liberation* (Berkeley, CA: Chardon Press, 1996), 51.

29. Larry Kessler, "Keeping Hope Alive," *Bay Windows*, December 5, 1996, 6-7. Reprinted by permission.

30. Ibid., 6.

31. See John Gallagher, "The New Crisis Facing AIDS Organizations: Adapt or Die," *The Advocate*, May 27, 1997, 35; see also Jeff Epperly, "Whither AIDS Service Organizations," *Bay Windows*, January 9, 1997, 6.

32. "Green Bay's Center Project, Inc. and AIDS Resource Center of Wisconsin Merge," *The Wisconsin Light*, March 13, 1997, 1; "Merger of ARCW and Center Project," Editorial, *The Wisconsin Light*, March 13, 1997, 4.

33. Frederic Ball, "AFSD Closes—Now What?," *Update*, March 5, 1997.

34. J. Jennings Moss, "Where's the Money Going?," *The Advocate*, April 1, 1997, 45; Paul Rudnick, "Now It's AIDS Inc.," *Time*, December 30, 1996, 86-87.

35. Peter Freiberg, "After 10 Years, ACT UP Now Fights Dwindling Membership," *The Washington Blade*, March 14, 1997, 1.

36. Matthew Sharp, "ACT UP: Ten Years on the Front Lines of an Epidemic," *Bay Area Reporter*, March 6, 1997, 1.

37.The General Membership of ACT Up [sic] Golden Gate, "Uncivil War," *SF Weekly*, March 5, 1997, 3.

38. Kai Wright, "ADAPS Are Struggling, According to New Study," *The Washington Blade*, July 24, 1997, 25.

39. It is not yet clear whether fears of the much-discussed "funding fatigue" are becoming a reality. See Peter Freiberg, "Early Signs of Funding Fatigue?," *The Washington Blade*, August 8, 1997, 12; "The Coming Sunset on AIDS Funding Programs," *Project Inform Perspective*, July 1997, 1; B.J. Stiles, "AIDS Funding Trends," *The Washington Blade*, August 29, 1997, 31, 33; "AIDS Walk Colorado Breaks $1.4 Million Mark," *The Urban Spectrum* (Denver), October 1997, 4.

40. Cynthia Laird, "Over 25,000 Walk for AIDS; Largest Event Ever Raises $3.5 Million," *Bay Area Reporter*, July 24, 1997, 14.

41. For an insightful analysis of the need to reenergize treatment activism, see John James, "AIDS Treatment Activism: Turning to Service," *San Francisco Bay Times*, April 3, 1997, 16; also Carey Goldberg, "How Political Theater Lost Its Audience," *The New York Times*, September 21, 1997, WK6; Michael Onstott, "Not Dead Yet," *POZ*, August 1997, 77; "Dying to Live: New Drugs Are Keeping Clients Alive Longer—and Raising the Stakes for AIDS Service Center's Eighth Annual Posada," *Pasadena Weekly*, December 6, 1996, 6.

42. Fred Kuhr, "World AIDS Day Seen as Reminder That Epidemic Is Far from Over," *Bay Windows,* December 5, 1996, 3; Michael Gregory Lauzier, "World AIDS Day," *Metroline,* November 27, 1996, 6; "Warnings to Young Dominate AIDS Day," *The New York Times,* December 2, 1997, A14; Cynthia Laird, "14th AIDS Candlelight March This Sunday," *Bay Area Reporter,* May 1, 1997, 14.

43. Tim Kingston, "Candles Lit Around the World," *San Francisco Frontiers,* May 22, 1997, 6; "Names Project To Cut Staff About 20%," *San Francisco Chronicle,* June 3, 1997, A22.

44. Lisa Krieger, "Fewer Panels to AIDS Quilt Signal Progress," *San Francisco Examiner,* June 4, 1997, A6.

45. Animal J. Smith is the author of *Burn the Quilt,* a "solo music theatre piece that takes a hard-hitting look at the culture of death and mourning." See Dennis Conkin, "Inflammatory Musical Bows: 'Burn the Quilt'," *Bay Area Reporter,* August 17, 1997, 27.

Epilogue

1. Advertisement, *Bay Windows*, May 22, 1997, 37. See The Medical Foundation, "Health Concerns of the Gay, Lesbian, Bisexual, and Transgender Community," 2nd edition, Massachusetts Department of Public Health, June 1997.

2. Carol Ness, " 'Brothers' Take Time to Give Back to 'Sisters'," *San Francisco Examiner,* November 21, 1996, A24.

3. "New Home for Gay/Lesbian Health Center," *The New York Times,* January 12, 1997.

4. See Editorial, "Parading Our Sympathies," *Bay Area Reporter,* September 11, 1997, 10; Cynthia Laird, "E. Bay Pride to Honor Diana Next Weekend," *Bay Area Reporter,* September 11, 1997, 7; Cynthia Laird, "Thousands March in Tribute to Diana," *Bay Area Reporter,* September 11, 1997, 6; Nancy Ford, "Coping with Loss," and "She Touched Us," *The Texas Triangle,* September 4, 1997, 16–17 features a photo of Houston's memorial to the princess, located at the corner of Montrose and Westheimer, the heart of that city's gay neighborhood; Jeffrey Clagett, "The Indelible Impact of a Princess," *Baltimore Gay Paper,* September 5, 1997, 16; Rick Gordon, "Diana Rescued Britain from Recent Mediocrity; What Happens Now?" *Baltimore Gay Paper,* September 5, 1997, 16.

5. Onno de Zwart, M.P.N. van Kerhof, and T.G.M. Sandford, "Anal Sex and Gay Men: The Challenge of HIV and Beyond," *Journal of Psychology and Human Sexuality,* 10(3-4), 1998.

6. Mary Chapin Carpenter, "The End of My Pirate Days," *Stones in the Road,* Columbia Records, Sony Music, 1994.

7. Jack Fritscher, *Some Dance to Remember* (Stamford, CT: Knights Press, 1990).

Index

Abba, songs of, 303-304
Activism, failure of gay, 246
Advertising, AIDS crisis, 74
Advocate, The, 192
   "End of AIDS crisis," 30,41,53
   on gay youth, 142
   Invirase marketing in, 54
   "Sex and Sensibility," 131
   on sex-obsessed culture, 135-141
African American
   AIDS among, 5,10,44
   AIDS programs for, 243
   community building among,
     255-256
Ageism, gay male community and,
   130-131
Agosto, Moises, 128
AIDS
   activism, decline in, 73
   as biomedical syndrome, 10-11,14
   burnout, 119
   CDC prevention interventions,
     213-214
   closing prevention programs,
     241-243
   crisis
     characterization of, 43,44,
       67-70,120
     end of, 28,29-32,39-53,
       68-71,75-76
     rural gay men, 97,108-109
   deaths
     in Australia, 17
     in United States, 17,47
   decentering of, 66
   eliminate acronym of, 72
   epidemic, ending of, 3-5,47
   as event, 10-11,14

AIDS *(continued)*
   fund raising, decline in, 73
   gay identity, impact on, 12
   geographic distribution of, 95
   infection rate, comparative,
     18,20,26
   meaning in Gay ghettos, 11
   narrative of, 199-200
   organizations
     in Australia, 16
     crisis construct, 73-74
     need for change, 271-274
     reconceptualizing, 244-245
   political resistance, first incidence
     of, 37
   prevention of
     moralism and, 261-264
     programs for, 214-217,
       219-224,234-238
     young gays and, 89
   projected infection rate
     of, 200-201
   reconceptualization of, 71-72
   in rural areas, 97-108
AIDS Action Committee (Australia),
   16
AIDS Action Committee (Boston),
   187,229,281,283
AIDS Benefits Counselors, 273
AIDS Candelight Vigil, 289
"AIDS Civil War," 280
AIDS Coalition to Unleash Power
   (ACT UP), 37-67
   history of, 285-286
   Golden Gate, 280,286
   need to revitalize, 287
"AIDS communities," 103
AIDS Control Program (Seattle), 42

Kaldor, John, 17
Katz, Mitch, 178
Kessler, Larry, on role of ASO's,
    283,284
Key West, gay community in, 96
Kramer, Larry, 127-129
    compared to Hitler, 139-140
    on drugs in gay community, 184
    on gay culture, 123,131-142,176
    on gay youth, 141,142
    as literary critic, 133-134
    on Lesbian responsibility, 137
Kuehn, Chuck, 278
Kushner, Tony, 164

Laguna Beach, gay community
    in, 96
LaHaye, Timothy, on gay culture,
    123
Lambda Legal Defense, 66
LaRouche Initiative, 80
Latin America, gay culture
    in, 245-246
Latinos, AIDS among, 5,10,44
Lauritsen, John, on gay culture, 139
Lavender Quill, 134
Lawrence, D. H., 133-134
Lazarus, symbol of, 5,8,12
"Learning from Each Other
    or Monogamy: Pleasures
    and Pitfalls," 217
"Leather Buddies," 205
Leavitt, David, 134
Lebowitz, Fran, on impact of AIDS,
    164
Leonard John, 277-278
Lesbian Avengers, 183
Lesbian and Gay Rights March
    (Washington), 127
Lesbian health issues, need
    to address, 276
Lesbian health movement, 248
Lesbian health services, unequitable
    resources for, 233-234

Lesbians
    sex panic impact, 177
    view of gay male culture, 137
Lesbians and gay men, divisions
    between, 111
Levi, Jeff, 66
Lewis, Lynette, 193-195
LGNY
    harm reduction, 235-236
    sex debates, 175
"Life After AIDS," 275
*Life Outside: The Signorile Report
    on Gay Men,* 143
Lobel, Kerry, on Peace Keepers, 259
Long-term nonprogressors, 19,22-23
    post-AIDS identities, 77,108-117
Longtime Companion, 78,92-93
Los Angeles, gay harassment
    in, 181-182
Los Angeles Gay and Lesbian
    Community Services Center,
    response to AIDS, 79-80,229
Loss, symbolic, 18,79
Lost generation, 80-81,84,90

Madison (Wisconsin), gay
    community in, 96
Mandatory testing, 66
Mann, Bill, 134
Mapplethorpe, Robert, 164
Mardi Gras party (Sydney), 189
Marijuana, gay drug use, 185-186
Market Street Gym, 253-254
Martin-Baro, Ignacio, 155
Masculinities, varieties of, 191
Mass, Lawrence, on oral sex,
    230-231
Matlovich, Leonard, 37
Maupin, Armistead, 164
McCauley, Stephen, 134
McInnes, David, 24-26
McQuaid, Peter, on circuit culture,
    191
"Men of Color Health Resources,"
    234

Men's Health, Crixivan marketing
    in, 54
Merck, marketing of Crixivan, 54,55
Metropolitan Community Church,
    37,46
    International Convention, 260
Meyer, Ilan, on gay identity, 203
Miami
    gay harassment in, 183
    gay male sex practices, 168
Milk, Harvey, murder of, 126,127
Minneapolis, gay male sex practices,
    168
Mirken, Bruce, 53
Mobilization Against AIDS, 37
Mohr, Richard, survey of
    harassment, 183
Moldanado, Carlos, 38
Monette, Paul, 134
Monogamy, 217-220
Moral panic
    emerging, 171-173,177
    role of scapegoating, 187
    tools of, 186
Moralism, AIDS prevention work
    and, 261-264
Morning Party, The, 184-185,224
"Morning-after-pill," 242
Morris, Mark, 164
Muir, Starla, on gay male sex,
    137-138
Muscle boy culture, criticism of,
    130,163,172
Muscle System, 253-254

Nabozny, Jamie, 100
Naked Escape, 190
Names Project, 74,265,290-292
Nation, The, on Promise Keepers,
    258-259
National Centre in HIV
    Epidemiology and Clinical
    Research, Australia, 17

National Gay and Lesbian Task
    Force
    Policy Institute, 53
    sodomy law repeal, 248
National Gay Rights Advocates, 37
National HIV Prevention Summit,
    211,282
National Lesbian and Gay Health
    Conference (Atlanta), 84,217,
    229,230,231-232
National Minority AIDS Council, 54
"Natural history of HIV," 39
Negotiated safety, 222-224
Neoconservatives, gays as targets
    of, 158-159
"New Puritanism," 172
New York City
    AIDS deaths, peak of, 9
    decline in AIDS deaths, 47,48,49
    gay harassment in, 173-177
    prevention activism, 247
    seroprevalence rate, 130
New York Lesbian and Gay
    Community Services Center,
    128,172
New York Times, The, 193,294
    on drugs in gay community,
    184,224
    on gay community, 128
    on gay sex debates, 175-176
New York Times Magazine, The, end
    of AIDS crisis, 30,41,50
Newsweek
    on end of AIDS crisis, 30,41,52
    on gay community, 128
Next, 142
Northwest AIDS Foundation, 42,276
Novir. *See* Ritonavir

Obituaries, AIDS deaths, 36-37,39
Odets, Walt, AIDS prevention, 212
"Old guard," 35
Open Hand, 293

Ritonavir, 29,52,55
Rituals, gay male need for, 260-261,
    289-290
Roche laboratories, marketing
    of Invirase, 54
Rodriguez, Richard, 164
Rorem, Ned, 164
Rosett, Jane, 37
Ross, Michael, 193-195,212
Rotello, Gabriel, 127-129,131,158,
    186-188,245
    on drugs in gay community,
      184-185
    on immorality, 263-264
Rubin, Gayle
    on sex wars, 173
    on sex panic, 169,179
    sex values, 218
Rudnick, Paul, 128
RuPaul, 128
Russian River area, gay community
    in, 96
Rustin, Bayard, 164
Ryan, Jim, 38
Ryan White CARE Act, 49,70

Sadownick, Doug, 134
SafeGuards Project (Philadelphia),
    237-238
Safer sex, 13,21
Saint-at-Large White Party (New
    York), 196
Same-sex marriage, sex debates, 167
San Antonio, gay harassment in, 183
San Diego
    gay harassment in, 183-184
    gay male sex practices in, 168
San Diego AIDS Foundation,
    closure of, 284
San Diego Gay Rodeo, 259
San Francisco
    AIDS death rate, 48
    AIDS infection rate, 18,26

San Francisco *(continued)*
    gay male sex practices
      in, 168,179-180
    gay deaths, peak of, 9
    seroprevalence rate, 130
    sex debates, 177-181
San Francisco AIDS Foundation,
    criticism of, 271-273
San Francisco Bay Area Couples,
    220
San Francisco Chronicle
    advertisements in, 74
    decline in AIDS death, 48
San Francisco Examiner, decline
    in AIDS deaths, 49
San Francisco Week, ADS Civil
    War, 280
Saugatuck (Michigan), gay
    community in, 96
Savage Dan, 41-42,161,162,
    275-276,278-279
"Savage Love," 41
"Save Our Children," 125
Scapegoating
    gay community, 131,187-197
    process of, 196
Schneider, Jason, on role of ASO's,
    281,284
Schoofs, Mark, on gay sex, 217-218,
    225
Seattle, seroprevalence rate, 130
"Second wave" infections, 32
"Segregated partner selection," 25
Select Body, A, 193-195
Semen exchange, importance
    of, 226-227
Seroprevalence rate, major cities,
    130
Sex
    among rural gay men, 99-101
    role in Gay culture, 132-133,
      135-138,152
    as survival strategy, 225

Critical Acclaim for Eric Rofes's Best-Selling Book,
Reviving the Tribe: Regenerating Gay Men's Sexuality and Culture in the Ongoing Epidemic

"The most important book yet written about the ongoing AIDS epidemic." —Urvashi Vaid, author, *Virtual Equality: The Mainstreaming of Gay Liberation*

"Anyone concerned with the mental or sexual health of gay or bisexual men—especially those interested in helping gay men thrive beyond survival—should read this book . . . Required reading for anyone who is gay or who is working with gay men in an attempt to help us enrich our lives." — *The Journal of Sex Research*

"This book is a must for every gay male . . . It gives us back the sense of self-esteem we so badly need. This is going to be the book to change the way we look at life." —*Impact* (New Orleans)

"I am strongly tempted to just write, 'Read this book, it's brilliant' 200 times . . . I can't recommend it highly enough. My experience of reading *Reviving the Tribe* was that of having doors kicked open in my head." —Greta Christina, *Frontiers* (San Francisco)

"Rofes's passion, insight, and candor serve both to witness the epidemic and define a path along which gay men can struggle, endure, and survive . . . recommended reading to everyone living in the era of AIDS." — *Focus: A Guide to AIDS Research and Counseling*

"No other book wrestles with the controversial issues of gay male existence in the 90s with so much courage and integrity." —*Southern Voice* (Atlanta)

"Clearly the most significant gay reflection on sexuality during the decades of AIDS." — *The Front Page* (North Carolina)

"An excellent book that may well turn out to be a seminal work on AIDS . . . *Reviving the Tribe* asks some of the most intelligent and insightful questions on the epidemic that I've read." —*Homo Xtra* (New York City)

"A brilliant and courageous work that will challenge readers and provoke intense thought, emotion, and discussion . . . An eloquent and critically needed voice for the regeneration of gay male identity and culture." —Ben Schatz, Gay and Lesbian Medical Association

"As *Tales of the City* was to the 70s and *And The Band Played On* was to the 80s, so *Reviving the Tribe* will be to the 90s: A lens through which we fearlessly scrutinize our communal culture and redirect our activism." —Rev. Jim Mitulski, MCC/San Francisco

Order Your Own Copy of
This Important Book for Your Personal Library!

DRY BONES BREATHE
Gay Men Creating Post-AIDS Identities and Cultures

_____ in hardbound at $49.95 (ISBN: 0-7890-0470-4)

_____ in softbound at $24.95 (ISBN: 1-56023-934-4)

COST OF BOOKS_____

OUTSIDE USA/CANADA/
MEXICO: ADD 20%_____

POSTAGE & HANDLING_____
(US: $3.00 for first book & $1.25
for each additional book)
Outside US: $4.75 for first book
& $1.75 for each additional book)

SUBTOTAL_____

IN CANADA: ADD 7% GST_____

STATE TAX_____
(NY, OH & MN residents, please
add appropriate local sales tax)

FINAL TOTAL_____
(If paying in Canadian funds,
convert using the current
exchange rate. UNESCO
coupons welcome.)

☐ **BILL ME LATER:** ($5 service charge will be added)
(Bill-me option is good on US/Canada/Mexico orders only;
not good to jobbers, wholesalers, or subscription agencies.)

☐ Check here if billing address is different from
shipping address and attach purchase order and
billing address information.

Signature_____

☐ **PAYMENT ENCLOSED: $**_____

☐ **PLEASE CHARGE TO MY CREDIT CARD.**

☐ Visa ☐ MasterCard ☐ AmEx ☐ Discover
☐ Diners Club
Account # _____

Exp. Date _____

Signature _____

Prices in US dollars and subject to change without notice.

NAME _____

INSTITUTION _____

ADDRESS _____

CITY _____

STATE/ZIP _____

COUNTRY _____ COUNTY (NY residents only) _____

TEL _____ FAX _____

E-MAIL_____
May we use your e-mail address for confirmations and other types of information? ☐ Yes ☐ No

Order From Your Local Bookstore or Directly From
The Haworth Press, Inc.
10 Alice Street, Binghamton, New York 13904-1580 • USA
TELEPHONE: 1-800-HAWORTH (1-800-429-6784) / Outside US/Canada: (607) 722-5857
FAX: 1-800-895-0582 / Outside US/Canada: (607) 772-6362
E-mail: getinfo@haworth.com
PLEASE PHOTOCOPY THIS FORM FOR YOUR PERSONAL USE.
BOF96